医疗口译实务教程

A Practical Guide to Medical Interpreting

主编 雷 静 王 展
参编 边慧媛 郭佳文 王昭鉴 张 缘

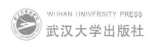
武汉大学出版社

图书在版编目(CIP)数据

医疗口译实务教程 / 雷静,王展主编. -- 武汉：武汉大学出版社,
2025.3. -- ISBN 978-7-307-24806-9

Ⅰ.R

中国国家版本馆 CIP 数据核字第 2024HS3196 号

责任编辑：吴月婵　　责任校对：鄢春梅　　版式设计：马　佳

出版发行：武汉大学出版社　　(430072　武昌　珞珈山)
（电子邮箱：cbs22@whu.edu.cn　网址：www.wdp.com.cn）
印刷：武汉邮科印务有限公司
开本：787×1092　1/16　印张：15.25　字数：340 千　插页：2
版次：2025 年 3 月第 1 版　　2025 年 3 月第 1 次印刷
ISBN 978-7-307-24806-9　　定价：59.00 元

版权所有，不得翻印；凡购我社的图书，如有质量问题，请与当地图书销售部门联系调换。

主编简介

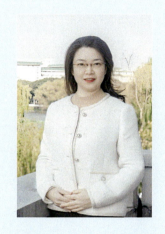

雷静，博士，教授，硕士生导师，中央民族大学外国语学院翻译系主任。目前已发表学术论文三十篇，出版专著三部，教材四部，译著十部。主持国社科中华学术外译项目一项、教育部等省部级项目四项、校级科研项目四项，获国家民委教学成果奖一项。担任教育部学位论文评审专家、全国商务英语翻译考试专家委员会委员，资深职业国际会议口译员。曾为国家领导人、国际机构、国家部委等提供上千场同传服务。2023年指导学生获得"外研社·国才杯""理解当代中国"全国大学生英语能力大赛口译赛项全国金奖，多次指导学生获得全国口译大赛国家级奖项等。

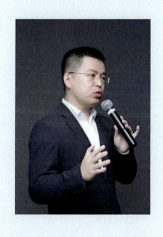

王展，现居上海，毕业于复旦大学，临床医学学士，外科学硕士。曾在华山医院担任临床医生，之后转做口译、咨询与教学工作。近几年，每年完成会议口译服务逾240场次，对医学会议口译有一定的造诣。主要从事医学领域的口译，服务的客户包括国内外顶尖医院、医疗监管机构以及跨国医药器械公司等；并主要从事医学口译教学，随着线上口译活动的盛行，特别独创了线上会议同传实践培训系统，能在短期内显著提升学员的能力。

序　言

欣闻最近小友王展与中央民族大学的雷静老师合作，一起编撰了一本教材——《医疗口译实务教程》，邀我为该书作序，倍感荣幸，心中也不禁泛起种种感慨。对于那些有志于进入英语口译领域或从事医学专业口译的大学老师、学生或者口译爱好者来说，这本《医学口译实用教程》尽管可能只是一本启蒙或引路的教材，却可以帮助大家省去很多时间，少走弯路，迅速成长。

我与王展相识于在复旦大学附属华山医院工作期间。王展毕业于复旦大学上海医学院，之后保送至骨科攻读硕士研究生学位。当时华山医院正在推进JCI国际医院标准，邀请国外同行专家来院指导，所以在学生中广征口译志愿者进行现场口译。王展在其中表现优异，之后跟随我参加了多场医学英语同传会议。而后，他更是越来越专注于医学专业口译，从临床医生转而成为一名医学口译从业者。他不仅勇于实践，在大量的口译活动中不断提升，而且愿意归纳总结，把实践中积累的心得提炼成为有益的经验，并分享给大家，帮助后来者茁壮成长。

我从改革开放伊始就在中华医学会上海分会从事医学口译。经历了四十载的口译生涯，再回首无数场的医学口译实践，我总结起来就是十六个字：滴水不漏，丝丝入扣；话如其人，画龙点睛。前八个字说的是在口译时译员不仅要完整传递信息，还要使用符合中文逻辑的表达，不说欧式中文，以免让听众费解；后八个字源自著名医学科学家吴阶平教授给我的评价，说的是为不同讲者译出不同风格，而学术点睛又最是让人难忘。

四十年前的条件远没有现在这么好，也缺乏各种专业参考教材，要购买一本新出版的《新英汉词典》都要专程回到五角场，到我们复旦大学里的新华书店里购买，与现在完全不可比。现在的出版物百花齐放，雷静老师与王展主编的这本《医疗口译实务教程》，结合了当今医学口译中的热门主题，从实践出发，兼顾医疗领域的知识与口译实践的理论技巧，按照专题分为多个单元展开，主体部分更是以小段的中英对照形式编写，以便读者阅读。读者既可视其为教材而循序渐进地学习，也可以视其为资料而有的放矢地参考。对于对医学口译感兴趣的外国语学院学生、口译爱好者及译员，本书不失为入门阶段及成长时期的营养来源，值得一览。

作为译员，不忘初心，一路而行，多年荏苒，在经历了大量的翻译实践后，也许心中才会泛起一丝"看山是山，看山不是山，而后看山又是山"的感悟，这也是任何一个专业由术而入道的天然过程。当然，我这些浅薄的认识只能是对严复先生提出的"信、达、雅"三原则的解读注释。严复老前辈在《天演论》的"译例言"中提出："译事三难：信、达、雅。求其信，已大难矣！顾信矣，不达，虽译，犹不译也，则达尚焉。"

现在再读，深有同感。作为有志成为专业口译或医学专业口译的后来者，我们一定不要忘记近代翻译老前辈们对我们的寄语，对自己的专业水准与职业追求要有一个可衡量的评判标准，并在平时实践中努力地去实现。不要过分担忧现代技术的迅猛发展对翻译市场的冲击，人工智能或机器翻译目前尚不能满足中端、高端翻译市场的需求。只要你能够占据高点，把自己的口译表现提高到"信、达、雅"的水准，那么你能够做到的不仅仅是翻译的基本信息传递，还将成为一名跨文化的知识传播大使，也必将成为我们中华优秀传统文化的传承者。

林建华

上海复旦大学附属华山医院

2024年9月

前　　言

随着新冠疫情的结束，人们对医疗口译的需求持续增长。在中国医疗口译市场快速发展的背景下，医疗口译相关的教程和适合高校师生的学习材料却未能跟上时代的需求。为了尽快改变现状，编者基于多年医疗口译的实践经验，推出这本创新、实用的教程，给对医疗口译感兴趣的老师、学生以及口译爱好者提供最贴近市场需求的内容。我们期望这本教材能够为中国医疗口译市场的良性发展带来新的活力。

本书分为理论介绍和医疗知识两大版块。理论介绍版块为前三个单元，主要讲解口译相关的基本概念、交传核心技巧以及同传核心技巧。医疗知识版块从第四单元开始，按各大医疗专题进行讲解，每单元的内容依次包括口译知识点、真实世界口译情境、中英对照篇章及分析和补充练习四部分。

本书的最大特色就是对当下最主流的医疗口译领域进行了梳理和介绍，涵盖了相关的术语和知识点，以及口译实战当中会接触到的现实场景和处理技巧。这些内容达到了理论与实践的高度融合，是目前市场上唯一兼具医疗领域知识与口译技巧实务的口译类教材。本书内容侧重向无医学背景的口译员快速简洁地介绍部分医学会议口译中所涉及的相关知识，注重实际应用，因此平衡了知识内容的组织层次、细致程度以及专业语言表述，故而有别于传统的医学教材及口译教科书。各章节的主题选择是基于编者的个人工作经历，并不能完全反映当前医学口译市场的全貌。本书无法详述细致的医学原理，还请读者按需整理资料，自我学习。

本书的受众是高校对医疗口译感兴趣的外语学院本科生、研究生以及口译爱好者。通过此书的编撰工作，编者希望能够为大学生和相关社会人士提供基础性的医学知识和口译技巧，使初学者能够较全面地了解医疗口译市场的实际需求和医疗领域的最新技术。

本书的撰写得到了相关人士的大力协助。中央民族大学的边慧媛老师、郭佳文同学、王昭鉴同学以及英国纽卡斯尔大学的张缘同学参与了本书理论介绍部分的编写工作。在此，对上述老师和同学作出的贡献表示由衷的感谢！本书的编排设计蕴含了两位主编的巧思和努力，如有不当之处，还望各位读者指正！

编　者

2024 年 8 月 19 日于北京

目 录

第一单元　基本概念 ··· 1
　第一节　口译历史概况 ··· 1
　第二节　口译与笔译 ·· 2
　第三节　口译的特点与分类 ·· 3
　第四节　译员应当具备的条件 ··· 5
　第五节　口译的标准 ·· 6
　第六节　英译汉和汉译英的异与同 ·· 7
　　一、英译汉 ··· 7
　　二、汉译英 ··· 8
　第七节　译前准备 ··· 9
　　一、核心内容 ·· 9
　　二、会务准备 ·· 10
　　三、身心准备 ·· 10

第二单元　交传核心技巧 ·· 16
　第一节　口译记忆 ··· 16
　　一、记忆机制 ·· 16
　　二、记忆方法 ·· 19
　第二节　口译笔记 ··· 22
　　一、为什么需要口译笔记 ·· 22
　　二、口译笔记的特点 ·· 22
　　三、口译笔记的记法 ·· 23
　　四、口译笔记讲解示例 ··· 24

第三单元　同传核心技巧 ·· 26
　第一节　视译 ··· 26
　　一、视译的概念 ··· 26
　　二、视译的分类 ··· 26
　　三、视译的原则与技巧 ··· 27
　第二节　同声传译 ··· 29

一、同声传译的特点与发展 …………………………………………………… 29
　　二、同声传译需要具备的素质 ………………………………………………… 30
　　三、同声传译的要领与技巧 …………………………………………………… 31

第四单元　糖尿病与血糖管理 ……………………………………………………… 36
第一节　糖尿病与血糖管理口译知识点 ………………………………………… 36
　　一、糖尿病知识概述 …………………………………………………………… 36
　　二、血糖知识概述 ……………………………………………………………… 37
　　三、糖尿病相关检查与监测 …………………………………………………… 37
　　四、糖尿病治疗 ………………………………………………………………… 38
第二节　真实世界口译情境 ……………………………………………………… 40
　　一、主题会议 …………………………………………………………………… 40
　　二、行业特点 …………………………………………………………………… 41
　　三、口译难点 …………………………………………………………………… 41
第三节　中英对照篇章及分析 …………………………………………………… 42
　　一、英译中 ……………………………………………………………………… 42
　　二、中译英 ……………………………………………………………………… 50
第四节　补充练习 ………………………………………………………………… 56
　　一、中译英 ……………………………………………………………………… 56
　　二、英译中 ……………………………………………………………………… 58

第五单元　心脏介入 …………………………………………………………………… 61
第一节　心脏介入口译知识点 …………………………………………………… 61
第二节　真实世界口译情境 ……………………………………………………… 64
　　一、主题会议 …………………………………………………………………… 64
　　二、行业特点 …………………………………………………………………… 64
　　三、口译难点 …………………………………………………………………… 65
第三节　中英对照篇章及分析 …………………………………………………… 68
　　一、英译中 ……………………………………………………………………… 68
　　二、中译英 ……………………………………………………………………… 77
第四节　补充练习 ………………………………………………………………… 85
　　一、中译英 ……………………………………………………………………… 85
　　二、英译中 ……………………………………………………………………… 87

第六单元　心脏瓣膜 …………………………………………………………………… 90
第一节　心脏瓣膜口译知识点 …………………………………………………… 90
第二节　真实世界口译情境 ……………………………………………………… 93

| 一、主题会议 …………………………………………………………… 93
| 二、行业特点 …………………………………………………………… 94
| 三、口译难点 …………………………………………………………… 94
| 第三节　中英对照篇章及分析 ………………………………………………… 95
| 一、英译中 ……………………………………………………………… 95
| 二、中译英 ……………………………………………………………… 104
| 第四节　补充练习 ……………………………………………………………… 109
| 一、中译英 ……………………………………………………………… 109
| 二、英译中 ……………………………………………………………… 110

第七单元　神经介入 …………………………………………………………………… 114
  第一节　神经介入口译知识点 ………………………………………………… 114
  第二节　真实世界口译情境 …………………………………………………… 117
      一、主题会议 …………………………………………………………… 117
      二、行业特点 …………………………………………………………… 117
      三、口译难点 …………………………………………………………… 117
  第三节　中英对照篇章及分析 ………………………………………………… 119
      一、英译中 ……………………………………………………………… 119
      二、中译英 ……………………………………………………………… 126
  第四节　补充练习 ……………………………………………………………… 133
      一、中译英 ……………………………………………………………… 133
      二、英译中 ……………………………………………………………… 135

第八单元　神经内科 …………………………………………………………………… 137
  第一节　神经内科口译知识点 ………………………………………………… 137
      一、癫痫 ………………………………………………………………… 137
      二、帕金森病 …………………………………………………………… 138
      三、阿尔茨海默病 ……………………………………………………… 138
      四、神经肌肉病 ………………………………………………………… 139
      五、脱髓鞘疾病 ………………………………………………………… 139
      六、罕见病 ……………………………………………………………… 140
  第二节　真实世界口译情境 …………………………………………………… 140
      一、主题会议 …………………………………………………………… 140
      二、行业特点 …………………………………………………………… 140
      三、口译难点 …………………………………………………………… 141
  第三节　中英对照篇章及分析 ………………………………………………… 142
      一、英译中 ……………………………………………………………… 142

目录

  二、中译英 ··· 151
 第四节　补充练习 ·· 157
  一、中译英 ··· 157
  二、英译中 ··· 159

第九单元　血液肿瘤 ·· 162
 第一节　血液肿瘤口译知识点 ··· 162
 第二节　真实世界口译情境 ·· 165
  一、主题会议 ··· 165
  二、行业特点 ··· 165
  三、口译难点 ··· 166
 第三节　中英对照篇章及分析 ·· 167
  一、英译中 ··· 167
  二、中译英 ··· 176
 第四节　补充练习 ·· 180
  一、中译英 ··· 180
  二、英译中 ··· 182

第十单元　实体肿瘤 ·· 185
 第一节　实体肿瘤口译知识点 ··· 185
 第二节　真实世界口译情境 ·· 188
  一、主题会议 ··· 188
  二、行业特点 ··· 189
  三、口译难点 ··· 189
 第三节　中英对照篇章及分析 ·· 190
  一、英译中 ··· 190
  二、中译英 ··· 198
 第四节　补充练习 ·· 206
  一、中译英 ··· 206
  二、英译中 ··· 208

第十一单元　骨科与运动医学 ·· 210
 第一节　骨科与运动医学口译知识点 ··· 210
 第二节　真实世界口译情境 ·· 212
  一、主题会议 ··· 212
  二、行业特点 ··· 213
  三、口译难点 ··· 213

第三节　中英对照篇章及分析 ·· 215
　一、英译中 ··· 215
　二、中译英 ··· 225
第四节　补充练习 ·· 229
　一、中译英 ··· 229
　二、英译中 ··· 231

参考书目 ·· 234

第一单元　基本概念

第一节　口译历史概况

　　翻译分为口译（interpreting）和笔译（translation）两种主要形式。口译的兴起与人类各民族间日益增长的交流需求密不可分，其历史或许可以追溯到人类语言逐渐分化成形的远古时期。① 自语言产生于人类世界以来，不同民族之间有着从事经济和文化活动的需求，此类需求依靠翻译完成。在尚未出现文字的时代，首先进行的翻译活动即是口译。随着使用不同语言的民族间往来的增加，翻译也逐渐发展起来。同时翻译本身也促进了不同民族间的贸易往来和文化交流。

　　作为人类跨文化沟通的重要桥梁和关键纽带，口译承载着连接不同文化背景的重要使命。在我国，口译这一专门职业的历史可追溯到两千多年前。古时，口译从业者被赋予了各种称谓，如"译""寄""象""狄鞮""舌人""象胥""通事""通译""重舌"或"九译令"，② 这些称谓不仅体现了口译工作的多样性，也见证了其在历史上的重要地位。《礼记·王制》中详细记载："五方之民，言语不通，嗜欲不同。达其志，通其欲，东方曰寄，南方曰象，西方曰狄鞮，北方曰译。"这一描述展示了口译在古代社会中的重要作用，无论人们来自何方，只要有口译的存在，就能够沟通心意，传递信息。《国语·周语中》则针对译员这一群体给出了定义，文中注解道："舌人，能达异方之志，象胥之官。"这表明译员不仅是语言的转换者，更是文化的传播者，能够准确传达不同民族、不同地域的意愿和心声。在《癸辛杂识后集·译者》中，口译工作被赋予了更深的内涵："译，陈也；陈说内外之言皆立此传语之人以通其志，今北方谓之通事。"这里的"译"不仅仅是简单的翻译，更是通过口译者的努力，让不同语言和文化背景下的人们能够互相理解，达到心灵的沟通。由此可见，口译在我国历史长河中扮演着不可或缺的角色，它不仅是语言之间的桥梁，更是文化交流的使者。随着时代的变迁和社会的发展，口译工作将继续发挥重要作用，为人类跨文化沟通贡献更多的力量。

　　我国的翻译工作在汉末佛教传入之前一直以口译为主，明代郑和下西洋之后，随着沿海的商品经济和对外贸易逐渐发展，西方文化也随之东渐，因此，口译得到了进一步发展，笔译也随之起步。清代翻译家严复于1898年提出了著名的翻译标准"信、达、

---

①　鲍刚. 口译理论概述[M]. 北京：中国对外翻译出版有限公司，2011.
②　梅德明. 高级口译教程[M]. 上海：上海外语教育出版社，2006.

雅",为我国现代翻译理论的发展奠定了基础。五四运动之后,我国得以广泛接纳众多西方著作与新思想,在这一转变中,翻译人员的贡献不可磨灭。改革开放以来,尤其是加入世贸组织之后,我国在经济、贸易、科学及文化领域的对外交流达到了前所未有的高度,翻译工作也迎来了空前的繁荣时期。这一时期中,无数杰出的笔译和口译人才崭露头角,他们的辛勤付出极大地推动了改革开放的进程。①

在西方,早在公元1世纪,基督教使徒保罗便强调了口译的重要性。随着时间的推移,口译工作逐渐受到重视。14世纪初,法国的杜布瓦提出了建立东方语言学校,旨在培养能与"异教徒"顺畅交流的口译人才。15世纪末,哥伦布发现新大陆后,更是派遣了大批印第安青年前往西班牙学习西班牙语,以培养更多的译员。

第一次世界大战后,口译工作的重要性更加凸显。1919年,为确保巴黎和会的顺利召开,第一批正式的译员被组织起来,其间涌现出许多杰出的口译人才,如参加巴黎和会的保尔·芒图、日内瓦翻译学院的创始人安托万·维洛门以及负责筹建联合国翻译处的琼·赫伯特等。第二次世界大战后,随着国际交往的日益频繁,口译工作迎来了前所未有的繁荣时期。重要的国际组织如联合国、欧盟等,均设有专门的翻译机构。与此同时,许多翻译院校相继成立,世界范围内译员的口译水平得到了显著提升。口译理论与技巧的研究也逐渐受到关注,口译工作逐渐走向专业化。1953年,成立了第一个口译工作者的职业性组织——国际会议口译员协会(英文简称AIIC),这标志着口译行业进入了一个新的发展阶段。

第二节　口译与笔译

翻译分为笔译与口译两种形式。在英语中,从事笔译的人被称作 translator,从事口译的人被称作 interpreter;在汉语中,翻译工作者一般被统称作翻译,口译人员也被称作译员。

目前研究翻译理论的文献大多聚焦于笔译领域,相比之下,对口译的深入研究显得较为不足。但这并不意味着口译的重要性逊色于笔译,或者口译的研究价值较低。实际上,口译作为翻译的一种基本形式,在各国间政治、经济、科技、文化等领域的交流中扮演着举足轻重的角色。从劳动强度来看,口译甚至可能超过笔译。此外,对口译人员的素质要求也丝毫不低于对笔译人员的要求,翻译工作者均需要具备扎实的语言基础、出色的应变能力以及深厚的专业知识。

口译与笔译之间既有较大的差别,又有着密切的联系。二者各有其不同的特点和要求。

在谈论口译与笔译之前,我们首先要了解口语与笔语。首先,口语作为口译的基础,具有先决存在性,其历史远早于笔语,所有民族语言的笔语形式都晚于口语形式。其次,口语的存留时间较短,因为口语依赖于声波振动传播,不易流传后世,而笔语可

---

① 齐涛云. 商务英语翻译教程(口译)(第三版)[M]. 北京:中国水利水电出版社,2022.

以长久保存。最后，口语的发布速度较快。因此，口语与笔语同样是重要的交流体系。①

笔译工作者通过"读"来深入理解原文，进而获取所需信息。译者拥有充足的时间去思考翻译中的难点，有时甚至会反复推敲某个词汇，正如严复所言："一名之立，旬月踟蹰。"在翻译过程中，笔译工作者可以借助词典和各类参考书籍，甚至寻求他人的帮助。因此，笔译要求译者不仅能够精确传达原文的含义，还要保证文字流畅、易于阅读，同时追求语言的生动性和感染力，尽量贴近原作风格。

相较之下，口译工作者则是通过"听"来快速理解讲话内容，并获取信息。译员需要在听完讲话后立刻用目标语言进行表达（交替传译），或者边听边译（同声传译），几乎没有时间进行细致推敲，更难以查阅工具书或寻求他人的帮助（尽管在特殊情况下可能偶尔为之，但这并不值得提倡）。因此，口译工作者的劳动强度在单位时间内远超笔译工作者。对于口译的要求，自然不能像笔译那样严格。虽然优秀的口译工作者能够译得既完整又准确，甚至生动传神，使会谈双方沟通顺畅，但这并非所有口译工作者都能达到的效果。

不过，口译工作者也有笔译工作者无法获得的优势，如可以借助讲话人的语调、表情和手势来理解原意。在口译表达时，译员还可以适当地添加一些解释来帮助沟通。正因为笔译与口译存在这些差异，有人甚至认为它们是两种截然不同的工作。虽然这种说法有些极端，但同时精通口译与笔译的译员的确难得。实际上，很多著作丰富的翻译家并不擅长口译工作，而一些杰出的口译人员也并未留下多少传世译作。

口译与笔译虽然形式有所不同，但二者的核心任务与性质是一致的，即用一种语言来重新表达另一种语言所承载的思想。两者的基本过程都是从理解原文到进行再表达。事实上，笔译中经常使用的技巧，如词类的转换、增词或省略、反译、具体化或抽象化，以及合句与拆句等，在口译中同样具有广泛的应用价值。对于那些笔译水平高超的人来说，只要他们具备良好的听力和口头表达能力，他们的口译质量往往也会非常出色。反过来，口译能力的增强至少会促进笔译速度的提升。因此，口译与笔译是相互促进的，而非相互牵制或妨碍。其中一种翻译能力的提高必然也会带动另一种翻译能力的提高。

第三节 口译的特点与分类

口译是一项独具特色的语言交际活动，其特殊性源于口头翻译工作所展现的一系列鲜明特点。

首先，口译是一项具有高度即时性的语言交际活动，要求译员在有限时间内准确地将源语言转化为目标语言。这不仅考验译员的语言功底，还要求其具备迅速的反应能力和出色的应变能力。换言之，口译作为一种高度即时的语言活动，对译员的语言素养、

---

① 鲍刚. 口译理论概述[M]. 北京：中国对外翻译出版有限公司，2011.

反应能力和应变能力有着极高要求。在现场口译中,译员须在准备不足的情况下迅速进入状态,进行双语切换和口译操作。尤其是在话题多变的场合,如记者招待会或商务谈判,译员难以准确预测话题走向,只能通过有限的预设进行判断,然而这种带有主观性的预判往往不够充分,是靠不住的,甚至可能导致风险。① 此外,由于口译的存在,信息的连贯性和传达速度也会受到影响,因此译员须尽力保持信息传递的快捷与准确,这就需要译员不仅要口才好,还要具备出色的应变能力,以应对各种突发情况。

其次,口译是一项极具挑战性和高压的工作,对译员的身心素质有着极高的要求。在进行口译时,译员须在长时间内保持高度集中的专注力,这不仅要求译员具备扎实的语言功底,还须拥有出色的记忆力和应变能力。在口译现场,译员必须全神贯注地倾听讲话人的发言,迅速理解并把握其中的要点,同时还要将其准确地翻译成目标语言,传达给听众。这一过程中,任何一丝分神都可能导致翻译失误,影响交流的顺利进行。有时口译场合显得尤为庄重肃穆,例如在国际会议和外交谈判中,对于经验尚浅的译员而言,正式场合的紧张氛围可能会带来较重的心理压力。这种压力不仅可能削弱他们的自信,导致紧张情绪滋生,还可能使他们在口译过程中出现频繁的口误。此外,现场瞬息万变的气氛也可能使译员反应变得迟缓,进而影响到他们口译水平的正常发挥。② 因此,口译还要求译员具备良好的心理素质和抗压能力。

最后,口译是以口头方式将一种语言所表达的思想内容转化为另一种语言的过程。这种转化形式使得口译与笔译在表达形态上存在明显差异。口译更加强调口语的流畅与自然,追求现场感,要求译员能够运用自然、流畅的语言进行即时传达,确保信息的准确与高效传递。

就口译的工作方式而言,我们可以将口译划分为两大类。其中,交替传译(consecutive interpreting)是当讲话人完成一句、一个意群段或整篇发言后,译员再将其内容翻译给听众的方式。这种方式也被广泛称作连续翻译、接续翻译或即席翻译。在交替传译中,译员通常会在现场直接翻译讲话内容,讲话与翻译交替进行,为听众提供实时理解的机会。

而另一种口译方式则被称为同声传译(simultaneous interpreting),它要求译员在讲话人发言的同时进行翻译。这种方式需要借助大会的传译设备,译员在口译箱里通过耳机收听讲话,并立即通过话筒将内容翻译给听众。由于译员的翻译几乎与讲话人的发言同步,故得名"同声传译"或"同步口译"。

此外,还有两种口译方式与同声传译较为相似。首先是耳语翻译(whispering interpreting),译员在听到讲话后,会立即轻声地将内容翻译给身边的一两个人。在这个过程中,讲话人持续发言,译员则不断翻译,通常会对原讲话内容进行一定的压缩与概括。

另一种是视译(sight interpreting),要求译员在查看文字材料的同时,将其内容口译

---

① 梅德明. 高级口译教程[M]. 上海:上海外语教育出版社,2006.
② 梅德明. 高级口译教程[M]. 上海:上海外语教育出版社,2006.

出来。这种翻译方式与其他口译种类的主要区别在于，它是通过阅读书面材料获取信息的，而不是通过听觉。视译通常要求译员持续阅读并翻译，而不是一句一句地进行。因此，这种翻译方式在某些方面接近同声传译。

第四节　译员应当具备的条件

口译是一项极具挑战、劳动强度高且涉猎领域广泛的职业，仅仅外语水平高超并不意味着译员足以胜任口译工作。一名合格的口译员须满足以下条件：

第一，口译员必须精通两种语言的互译，并最好掌握一两门外语。这种精通不仅体现在对基础词汇的掌握上，还需要译员深入理解和记忆各领域的专业词汇。对于口译员来说，词汇量越丰富越有利，特别是其英语认知词汇量应达到1.5万以上。此外，外语听力的优劣直接关系到外译汉的质量，因此口译员应努力提升听力水平，以求接近或达到母语听力水平。同时，良好的外语口头表达能力也是汉译外的关键，口译员应具备敏锐的语感和丰富的语言经验，能够熟练驾驭语言。

国际口译界普遍认为，口译员应将外语译成自己的母语，而不是将母语译成外语，在同声传译中更应如此。这更说明了语言熟练程度对口译的重要性，因为一般认为一个人掌握得最好的是母语。然而，由于汉语的独特性，真正熟练掌握汉语的外国人并不多。因此，中国的口译员不仅需要承担外译汉的任务，还要承担汉译外的任务，这对他们的语言熟练程度提出了更高的要求。

第二，广泛的知识面对于口译员来说至关重要。译员只有具备丰富的知识，才能更好地理解和表达所译内容。对于所译内容的相关知识一无所知或知之甚少，仅凭语言能力进行翻译将非常困难，甚至无法完成。虽然个人的精力有限，无法知晓所有知识，但合格的口译员应尽可能多地涉猎百科知识，包括经济、政治、外交、时事、历史、地理、科技、文化、宗教和习俗等领域。译员对于自己经常涉及的领域，更应深入了解。例如，从事商务口译的人员应熟练掌握商务知识、方针政策、具体做法、商品市场以及会议或会谈的背景和目的等。

第三，口译员须具备抗压能力。口译员在工作中往往处于高度紧张的环境，不仅要即时准确地将源语言转化为目标语言，还要面对各种突发状况，如发言人的语速过快、口音独特、信息密集等。[1] 此外，现场环境可能充满不确定性，如技术故障、噪音干扰等，这些都可能对口译员的工作造成干扰。因此，口译员必须具备强大的抗压能力，能够在压力下保持冷静、专注，迅速作出反应，确保口译工作的顺利进行。

第四，口译员须具备强大的记忆力，无论是长时记忆还是短时记忆。[2] 长时记忆要求译员能够记住大量的词汇和知识，并能够迅速理解和表达。而短时记忆对于口译员来说尤为重要，因为大部分口译并不是以句子为单位进行的，而是以段落为单位。如果短

---

[1] 梅德明. 高级口译教程[M]. 上海：上海外语教育出版社，2006.
[2] [瑞士]让·艾赫贝尔. 口译须知[M]. 孙慧双，译. 北京：外语教学与研究出版社，1982.

时记忆能力不足，译员将无法胜任口译工作。对于同声传译员来说，瞬时记忆能力也至关重要。记忆力虽然与先天遗传有关，但通过后天的训练可以得到增强。对原话的理解越透彻，就越容易记住；如果理解不透或抓不住逻辑关系，仅凭强记将会使口译工作变得非常困难。口译记忆还可以借助辅助手段，如口译笔记等。笔记的方式和数量应根据个人的条件和习惯而定。

在口译过程中，敏捷的反应能力也是必不可少的。国际会议同声传译员每小时需要翻译约9000个英文单词，而交替传译员每小时也需要翻译约5000个单词。这样的速度要求译员几乎像条件反射一样将一种语言迅速译成另一种语言。然而，敏捷并不意味着匆忙。当遇到个别未听懂或未听清的词汇时，译员应保持冷静，根据上下文和自己掌握的知识迅速作出判断并表达出来。在翻译过程中遇到难点时，译员也应冷静处理，以灵活的方式传达原文的精神。

第五，译员须口齿清晰。这意味着译员说话应干脆利落，避免重复和啰嗦，同时要避免使用不必要的口头语。语调应自然生动，既不要过于拘谨，也不要装腔作势。语速要适中，停顿要自然。声音大小应适中，确保听众能够轻松听清译员的话。

当然，认真严谨的工作态度也是口译员不可或缺的素质。在口译过程中，即使偶尔未听清个别词汇，译员也不能随意编造或增减原话内容。合格的译员不仅在翻译时要保持认真态度，还应积极为口译任务作好译前准备。

第五节　口译的标准

口译的核心是意译，但这并不代表译员可以随意翻译或者仅仅传达源语大意。意译强调的是在保持原话内容完整、精神准确的基础上，不拘泥于语言形式。这自然就涉及口译应当遵循的标准与要求。笔译历来多以严复提出的"信、达、雅"为标准，尽管学者对此有着各种看法，但翻译活动基本上仍围绕这一框架展开。然而，口译与笔译在工作特性上存在显著差异，因此口译应有其独立且符合自身特点的标准。

为了更直观地理解，我们可以借鉴严复的提法，稍作调整，将"信、达、速"作为口译的三大标准。

具体来说，"信"即要求译员忠实于原话的内容与精神，不得随意增减、改变或编造。必要时，译员可以适当压缩或提炼原话内容，甚至进行适度解释，但语言风格应尽可能贴近原话风格，保持其原有的严肃、活泼、通俗或正规的特点。

"达"则强调译出的语言应流畅自然、易于理解，不拘泥于原话的词汇和结构，而是用符合目标语言习惯的表达方式来传达原话的内容。译员应避免拖沓和重复，确保译出的语言干脆利落。

"速"则是口译特有的要求，它体现了口译工作的高效性。交替传译时，译员需要快速准确地传达讲话人的内容，其语速应略快于讲话人，且在讲话人停顿时应立即开始翻译，以缩短时间差，确保翻译的连贯性和效率，使翻译准确而流利。

这三大标准——信、达、速——共同构成了口译的完整统一要求。其中，"信"是口译的基础和核心,而"达"和"速"则是在"信"的基础上进一步提升口译质量的关键,只有在三者都得到满足的情况下,我们才能称之为成功的口译。然而,这三条标准的权重并非等同,"信"无疑是第一位的,而"达"和"速"则是在"信"的基础上追求更高水平的口译表现。

第六节　英译汉和汉译英的异与同

前文提及,鉴于汉语的特殊性,我国的口译员不仅要将英语译成汉语,还要将汉语译成英语,这双重任务使得口译工作更具挑战性。尽管这两种口译任务都涉及英语与汉语之间的转换,但它们各自的特点和难点却大相径庭。口译员必须洞察这两种口译任务的核心差异,明确自己的提升方向,才能不断进步,更出色地完成口译任务。通过了解各自的关键点,译员能够更有针对性地提升自己的口译能力,确保在各种场合都能游刃有余,准确无误地完成口译工作。

一、英译汉

英译汉口译尤其注重听辨。英译汉的关键在于通过听取英语话语来捕捉信息,理解原话内涵,并用汉语将译文流畅表达。虽然每位译员对汉语的掌握程度不尽相同,但汉语作为我们的母语,译员自小学至大学都有深入学习和使用的基础。一般来说,中国译员能够较为熟练地运用汉语表达思想。而且,与笔译相比,口译译员不必过分雕琢词句,只要理解原话,用汉语表达通常不会有太大困难。然而,口译的难点在于准确理解原话,这不仅是英译汉的关键,也是译员容易遇到挑战和问题的环节。因此,译员必须高度重视英语听辨能力的训练。听辨能力的提升涉及多个方面,敏锐的听觉固然重要,但词汇量、知识面和语感也是不可或缺的要素。通过系统的听辨训练与大量的实践,译员的听力水平必将得到显著提升,从而更好地适应口译工作的需求。

译员在日常学习中应充分利用各种机会进行英语听力训练,做到精听与泛听相结合。在精听练习中,译员应努力分辨每一个词甚至音节,特别注意发音相近的词和连读现象。对于难以听清的部分,可以反复听取,直至能够准确理解。值得注意的是,译员不应期待总是听到"标准""规范"的英语。许多外语院校及其专业的学生往往更侧重于练习"标准音"的听辨,对于非课堂模拟环境中常见的噪声、语音变体等因素所带来的变化,他们往往不太适应,必须确保每个发音都清晰无误才能完成听辨。然而,对于译员而言,不应该过分追求发音的完美,而应该将理解作为首要任务。即使在源语中存在噪声干扰、语音畸变(如口音差异、电子线路传播失真等)的不利条件下,译员也应该能以较高的效率进行听辨,完成准确传递源语信息的任务。① 英语作为国际通用语言之一,其使用者遍布世界各地,各地的英语口音、用词习惯等都有所不同。因此,译员在平日训练中应有意增加对各种口音的英语材料的听取,以提高对不同口音的适应能力。

---

① 鲍刚.口译理论概述[M].北京:中国对外翻译出版有限公司,2011.

面对以非英语为母语的讲话者，如南亚人、东南亚人等，他们的英语发音可能带有母语特色，译员应保持冷静，通过训练使自己适应这些不同的口音，而不是期待对方改变讲话方式。任何不良情绪都可能影响翻译质量，甚至造成不良影响。

精听练习应分阶段进行，每阶段的关注点应有所不同。虽然最终目标是能够清晰分辨每个词甚至音节，但在初期阶段，译员应首先把握整体意思，再逐步深入细节和单个词汇或音节的听辨。这种"先理解后辨音"的方法才是口译听辨练习的正确途径。过于关注单个单词容易忽视整体结构和逻辑关系，从而影响对听力文本的理解。

此外，泛听练习同样重要。泛听有助于提高译员的语感、增加语言经验、熟悉不同口音。除了听取录音资料，译员还可以通过收听英语广播、观看英语电视节目等方式进行泛听练习。这些练习不仅有助于译员提升英语听力能力，还能使译员在口译现场更加从容应对各种情况。

坚持训练是提高听辨能力的关键。随着时间的推移，译员的听辨能力必将得到显著提升，口译工作也将变得更加得心应手。

二、汉译英

在汉译英口译中，表达能力尤为重要。汉译英的过程首先是听汉语以获取信息，然后转化为用英语进行表达。尽管我们不能保证中国译员在汉语表达上能做到毫无瑕疵，但他们听懂汉语并不成问题。然而，如果说中国译员在听英语时可能会遇到困难，那么他们用英语表达的难度可能更大。因此，中国译员在汉译英中的主要挑战并非在于听辨和理解，而在于英语表达。

英语表达能力是汉译英的核心。这种能力的提高并不能一蹴而就。严格来说，一个人在成为译员之前就应该基本掌握英语表达能力，否则他就没有资格担任译员。然而，表达能力的提升是一个持续的过程。为了更好地完成口译任务，即使是职业译员也必须不断努力。

表达能力受到多种因素的影响。虽然词汇量是基础，但仅仅拥有大量词汇并不足够，更重要的是译员能够灵活运用这些词汇，做到脱口而出。要实现这一点，大量的基本功训练是必不可少的。译员需要经常朗读有代表性的讲话，并熟练背诵常用的表达方式和句型。此外，为提高表达能力，译员还应练习用英语演讲。要想成功翻译他人的讲话，译员自身首先应具备自如的英语表达能力。

在表达时，译员可以选择使用英音、美音或其他英语国家的口音，但并不要因为听众的不同而特意改变口音。然而，重音的处理尤为重要，包括单词重音和句子重音。从语音角度来看，英语是一种重音语言（stress language），掌握好重音有助于听众更好地理解译员的翻译。对于非重读音节，译员可以适当模糊处理其发音，过于清晰地发出每个音反而会分散听众的注意力，不利于思想的表达。译员的语音语调越地道越好，但是也并不需要像播音员那样完美，译员的发音能达到正确、自然、流畅的效果为佳。此外，译员的语调生动程度和表情生动程度一般不应超过讲话人，更不应过多使用手势，以免产生喧宾夺主或哗众取宠的不良效果。

第七节 译前准备

口译涵盖的主题包罗万象，口译员难以做到样样精通。为确保口译工作的顺利进行，充分的译前准备非常有必要，可以说是不可或缺的一环。从广义的角度来讲，译前准备其实是译员在努力成为优秀口译者的道路上长期积累知识与素质的过程。口译员在日常生活中应当养成良好的学习习惯，保持对社会的浓厚兴趣，广泛涉猎各个专业领域，以此扩大自己的知识面并提升理解能力。同时，译员还需要不断地积累和更新自己的词汇库和表达方式，进行语言与专业知识的长期积淀。

本节聚焦于狭义上的译前准备，即口译员在接到任务后所进行的一系列准备工作。译前准备要尽可能考虑周详、方法恰当。接下来，本节将通过核心内容、会务准备和身心准备三个方面介绍译前准备的基本原则，然后通过案例展示这些原则在不同类型会议中的具体应用。

一、核心内容

尽管口译的成功在很大程度上依赖于译员平时的积累，但每一场会议之前的"紧急备战"同样至关重要。就核心内容准备而言，译员除了需要了解讲者本人情况，了解讲者国家的概况[1]，还需要着重拓宽并深化对特定主题的理解。然而，译员在会前准备过程中常常会面临时间紧迫的情况。如果译员可以在会前拿到会议目的、议程、主题，以及发言稿等详尽信息，并有足够的时间去消化和吸收这些资料，那么核心内容的准备会相对容易一些。然而，实际情况往往并非如此，译员通常只有一两天甚至更短的时间进行准备，他们可能面临信息不足或过多、内容过于专业或过于宽泛的难题。因此，译员在准备时必须采取有效的方法，如制订准备计划，明确内容的优先级等。

作此类准备时，译员不妨记住下述这些原则：
1. 确定关键信息；
2. 对于关键信息，力争"知其然，亦知其所以然"；
3. 充分利用各种资源，加强对特定主题的理解；
4. 不忽略细节准备。

在准备不同类型的会议翻译时，可获取的资料类型各异，译员应基于上述原则，根据会议类型制订个性化的译前准备方案。无论准备哪种类型的会议翻译，译员都应特别注意将可能遇到的困难词汇，如专有名词和术语等整理成词汇表，以便在会议翻译期间随时查阅使用。这样，译员不仅能够更好地应对各种挑战，也能确保翻译的准确性和流畅性。

---

[1] ［瑞士］让·艾赫贝尔. 口译须知[M]. 孙慧双，译. 北京：外语教学与研究出版社，1982.

二、会务准备

会务准备涉及会议的时间、地点、联络人、设备以及会场坐席安排等多方面关键细节。有关会合时间，译员最好提前 15~30 分钟到达指定地点，这样不仅可以为通行预留充足的时间，还能应对可能的突发情况，避免迟到所带来的慌乱和压力。关于会合地点的选择，译员可以选择直接到会场与代表团会合，或在代表团的下榻酒店或其他出发地点与代表团碰头，后者更有助于译员在会前与代表团成员相互熟悉，为后续的沟通打下良好基础。如果在会议准备过程中遇到疑问或需要澄清的问题，会前会合则为译员提供了更多与代表团成员交流的机会。译员会前应尽可能详细记录联络人信息，包括主管官员、司机以及对方联络人的联系方式等，以备不时之需。

在设备方面，译员应与会场设备人员密切配合，在会前测试麦克风音质，确保没有杂音和干扰。麦克风的摆放位置也至关重要。如果译员和发言人使用不同的落地麦克风，为了保证能够清晰听辨，建议译员将麦克风置于发言人麦克风的侧前方。例如，在某次行业协会年度答谢会上，麦克风位置不当导致译员未能听清大使的开场发言，这种尴尬局面完全可以通过会前的设备核实和测试来避免。译员可以根据个人偏好选择麦克风位置，但关键是要在会前测试音效，确保位置既方便译员听清发言又不妨碍受众。

对于涉及多人发言的研讨性会议，发言人坐席的安排也是译员必须关注的一个细节。发言人如果是坐着发言的，译员就可以要求主办方将其安排在紧邻发言人的位置，这样既能降低听辨压力，也便于译员在需要时向发言人请教技术问题或澄清疑点。

三、身心准备

口译工作的特性使得译员必须长时间维持高度集中的专注力。在进行口译时，译员的大脑要同时处理多项任务：一方面，要深入理解发言的核心要点，捕捉其中的细微差别，不论是涉及深奥的科技内容、复杂的法律条文，还是微妙的外交辞令；另一方面，还要进行笔记记录，这一过程本身就要求译员具备出色的逻辑分析和整理能力。同时，译员还须分出部分精力用于记忆，以便随时唤醒笔记中的内容与逻辑结构。最后，译员还须将存储的信息和逻辑关系以符合目标语言习惯的方式重新组合并表达出来。简而言之，口译过程中，译员的大脑就像是一个多功能的处理器，要同时完成多种任务，且每个步骤都必须在短时间内迅速完成，形成连续的循环，这无疑是对体力和脑力的极大挑战。

此外，口译工作还常常面临其他诸多挑战。例如，当译员服务的对象是精力充沛的政界或商界领袖时，工作难度会进一步增加。这些领导人的日程往往安排得十分紧凑，从早餐会到跨时区飞行后的会议，再到晚上的招待会，几乎整天都在忙碌。译员不仅拼智商、情商，更拼的是体力。面对这样的工作强度，译员如果体能跟不上，就很难保证翻译质量的稳定。因此，译员在会前可以做一些呼吸练习来放松身心，准备一些小零食来补充能量。更重要的是，译员要在平时就注重身心的锻炼，避免接受工作条件恶劣的任务，以及防止过度超时服务等。

同时，译员也要学会保持工作与生活的平衡。在翻译任务繁重时，过度透支身心并非长久之计。在实践中，译员会遇到各种不同类型的会议，每一种都有其独特的挑战和要求。下文将通过分析几种常见的会议类型，来具体说明译员应如何在口译工作中应用上述原则。

(一) 礼节性拜会[①]

对于译员而言，礼节性拜会这一环节既带有便利性，又充满挑战性。其便利性在于，此类会谈通常不涉及对实质性问题的深入探讨，因此译员无须过分专注于对某一议题的深入挖掘。然而，其挑战性则在于会谈内容的不确定性，会谈内容可能涉及广泛而多样的主题，涵盖多个领域。礼节性拜会可能出现在多种场合，如新领导上任时，双方须进行初步认识与交流；或是在工作交接之际，双方要回顾过去并展望未来；抑或是在政商领袖访问时，利用短暂的会面机会以了解当前动态，巩固双方关系。

在准备此类会议时，由于缺乏明确的议题清单作为指引，译员须依据准备时间的充裕程度，按照重要性和紧急性原则，为自己制定一个重点搜索清单。这份清单实质上是一个有序的、有重点的搜索计划，它能够帮助译员将有限的精力集中于关键内容，避免在信息的海洋中迷失方向或因遗忘而忽略对重要领域的了解。

以具体实例来说明搜索清单的制定过程。假设一位译员接受了拜访政府部门的会议翻译任务。在向客户索要背景资料时，译员得到的回复相当笼统，仅提到会谈将涉及一些税收和关税问题，而没有具体的讨论要点。这种情况可能由两个原因造成：一是客户对会议的重视程度不够，认为只是礼节性拜访，无须深入讨论，因此没有提供详细信息；二是客户对翻译工作的性质存在误解，认为译员凭借经验就能应对一切，不必过多准备。然而，这种误解在客户中并不少见。

面对这种情况，译员不应被动等待或敷衍了事，而应主动向客户追问必要的基础信息。例如，关于税收或关税的讨论是针对哪些服务或产品。这是一个关键信息，但客户并未明确说明，因此译员必须主动追问。在掌握了这些基础信息后，译员便可以列出搜索清单，充分利用有限的准备时间，确保会议的顺利进行。

上述礼节性拜会的搜索清单包括以下内容：

1. 双方简历

简历可帮助译员大致了解可能涉及的主题，在进一步搜索时知道用哪些主题词，译员还可以从教育、职业背景推测发言人可能的讲话风格等。

2. 特定商品或服务的关税

了解双方在此问题上的具体诉求和分歧。关税属特定领域，译员最好能够掌握该领域高频出现的词汇和用语的双语表达。

3. 两部门近期的高层互访

特别注意高层官员人名或签署/谈判的重要协议名称等。这些虽然不是什么实质性

---

① 齐涛云. 商务英语翻译教程(口译)(第三版)[M]. 北京：中国水利水电出版社，2022.

的内容，但不能凭借逻辑记忆的人名或协议名有时会意外地给译员造成困扰。

4. 会谈双方团长的近期发言

可借此了解双方近期的工作重点或关注重点，这或许会是闲谈时的话题。

5. 扩展阅读

若时间还有富余，译员可就搜索过程中发现的兴趣或热点领域作更深入的探究，这也是译员平时积累的一部分内容。

(二) 商务谈判型会议①

商务谈判型会议最主要的特点就是内容比较敏感，译员在会前往往难以获取大量实质性的资料。当面临时间紧迫且资料匮乏的困境时，译员应如何妥善准备？下文以"跨国并购谈判"为例，简要说明短时间内的准备方法。

第一步，需要搜索的关键条目包括：首席谈判人员简历，谈判双方立场、分歧及目标，公司并购的关键商务和法律术语，公司并购合同范本，两家公司（并购方和被并购方）的主要业务概况，两家公司所属的行业的发展概况等。

第二步，译员需要借助网络搜索。在掌握主谈人员的基本情况时，译员除了查阅简历之外，还可以重点观看双方在各种场合的发言和访谈视频资料。这样译员不仅可以加深了解服务对象所关注的核心议题和基本观点，还能通过从各种渠道收集到的信息，大致掌握双方的立场、分歧和目标等关键要素。然而，译员的工作并不止于此，他们还需要进一步挖掘这些立场、分歧和目标背后的深层次原因。例如，从公司的历史沿革、企业文化、所在国的文化习俗和法律环境等多个维度，去探究这些关键信息的形成背景。虽然谈判本身可能并不涉及这些深层次的讨论，但对这些议题的深入理解对于译员把握双方的逻辑思维、捕捉言外之意具有至关重要的作用。搜索阶段同样是一个梳理思绪的过程。在这个过程中，译员可以凭借个人经验进行信息的筛选与整合；同时，译员也可以主动向会议方提出疑问，以获取更多基础且必要的信息。在得到客户许可的情况下，译员还可以联系曾处理过类似议题的同事，从他们那里获取更多的信息支持，这样就能够更全面地掌握情况，为接下来的翻译工作作好充分准备。

第三步，需要选择会合地点，译员决定在代表团下榻的酒店与其会合。在乘车前往会场的途中，译员可以基于现有知识储备，向代表团团长和主题专家提出一些更为专业和细致的疑问，这些疑问涵盖了搜索问题清单中尚未得到解答的部分。提问不仅是一门技巧，更是一种重要的学习方式。恰当的问题能够激发客户的回答兴趣，同时也是客户评估译员工作态度和专业能力的重要依据。

(三) 技术类交流会议 ②

此类会议的一大突出特点便是其高度的专业性。因此，译员在紧迫的时间里建立起

---

① 齐涛云. 商务英语翻译教程（口译）（第三版）[M]. 北京：中国水利水电出版社，2022.
② 齐涛云. 商务英语翻译教程（口译）（第三版）[M]. 北京：中国水利水电出版社，2022.

必要的专业知识体系尤为关键。以某译员为航空航天代表团提供口译服务为例，他在会前获得了日程安排以及一系列相关部门网站的链接。虽然日程表仅列出了会议时间和单位名称，但这些链接却为译员提供了会谈机构的网络资源。由于会议准备时间只有一天，译员在正式搜索之前，先根据日程安排和会见单位的信息，对受众及可能的议题进行了初步分析，以明确搜索的重点方向。

在准备会见的过程中，译员首先要识别出会见机构的不同类型，这包括政府部门、基础研究机构、应用研究机构以及国家重点项目工程办公室等。同时，译员还须根据议题进行分类，涵盖地球科学、空间科学、航天科学等基础研究，以及资源、环境卫星、空间实验等应用技术，还有航天、航空工业的产业政策及技术标准。根据这些信息，译员可以预测可能的议题，如双边科技合作框架、知识产权、出口管制、国会态度、标准及规范以及已开展的合作等。

参与这类会议的人员主要是科学家和工程技术人员。因此，译员要重点准备三方面的内容：一是迅速识别各学科的重点会谈领域；二是理解合作领域涉及的科学、技术基本原理；三是掌握特定领域的术语及概念的双语表达。

在应对此类口译任务时，译员要有效利用各种资源。首先，译员可以依赖过往经验和网络资源，包括之前相关会议积累的资源、相关部门网站的内容以及特定领域的权威报告等。其次，译员可以向会议方追问访问意图、双方的合作项目及存在的问题，以及是否有计划中的合作项目等内容。再次，代表团成员也是宝贵的资源，译员要尽可能在会前和会议间隙多向他们提问并寻求解答。最后，现场资源同样不可忽视，例如主办方直接用英语介绍的展板内容，以及会场上的专家。译员应利用这些资源快速充电，并在必要时争取专家的帮助。

总之，译员在准备和参与此类会议时，需要全面考虑不同机构类型、议题分类以及人员特点，并有效利用各种资源，以确保口译任务的顺利完成。

（四）高级别会议——筹备会议[①]

此类会议通常涵盖的议题广泛而敏感，从贸易救济到数据保护，再到市场准入等，每一个议题都关乎双方的核心利益。以中美商贸联委会筹备会议为例，这种会议不仅议题众多，而且涉及双方多个政府部门，要协调各方立场，确保谈判的顺利进行。这些议题都是双方期待对方解释或承诺的关键领域，内容往往十分敏感，译员在会前往往难以获得详细的资料，这无疑增加了翻译的难度。此外，会议气氛有时也会变得紧张，因为双方都希望能在谈判中取得优势，这可能导致讲者语速加快、情绪激昂，双方甚至出现紧张的对峙局面。在这种情况下，译员要保持冷静，准确传达双方的意图和立场。为了应对这种挑战，建议译员尽早开始准备，通过查阅相关资料了解议题背景和现状，确定翻译难点，并主动向相关负责人员追问细节，如是否有涉诉案件及其具体情况，以便更好地掌握背景信息。同时，译员还须掌握各领域专门术语的双语表达，确保翻译的准确

---

① 齐涛云. 商务英语翻译教程（口译）（第三版）[M]. 北京：中国水利水电出版社，2022.

性和专业性。总之，此类会议的翻译工作不仅要求译员具备扎实的语言功底和专业知识，还要求他们具备高度的应变能力和心理素质，以应对可能出现的各种复杂情况。

（五）政府领导率领的贸易、投资代表团会议①

例如，美国某州州长率领了一个由多个行业部门的企业代表组成的贸易、投资代表团访问北京，行业涵盖酿酒业、旅游业、制造业和运输服务业等。此类翻译任务难度颇高，因为涉及的企业行业众多，要查阅的网站内容繁杂；而且代表团中的企业多为中小企业，提供的产品或服务较为专业和冷门，难以记忆和理解。此外，代表团规模庞大，部分成员离译员较远，如果发言声音小或语速快，会给译员带来额外的压力。

州长此次出访的目的主要是推介该州的投资和贸易机会，吸引外资，并帮助州内企业拓展在华的贸易和投资机遇。因此，译员在准备阶段要进行深入细致的工作。首先，译员应确定搜索重点，包括州情、推介项目、双方往来历史、团长信息以及企业产品服务等。其次，译员可以仔细浏览客户提供的资料以及州政府和企业的网站，特别关注施政方案、新闻公报和公司历史等内容。最后，译员在会前要主动与企业代表进行接触和沟通，了解他们的口音、发言要点和疑问，以便更好地进行翻译。

值得注意的是，政府率领的贸易代表团往往人员众多，开场自我介绍常常会给译员带来挑战。成员姓氏和公司名称各异，有些还难以记忆，而且每个人介绍自己和产品时速度非常快。为了应对这一问题，某使馆商务处采用了一种有效方法：按照企业宣传册子的顺序安排代表团成员的坐席。这样，译员只须按照宣传册子的顺序进行翻译，无须费力将名字、面孔和产品一一对应。对于未来可能遇到的类似情况，译员也可以采用这一办法，与主办方沟通，以减轻翻译过程中的负担。

（六）技术研讨会②

技术研讨会是技术人员在集中场地针对特定技术主题进行交流与讨论的会议，通常包含主题演讲及专题讨论等环节。

这样的会议，相较于其他技术性交流会，对内容的专业性要求更高。特别是在专业领域日益细分的今天，即便是同一领域的技术人员，若各自专注于不同的研究方向或子领域，可能也会难以理解对方的工作内容。因此，对于语言专业出身的译员而言，翻译技术研讨会所涉及的高度专业的会议内容无疑是一项巨大的挑战。

专业术语的复杂性和多样性，是技术研讨会专业性的一个重要体现。有时，仅仅一场研讨会就会涉及数百个专业术语，或者一张主题演讲的幻灯片就罗列出数十个术语。这些术语，有的构词复杂，难以记忆，如医学领域的"uvulopalatopharyngoplasty"（悬雍垂腭咽成形术）、"costochondritis"（肋软骨炎）等；有的则与其字面意义大相径庭，如法律领域的"attorney in fact"一词，译者很容易望文生义，直接译为"事实律师"或"实际

---

① 齐涛云. 商务英语翻译教程（口译）（第三版）[M]. 北京：中国水利水电出版社，2022.
② 齐涛云. 商务英语翻译教程（口译）（第三版）[M]. 北京：中国水利水电出版社，2022.

律师"，但实际上经过查证，译者应该知道该词是指"委托代理人"。再如"die without issue"这一表达，实际上是指"去世时无子嗣"。此外，研讨会还常使用缩略型术语，如石化行业的"BTX"和"HDS"等，在翻译这些缩略语时，译员有时可以直接移植到中文中使用，有时则要先还原其英文全称再进行翻译。缩略语有不同的翻译方式，有些习惯于移植到中文直接使用，如"BTX"（不必译成"苯-甲苯-二甲苯混合物"）；有些则要先还原英文全称再转换成中文，如"HDS"（英文全称hydrodesulfurization，中文译成"加氢脱硫"）。因此，译员必须熟练掌握这些术语的中英文表述，以便在口译现场能够迅速、准确地进行转换。

由于技术研讨会上的讲话人通常没有事先准备好的讲稿，译前准备显得尤为重要。译员主要围绕会议议程和演讲幻灯片进行准备，从议程中提取关键词，并通过互联网搜索建立初步的背景知识框架。对于幻灯片，译员要深入学习，确定术语的准确表述，理解技术背景知识，并在不确定或无法理解的地方做好标记，以便在适当的时候请教演讲嘉宾或其他专家。

除了对议程和幻灯片的准备，译员还应特别关注计量单位的使用习惯，并进行中英文转换训练。如果时间允许，译员还可以进一步学习其他会议资料，如嘉宾简介、参会机构简介等，以增强对会议内容的了解。

会议组织机构如果安排彩排，这对译员来说是一个极好的机会。在彩排中，译员可以提前熟悉演讲内容和演讲者的讲话风格，以便在口译现场更快地进入状态。即使没有彩排，译员也应积极争取与演讲者进行简短沟通，解决译前准备中的疑问，并约定会议现场的交流方式。

会议当天，译员应提前到达会场，确认口译工作条件，检查设备，并再次熟悉演讲内容。对于译员来说，克服紧张情绪、抓住讲话人的思路、调整好自己的情绪和声音、控制好表达节奏，都是确保口译工作顺利进行的关键。好的开始是成功的一半，一旦进入状态，译员就能更加专注于口译工作，应对各种挑战。

第二单元　交传核心技巧

第一节　口译记忆

在口译过程中，译员必须一边理解源语内容，一边对关键信息等进行储存。[①] 想要准确地进行口译工作，译员务必确保能够记住源语内容，而这主要依赖于两种记忆途径：大脑记忆与笔记。这两者之间，应确立一种以大脑记忆为主导，笔记记录为辅助的协作关系。实际上，大部分源语内容需要依靠译员的大脑进行记忆，而口译笔记仅仅起到辅助作用。尽管记忆力在很大程度上受先天遗传的影响，但译员完全可以通过后天的专项训练来提升记忆能力。本单元将首先介绍大脑记忆的工作原理，并在此基础上介绍几种在口译实践中广泛运用的记忆方法。

一、记忆机制

（一）瞬时记忆

瞬时记忆，亦可被称作"感觉记忆"或"感觉登记"，它描述的是外界信息在接触人的感觉器官后，如何在极短的时间内被迅速登记并暂时储存的过程。无论是听觉、视觉、嗅觉、味觉还是触觉，只要这些信息接触到了我们的感官，它们都会被记录。值得注意的是，这些信息大多处于原始的、未经加工的状态。如果我们不给予足够的关注，它们会迅速消失，因为瞬时记忆的容量虽然大，但保持的时间却非常短暂，通常只有几秒钟。

无论是谁，只要感官功能正常，身处某个环境时，都会不自觉地接收大量的瞬时记忆信息。比如，在机场等待飞机时，你可能会一边看着窗外的风景，一边感受着座椅的舒适度、机场的温度，同时听着周围的声音。这些感觉都是存在的，它们会被暂时储存为瞬时记忆信息。但有时候，你可能被窗外的风景深深吸引，以至于几乎感觉不到其他的事物。然而，一旦机场的广播响起，你可能会立刻将注意力转向广播，想要确认是否有关于你所乘航班的消息。这充分说明，我们随时都能感知到周围环境的变化，并能从海量的瞬时记忆信息中筛选出重要的信息，并给予更多的关注。通过对这些重要信息进一步加工，它们会在我们的大脑中留下更深的记忆痕迹，从而延长其保持时间，进入短时记忆乃至长时记忆。

---

① 鲍刚. 口译理论概述[M]. 北京：中国对外翻译出版有限公司，2011.

对于口译员来说，他们在口译现场接收到的瞬时记忆信息非常丰富，包括讲话人的肢体语言、幻灯片文本等视觉信息，但最为关键的还是讲话人的声音信息。一般而言，译员在听辨后，会将听到的语音存储在大脑感知记忆的储存仓里，等待着下一步处理。① 然而，由于语言的特性，并非每个信息单位，比如每个词、每个句子，在构建意义时都同等重要。因此，口译员必须在极短的时间内判断出哪些信息重要，哪些次要，甚至哪些无用，并据此有效地分配注意力，进一步加工那些高度相关的信息，使其从瞬时记忆转化为短时记忆或长时记忆。

讲话人有时会语速飞快、连读吞音，或带有浓厚的口音，甚至使用古语、俚语或深奥的行业术语，有时他们使用的语言还不是口译员的母语。在这种情况下，口译员若想迅速判断各信息单位的重要性，就必须具备出色的源语语音听辨能力。如果口译员不能在短时间内准确辨识出讲话人使用的词、句子等信息单位，那么他就无法判断其重要性，更无法对重要信息进行额外加工处理。这样，讲话人的声音信息就会像其他瞬时记忆信息一样，保持在未加工的状态，并在几秒钟后消失。

因此，瞬时记忆不仅是口译交际的基础，也是口译过程的信息源头。而口译员良好的源语语音听辨能力，则是确保讲话信息从瞬时记忆顺利转化为短时记忆和长时记忆的关键前提。

(二) 短时记忆

短时记忆是指个体在接收外界刺激信息后，能在几分钟内保持的记忆状态。这种记忆类型的容量是有限的，一般为 7±2 个组块(chunk)。举例来说，我们要拨打一个电话号码时，在电话簿中查找并读一遍，就可以立即根据短时记忆拨出这个号码。但打完电话后不久，这个号码可能就会被我们遗忘，这就是短时记忆的典型特征。

短时记忆在整个记忆系统中扮演着中转站和信息处理中心的角色。一般而言，短时记忆的持续时间在 1 分钟左右。② 一些信息在短时记忆中很快就会被遗忘，而另一些信息则可以通过反复回忆和复述，从而加深记忆痕迹，最终转化为持久性更强的长时记忆，成为我们长期储存的知识。

组块是短时记忆的基本单位，它可以是一个数字、字母、单词或音节等单独的信息，也可以是这些信息的集合或组合，比如一组数字、一句话、一个段落或者整个篇章。尽管从数量上看，短时记忆的容量是有限的，但由于组块内容的灵活性和可扩展性，实际上短时记忆的容量在一定程度上是可以扩展的。

例1： 读一遍以下两组数字组合，看看能记住几个。

1. 147483，395191，593045，720467，906389，874839；
2. 19491001，2024，135791113，12345678，0601，12315，666666，13511145678

---

① 梅德明. 高级口译教程[M]. 上海：上海外语教育出版社，2006.
② 鲍刚. 口译理论概述[M]. 北京：中国对外翻译出版有限公司，2011.

(你的手机号),20010823(你的出生年月日)。

对于第一组数字组合,由于其结构毫无规律,人们往往难以在单次阅读后记住超过两个数字。这是因为每一个数字都需要占用一个组块,而整个组合包含12位数字,远远超出了大脑短时记忆能够处理的7±2个组块的最大限度。相比之下,第二组数字组合由于其内在的规律性,使得人们能够更轻松地记住3个以上的数字。只要识别出这些数字组合的构造规律,记忆整个组合就只占用一个组块,理论上讲,人们能够记住的组块数量就可以达到7±2个。这种将小信息单元组合成更大信息单元,以扩展单个组块信息容量的方法,我们称之为组块化。

在口译实践中,译员往往需要即时记忆长达3~5分钟甚至更久的讲话内容。为了将这些内容保存在短时记忆中,译员必须对讲话内容进行组块化处理。这个过程涉及对信息的深入分析,以找出或建立信息单元之间的联系,属于对信息的深度加工。这样做不仅可以增大组块的容量,还能加深这些信息在大脑中的记忆深度,延长其保持时间,从而满足口译现场的实际需求。许多译员都有这样的体验:尽管在口译过程中表现得相当出色,完整准确地传达了讲话内容,但在口译结束后,要想全面回忆起自己所翻译的内容却相当困难。这是因为部分翻译内容会转化为长时记忆,而其余部分则会从大脑中消失,为后续的口译活动腾出记忆空间。

(三)长时记忆

长时记忆,作为大脑持久储存信息的核心手段,其保留期限从几分钟到数天,甚至伴随终生。长时记忆包括了个人认知经验、语言技能、百科知识等。自孩提时代起,我们每天都在经历新的事物,学习新的知识,其中许多都被深深刻画在长时记忆的画卷中。这种记忆的容量之大,几乎无法估量。

而在口译领域,长时记忆中的语言知识,特别是语音知识尤为重要。它不仅是口译员进行语音听辨的基础,更是判断讲话人声音信息重要性的依据。对于优秀的口译员来说,其长时记忆中应储备丰富的语音知识,既要能识别标准发音,也要能辨别各种口音的英语,包括非洲、拉美、南欧、东南亚、中东等地的口音,以及元音的细微变化、辅音的清浊转换等。此外,译员还要熟悉讲者的不同的音质、发音位置以及讲话习惯,如口语中的连读、略读等。

同时,长时记忆中的百科知识对于口译员准确理解讲话内容也至关重要。讲话人往往学识渊博,除了会议主题,还常常旁征博引。虽然译员可以针对会议主题进行译前准备,但讲话人即兴提及的其他领域内容却难以预测。因此,译员平时须广泛涉猎各类知识,包括政治、经济、人文、科技、商贸、法律、历史、地理、国际知识、民俗风情及生活常识等,努力成为跨学科的"杂家"。每次口译任务前,译员还须认真准备,通过阅读会议文件、收集相关资料、整理词汇等方式,丰富自己的长时记忆知识库。此外,长时记忆中的丰富知识还有助于译员在口译现场对讲话人信息进行高效的组块化处理。例如,对于常见的日期、数字组合等,人们往往能迅速将其作为一个整体记忆,这得益于长时记忆的积累。听到"跨太平洋战略经济伙伴关系协定"这样的专业术语时，熟悉该术语的译员只需占用一个组块进行记忆，而不熟悉的译员记忆该短语可能会占用5~6个组块（跨太平洋—战略—经济—伙伴—关系—协定）。因此，译员平时应积累大量的预构置语块（prefabricated chunk），以提高口译的效率和准确性。

有些人认为口译是年轻人的职业，因为随着年龄增长，人的记忆力会减退。然而，这种看法忽视了长时记忆在口译中的重要作用。即使现场记忆能力有所下降，丰富的长时记忆仍能帮助译员高效处理信息，保持出色的口译表现。一些联合国高级译员退休后之所以仍被返聘，正是得益于他们长时记忆中的丰富知识库。

二、记忆方法

在口译过程中，译员所调动的记忆方式并不是单一的长时记忆或短时记忆，而是二者的有机组合。① 前文提到，如果译员拥有庞大的长时记忆知识库，在口译现场就能更高效地进行信息组块化处理，从而显著提升口译现场的记忆效果。然而，这种知识库的积累是一个漫长而持续的过程，需要长时间的积累和努力。即便如此，译员在口译现场仍可能遇到一些不熟悉的新信息。因此，除了在日常充实长时记忆知识库，译员还须掌握现场记忆的技巧来增强对新信息的记忆效果，使新信息在口译现场的工作记忆中保持足够的时长。记忆效果是指大脑对信息进行加工处理后留下的记忆痕迹。信息加工得越深入，记忆痕迹就越深刻，记忆效果也就越佳。而记忆方法实际上指的就是对信息进行加工处理的方式。接下来，本节将梳理几种人们常用的记忆方法。我们首先通过一个有趣的心理学实验来了解一下。

（一）一个心理学实验

例2：表2.1中列出了16个词，在1分钟内，看看你能按顺序记住多少词。②

表2.1

1 树（tree）	9 猫（cat）
2 电灯开关（switch）	10 保龄球（bowling）
3 椅子（chair）	11 球门（gate）
4 汽车（car）	12 鸡蛋（egg）
5 手套（glove）	13 女巫（witch）
6 手枪（pistol）	14 戒指（ring）
7 骰子（cube/dice）	15 薪水（salary）
8 溜冰鞋（roller-skate）	16 鲜花（flower）

① 鲍刚．口译理论概述［M］．北京：中国对外翻译出版有限公司，2011．
② 齐涛云．商务英语翻译教程（口译）（第三版）［M］．北京：中国水利水电出版社，2022．

有心理学研究者曾做过一个简单的记忆实验，给不同的人1分钟时间，不让他们使用任何外在工具，仅凭大脑按既定排序记忆表2.1中的16个词。实验发现，记忆效果的个体差异非常明显。有人仅能记住5个或更少，绝大部分能记住5~10个，少数人能记住11~13个，也有人可以按顺序全部准确记忆。进一步分析参与者对自己记忆过程的描述，研究人员发现，记忆方法的不同直接导致了记忆效果的显著差别。

在实验中仅能记住5个及以下词汇的人大都采用了简单重复法，即在一分钟内反复诵读这些词条，大脑却没有对这些词条进行积极加工。有些参与者意识到自己的记忆能力有限，因此选择集中诵读前5个词条，并且能记下这5个词条。另一些人集中诵读前16个词条，每个词条诵读的次数都不够多，结果能记住的还不到5个。

一名参与者把16个词条按顺序准确地全部记住了，是因为这个参与者把16个词条串联起来，编成了下面的故事：

  大树上安装着电灯开关，树下有把椅子，椅子在一辆汽车里，"我"坐上汽车，戴上黑手套，拿上手枪，开车到了一个赌场。"我"先用骰子赌博；又穿着溜冰鞋溜冰，溜冰鞋被设计成了猫的形状；还打了保龄球，球门下的球瓶是用鸡蛋来代替的。鸡蛋打破后，女巫出现了，使用她的戒指施展魔法，"我"不得不把所有的薪水都拿出来买鲜花送给了她。

这名参与者一边用故事串联这些词条，一边想象它们构成的画面场景。这样，本来相互孤立的16个词条在故事里形成了联系。故事由时间线索贯穿始末，空间场景从"大树下"转换到"赌场"等空间，这使用的是"逻辑记忆法"。在大脑中想象这些事物构成的画面和场景，这使用的是"形象记忆法"。编故事时融入某些个人经历，想象场景时把自己熟悉的图像放置其中，把自己设想为主人公，这些都是"关联记忆法"的常用技巧。该实验参与者在记忆过程中采用了多种方法，对接收到的信息进行多种积极的加工处理，记忆效果很好。

"简单重复法""关联记忆法""逻辑记忆法"和"形象记忆法"是四种常用的记忆方法，是对信息进行加工处理的四种方式。

(二) 简单重复法

简单重复法是指通过反复诵读或默读信息来记忆的方法。然而，这种方法本质上是一种较为被动的记忆方式，因为它并不涉及大脑对接收到的信息深度且主动的思考加工，因此简单重复法的记忆效率往往不高，效果相对有限。很多常常抱怨自己记忆力不佳的人，可能正是习惯了这种记忆方式。

(三) 关联记忆法

关联记忆法通过连接大脑中已有的知识与新接收到的信息，对信息进行加工处理，从而达到记忆的目的。关联的形式灵活多样，例如，当译员听到关于某个议题的观点时，他们可以调动长时记忆库中关于同一议题的相似或相反观点进行对比。例如，听到美国官员提到以下观点：You know, historically, United States is the greatest emitter. But this year China surpassed us. We cannot look at per capita basis. We have to look at absolute emission。译员可以立刻联想到中国政府对这一问题的看法，即中国人口基数大，每个中国公民都有权利享有较高的生活水平，因此碳排放不能只看总量，要看人均。[1]

在口译现场，如果难以在短时间内从长时记忆中调出可以进行直接比较的知识，译员还可以基于个人的认知经验对接收到的信息作出个人化的评价，比如判断自己是否赞同其中的观点。这种简单的回应，也能加深该信息的记忆痕迹。

关联记忆法使用频率高、应用范围广，通常用来对完整信息的局部进行加工处理，并且常常与"逻辑记忆法""形象记忆法"等其他记忆方法结合使用。

（四）逻辑记忆法

语言是有逻辑的。词与词能依据其含义之间的关联被编织成连贯的句子。句子与句子之间，则通过句法规则和语义联系，编织成能够表达相对完整意思的意群。意群再通过整体的行文结构和逻辑框架，形成完整的语篇。这些连接手段，无论是词语的意义、句子的句法或语义关系，还是行文结构，都属于语言逻辑的范畴。

接收讲话信息时，如果我们能积极地分析和识别这些信息中不同层次的语言逻辑关系，就能将原本零散的词、句、意群串联成相互关联、逻辑缜密的有机整体。这种对语言逻辑关系的分析识别过程，也是对信息进行组块化处理的过程。这种基于语言逻辑关系的记忆方法，被称为"逻辑记忆法"。

（五）形象记忆法

形象记忆法，又称视觉化记忆法，其核心在于将接收到的意义或内容转化为大脑中的生动形象和图画，以此来增强记忆效果。这种方法不仅适用于记忆人物、事物、空间和景象等静态的、描述性的信息，同样也可用于记忆故事、动作等动态的、发展的内容。在记忆静态信息时，形象记忆法就像一台相机，在大脑中捕捉并存储下清晰的图像。而在记忆动态信息时，它像一台摄像机，将动作的变化、故事情节的展开"录制"成电影片段，存储在脑海中。通过这种方式，信息变得更加生动、直观，从而更容易存储在大脑中。

（六）结语

关联记忆法、逻辑记忆法和形象记忆法作为三种高效而积极的信息处理方式，有助于对信息进行更为精细的整合与分类，进而扩充记忆的容量，并加深记忆的烙印，使信息得以长久保留。其中，逻辑思维主要在左脑运作，而形象思维则在右脑展开。因此，在口译实践中，译员应灵活结合各种记忆方法，使大脑的左右两侧同时运作，从而达到

---

[1] 齐涛云. 商务英语翻译教程（口译）（第三版）[M]. 北京：中国水利水电出版社，2022.

最佳的记忆效果。

第二节 口译笔记

一、为什么需要口译笔记

口译笔记可以减轻大脑的记忆负荷。口译研究领域的知名专家、巴黎高等翻译学院的教授吉尔(Gile)提出了交替传译的认知负荷模型理论。该理论认为人的注意力是有限的。因此，译员在口译过程中要同时处理多项任务时，必须科学、合理地分配注意力。记笔记可以显著减轻译员短期记忆的负担。通过记录关键信息、数字、人名以及逻辑脉络，译员能够大大降低大脑的记忆压力。

适当地做笔记可以辅助译员激活记忆。译员一边理解原文逻辑，一边在笔记上留下痕迹，同时其大脑内会保持分析的过程。根据认知心理学的观点，有时短时记忆中的信息并未被忘记，只是很难被提取。当译员回顾笔记，然后重新组织语言进行翻译时，这些笔记便如同路灯一般，引导译员迅速定位并激活相关记忆。口译笔记中的关键词和表示逻辑的符号、箭头等，能够在译员进行笔记识读和口译的时候迅速激活译员的记忆，帮助译员回忆起听到的信息，辅助口译输出。

笔记还可以辅助改善译文。成熟的口译笔记不仅会呈现原文的信息关键点，还会体现原文的逻辑结构，而且这个逻辑结构是经过了译员大脑分析、提取和精炼之后的逻辑结构，是在理解的基础上对原文的重新整合。因此，做笔记并非是对原文信息的机械式记录，而是对原文深层结构的解析，是经过了理解和分析之后的逻辑和信息再现。这样的笔记往往会对口译的最后输出阶段起到积极的作用，甚至能够改善译文。尤其是当原文的表层逻辑条理不够清晰的时候，建立在深层理解基础上的笔记往往会帮助译员输出逻辑条理更加清晰的译文。

二、口译笔记的特点

口译笔记具有其独特性，它不同于课堂笔记和会议记录。口译笔记的核心价值在于即时应用，而不是为日后回顾或查证使用。由于口译工作具有即时性，译员在翻译时仍能清晰记得讲话的内容，因此译员不必把全文记录下来，而只需要作些简单标记，达到提示的目的。①

在交替传译过程中，如果译员能仅凭记忆力，完整无误地翻译讲者所说的全部内容，那就不需要记录。然而在实际操作中，一般译员很难做到这一点。在一些重大场合，如国际会议上，讲者不可能每说一句话就暂停等待翻译，而是会讲一段话才停顿，以保证意思的连贯和完整。有时，讲话还涉及一些较复杂的数字、人名、地名等元素。在这些情况下，如果完全依靠脑记而不作记录，往往会将重要内容漏译或错译，有时甚

---

① [瑞士]让·艾赫贝尔.口译须知[M].孙慧双,译.北京：外语教学与研究出版社,1982.

至会造成很大损失。因此，口译笔记作为交替口译中的一项核心技能，其作用不容忽视。它不仅可以帮助译员记录部分讲话内容，减轻记忆的负担，还能辅助译员整理信息，确保口译输出的准确性和完整性。

做口译笔记不是像速记一样进行简单的符号转换，不是像听写一样记下每个单词甚至包括标点符号，也不是像课堂笔记一样只记录重点信息。口译笔记有快速性、条理性、精练性、独特性这四大特点。

口译活动的快速性体现在它要求译员做到"一心多用"。译员应当以脑记为主、笔记为辅，遵循"三分记七分听"的脑力分配原则，在做笔记时，译员应尽可能花费最少的时间和精力做最高效的记录，甚至力求做到"自动输出"的程度。译员无须为了追求笔记的"美观"而牺牲时间和精力，因为口译笔记只起到即时提醒的作用，口译工作结束后，译员往往自己也无法回忆起笔记的内容。

口译笔记应具备条理性。口译笔记不是文字信息的罗列和堆砌，而是关键信息和信息之间逻辑关系的有机呈现。逻辑显化、条理清晰的笔记能有效地辅助口译输出，而缺乏内在联系的符号或文字堆砌则会给译员增加辨识负担，阻碍口译的连贯进行。

译员做笔记主要运用符号、缩略语等手段，精准凝练地记录讲话内容。随着练习的增加，译员逐渐会"条件反射"地记录下必要信息，略去可以省略的信息，合理协调笔记和脑记的分工。注意笔记应准确记录信息并易于辨认，不能为了追求速度牺牲准确性和易读性。读不懂或记录有误的笔记还不如没有笔记。

每一份口译笔记都具有其独特性。笔记是译员为了保证口译顺利进行，对讲话进行的概括性记录。口译笔记有别于听写和速记，仅为译员当场顺利完成口译提供提示和帮助。口译活动一旦完成，笔记也就失去了作用，所以口译笔记往往具有个性化和独特性。不同的译员记口译笔记的习惯不尽相同，有的译员习惯多用笔头记录，有的则更多依靠短时记忆；有的译员习惯多使用源语记录，有的则更偏向于使用译入语记录。即使是同一名译员，其口译笔记也会根据其对讲话内容的熟悉程度发生动态变化。学习口译笔记切忌生搬硬套。但需要注意的是，优秀译员的笔记呈现出的基本格式和遵循的基本原则往往是共通的。

三、口译笔记的记法

从内容上来说，口译笔记主要记录主要信息、逻辑结构、关键细节这几个方面的内容：

（一）主要信息

译员一般会采用记关键词的方法记录讲话的主要信息，但关键词的目的是提示译员原文的"意思"(sense)，而非具体的文字形式。因此译员并不是原封不动地记下原文词，而往往通过字符(文字、符号、图形等)来记录信息。

（二）逻辑结构

口译笔记的关键是理解，译员记笔记也是一个主动分析和理解的过程，在笔记中记录逻辑有利于译员对讲话整体结构的把握，记录下的逻辑关系符号能提示译员一系列意思之间的关联，从而有助于输出逻辑条理清晰的译文。

(三) 关键细节

讲话中出现的一些具体信息和关键细节，包括人名、数字、专有名词、专业术语等，往往难以通过联系上下文的方法进行理解式记忆，需要译员用笔记录下来。

从格式上来说，掌握正确的记录格式非常重要，记笔记的原则是要简明醒目，一目了然。译员在现场一般使用小于32开本可上下翻动的小型活页记事本，纸张质量要好，单面使用，避免透过纸的字迹影响辨认，行距要宽，字体要较大。每做一场新的口译最好把前面的记录撕掉。

口译笔记的基本格式要满足以下几点：

第一，做到少字多意：译员在口译过程中需要将大量的精力分配给脑记，笔记是一种必要的避免信息丢失的手段，作用在于辅助和激活脑记。口译笔记不是听写，不求记全，而是尽量使用最少的文字或符号来表现最丰富的含义。除了字词以外，译员可以灵活使用各种符号、箭头、缩略语等，框架性地提示内容之间的逻辑关系，使笔记更为简练。

第二，做到少横多竖：与其他笔记不同的是，口译笔记采取竖记的形式，每行最多记录三到四个意群，意群之间往往用斜线隔开。竖写笔记的目的在于方便译员一眼扫视，迅速读出。此外，纵向延伸的笔记还可以帮助译员对原文结构进行处理，显化信息之间的逻辑关系，进一步帮助译员输出译文。

第三，做到明确结束：每次记录完一段在开始翻译之前，都要在下方画一道横线或斜线，表示一个层次的完结。这样不会在翻译时看串行或漏译，并且避免和下一段记录混在一起。否则，很可能在翻译下一段时，一时找不到句子从何处开始，因而乱了阵脚。

四、口译笔记讲解示例①

段落1：文明之间的交流互鉴使世界更加多彩。我们要有开放的心态，多倾听不同文明的声音，从不同文明中寻求智慧、汲取营养。本次研讨会真是大咖云集，有来自中国、美国、俄罗斯、英国、菲律宾等国家的近50位顶尖学者。我们真心希望每位嘉宾都能畅所欲言，一起为打造一个和平、安全、繁荣的世界贡献力量。(见图2.1)

段落2：中华文明自古崇尚自然，热爱自然。大熊猫是来自800万年前的地球物种明星。中国辟出2.7万平方公里山林，成立大熊猫国家公园。近2000只野生大熊猫在这里自由生活、繁衍生息。(见图2.2)

段落3：Innovation stands as the beacon guiding humanity's relentless pursuit of excellence. It ignites creative sparks, shatters boundaries of possibility, and reshapes our world for the better. Let us embrace this spirit with open arms, fostering a culture of curiosity, experimentation, and collaboration, as we work towards a future where innovation

---

① 齐涛云．商务英语翻译教程(口译)(第三版)[M]．北京：中国水利水电出版社，2022．

thrives, and the limits of what is possible are continually pushed further. (见图 2.3)

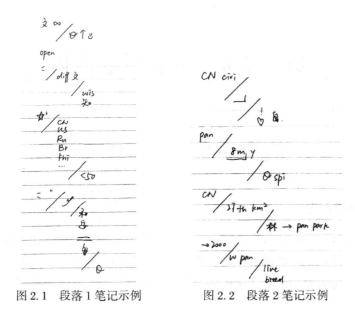

图 2.1　段落 1 笔记示例　　图 2.2　段落 2 笔记示例

段落 4：Ladies and Gentlemen, distinguished guests, in this pivotal moment, we stand united in addressing the formidable challenges that threaten our global health. From pandemics to chronic diseases, these issues transcend borders and require concerted efforts from all corners of the world. Our mission is clear: to foster international cooperation, foster innovation, and increase investments in healthcare solutions that promote wellness and resilience for every individual on this planet. (见图 2.4)

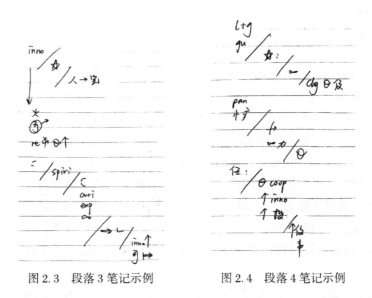

图 2.3　段落 3 笔记示例　　图 2.4　段落 4 笔记示例

25

第三单元 同传核心技巧

第一节 视 译

一、视译的概念

在正式的场合，一些发言人会按照预先准备好的演讲稿进行演说。这些演讲稿通常语言富有文采，逻辑比较缜密，但是讲者的语速会较快。相较于即兴发言，这种类型的演讲可能较难被理解和记忆。在这种情况下，译员可以向发言人索取讲稿，进行视阅口译，即视译。

视译过程中，译员一边阅读讲稿，一边进行快速翻译，这对翻译者的阅读理解能力提出了较高要求，特别是未经预习的即时阅读能力。翻译时须确保语言连贯流畅，避免频繁"回溯"。在翻译现场，译员还须注意讲者可能临时加入的例子，灵活地进行无稿翻译。[①]

视译是同声传译的重要训练方法和工作方式，但是在交传中译员也会经常遇到需要做视译的场景。比如客户通过屏幕展示某个文本，为了节省时间，有时会要求译员直接把文本内容翻译给现场听众，这种情况下就需要译员有较强的视译能力。此外，视译练习对于提升多项交传技能也很有帮助。

二、视译的分类

根据具体的工作状态，视译可细分为视阅口译（sight translation）和视听口译（sight interpreting），前者要求译员靠"sight"接收源语信息，边看边译；后者要求译员靠"sight"和"listening"同时接收信息，但"视"是信息输入的主导方式。就工作强度而言，视阅口译比视听口译的要求相对低些，因为后者还要跟上发言人的语速，这种工作模式其实就是有稿同传。此时的视译常指同传译员拿着讲话人的发言稿，边听发言，边看原稿，边进行传译。视译训练作为同声传译前的初阶练习，旨在使学员学会断句并迅速作出反应，提高口头表达能力。口译硕士专业通常安排一个学期的视译课作为同传预备课程。同传课中还有专门的有稿同传练习，旨在进一步强化视译技能，提高教学效率。

在非同传场合，视译也相当常用，如导游用口译的方式边看工艺品介绍，边译给游

---

① 冯庆华，梅德明. 英语口译教程[M]. 北京：高等教育出版社，2008：318.

客听；边看合作文件，边译给客户听的商务口译；边看治疗方案，边译给病人听的医疗口译；边看司法报告，边译给控辩双方听的法庭口译。视译要求译者在准备时间短甚至没有准备时间的情况下快速地将书面符号转换成口头信息，因此译者必须快速理解文本内容，并克服文本造成的视觉干扰，能边看边译。普通场合的视译和同传场合的视译共同点是两者均有稿件，不同点就是后者还要兼顾演讲者的说话速度，是视译的高级形式。某些时候，译员还须应对一些特别的挑战，如出现演讲者不按照讲稿发言而出现更换语句或段落顺序、总结要点、省略信息甚至临场发挥的情况。当然正式场合的发言力求严谨性，因此这种情况出现的频率不高。本节主要关注将书面稿变为口头表达的视阅翻译，即普通情况下的视译。

三、视译的原则与技巧

（一）顺句驱动

笔译中，译员可看完一个章节，仔细思考后再开始翻译。而视译时，随着视幅（eye span）的推进，信息源源不断涌入，这就要把先看到的信息迅速处理，才能继续处理其他接踵而至的信息。参考同声传译的技巧，可把"顺句驱动"作为视译的核心原则，即按照所看到的原文的顺序，不停地将句子切成"亚单元"，在考虑其连贯性和可接受性的情况下，将这些"亚单元"连贯地表述，使之成为与源语意思相同的目标语。

（二）视译技巧

视译是基于书面文字的口译，输入的是视觉信息，产出的是意思忠实于源语的句子。译员要出色完成任务，译前准备很重要，在时间允许的情况下，可通读书面材料全文，了解其写作框架及大意，对专业术语、数字以及货币、面积等单位进行标注。根据"阅读+记忆+整合+产出"的工作模式，视译主要使用断句及衔接两类技巧。

1. 断句。

断句是以适当的意群或概念为单位，将句子进行切割处理，分成意义相对独立的"亚单元"以方便用目标语表达，其出发点是"断好才可接得更好"。断句更多地针对英文长句，由于英语句式为"树形结构"，较为正式的视译材料中一句话有几十个单词的情况很普遍，因此合理断句很关键，是顺句驱动的首要条件。

例1：More private schools in Britain are posting ads / in foreign newspapers, / redesigning their websites / in multiple languages/ and taking part in various recruiting fairs worldwide / where they promise to provide language training / and the right mix of course work / and extracurricular activities / to enhance college applications. ①

视译为："很多英国的私立学校把广告刊登在/国外的报纸上，/或重新将网站设计成/多语种版本，/还参加各类招生推介会，/并且他们承诺提供语言培训，/精

---

① 齐涛云. 商务英语翻译教程（口译）（第三版）[M]. 北京：中国水利水电出版社，2022.

心准备课程/及安排丰富的课外活动/来吸引学生申请。"

学员可快速扫描，将长句切分成多个语意单元，理清相互之间的逻辑关系，找准主语、谓语、宾语等核心成分及其他补充成分，就可依据"顺句驱动"的原则快速视译（参见例1的断句）。

2. 句间衔接。

从例1可看出，由于英语和汉语在句子结构及表达习惯上的差异，很多情况下，译员在整合过程中要对目标语进行润色，使译文既遵守"顺句驱动"的原则又能流畅自然、符合逻辑。译员通常可采用重复、增补、省略、反说、词类转换等技巧，使信息上与源语基本等值。这些技巧在英译汉或汉译英中都适用，如以下实例。

例2：中国是一个有五千年文明历史的国家，从历史文化来了解与认识中国，是一个重要的视角。①

视译为：China is a country with 5,000 years of civilization. Therefore, to approach China from its history and culture forms an important perspective.（增补 therefore，使逻辑关系更明确）

例3：I would like to assure you once again that we are not insensitive to the problems of developing nations.②

视译为：我想再次向你保证，我们关心发展中国家的问题。（把英文中的 not insensitive 反说，直接译成"关心"）

在篇章视译中，需要以上几种技巧的综合使用，以使译文完整顺畅。

"顺句驱动"的策略使译员能够一直向前，避免回溯已翻译的内容，提高了翻译效率。译员灵活运用断句及句间衔接等技巧，能确保译文在保持源语顺序的基础上，实现语义的精准传达，使译文更加自然流畅。

与笔译中追求的"信达雅"标准相比，视译是一种准备时间有限、以口头表达为主的翻译方式，我们不必在视译中过于追求"雅"的标准，而应更侧重于"准确、流畅、简洁、易懂"。其中，"准确"意味着译者能读懂原文意思并能准确表达；"流畅"则要求译文摆脱源语结构的束缚，让译文表达顺畅；"简洁"强调抓住原文的核心，避免冗长繁复的表述；"易懂"则是为了方便听众理解。

在实际操作中，视译还须遵循一些具体要求，如不重复翻译句子或回溯，不过长停顿，不说多余的词句，不用拗口的表达，避免翻译腔等。同时，因为听众更注重的是整体意思的理解，所以译者在视译过程中可以适当添加衔接词来突出逻辑关系，或以个人转述（paraphrasing）的方式表达原意。

---

① 齐涛云. 商务英语翻译教程（口译）（第三版）[M]. 北京：中国水利水电出版社，2022.
② 齐涛云. 商务英语翻译教程（口译）（第三版）[M]. 北京：中国水利水电出版社，2022.

第二节 同声传译

一、同声传译的特点与发展

同声传译，英语叫作 simultaneous interpretation，也叫作"同声翻译"或"同步翻译"，译员们将其简称为"同传"。同声传译的难度比交替传译要大得多。① 无论是其英语名称还是其汉语名称，表面含义似乎都是"在讲话的同时立即将其译出"。但这种理解是形而上学的，并不完全符合同传实际情况。同声传译的本质在于，当发言人开始讲话时，译员在很短的时间内即开始翻译，形成了一种讲话与翻译几乎无缝衔接的同步状态。翻译人员在听取讲者发言的同时，要实时将其转化为另一种语言进行表述。因此，同声传译要求翻译人员具备同时处理"听"与"说"两项任务的能力，确保信息的及时传递和准确转达。讲者全部讲完后，译员也很快结束传译。同声传译不是真正的"同声"，因为译员必须先听到一部分原话而后才能译出来，不可能在听到话的同时就把同样的内容表达出来（读讲稿的同传例外）。译员所译的实际上是刚刚听到的话，而耳内听的却是马上要译的话。

同声传译一般用于大型国际会议进行过程中若干种工作语言的相互转换。讲话人使用一种工作语言发言时，要求同声传译人员几乎同步译成其他工作语言，使所有与会者都可以听到自己熟悉的语言。同声传译人员从听到说的时差极短，与讲话人的时间差仅在半句到一句之间。英汉两种语言句型结构极不相同，这给同声传译造成更大困难。

比起交替传译，同声传译要年轻得多。直到第二次世界大战结束，交替传译一直垄断着口译舞台。但这种口译方式有一个明显的缺点：它使交流花费的时间几乎延长了一倍。如果与会人员操三种或更多的语言，需要进行语言之间的接力口译，花费的时间还要更长。随着国际交往日趋频繁，工作节奏日益加快，人们必然要探求一种既不多费时间，又能达到交流目的的口译方式。同声传译正是在这种背景下产生并发展起来的。

同声传译也是科技发展的产物。同传需要效果良好的现代化设备。译员在隔音良好的同传室（interpreting booth）中工作，从耳机中听到讲话后，通过麦克风向听众传译。同传室中的接听系统有几个不同的频道，可以接听不同的语言，有时译员无力直接翻译讲话人的语言，需要接听另一个同传室中传来的自己所掌握的语言再进行传译，形成三种甚至更多语言接力传译的局面。而听众席上的耳机也有不同频道，可选择各自需要听的语言。

据说国际商业机器公司（IBM）在第二次世界大战前已获得同传设备的专利权。但同声传译正式登台亮相是在1945年第二次世界大战结束后，用于在纽伦堡军事法庭审讯纳粹战犯。1946年伦敦举行联合国第一次大会筹备会时也试用了同声传译。起初不少人对同声传译的准确性持怀疑态度，经过多年实践，人们终于对同声传译建立了信

---

① 王逢鑫. 高级汉英口译教程[M]. 北京：外文出版社，2004：410.

心。现在同声传译已在国际会议上得到广泛使用。世界主要国际组织如联合国、欧盟等在其举行的各种会议上均采用同声传译，会议口译（conference interpreting）几乎已成为同声传译的同义词。

改革开放以来，我国对外交往日益增多，各种国际会议、研讨会、报告会等大多采用了同声传译。同传已逐渐为人们所熟悉并接受。1979 年起，联合国与我国政府在北京外国语大学合办的 13 期译训班，为我国培养了第一代同传精英。后来，欧盟每年从我国选收学员进行同传培训。由于同传工作挑战性大，接触新事物广，报酬丰厚，对外语水平高的年轻人吸引力很大，他们中间形成了一股同传热。北外、上外等外语专业院校相继成立了高级翻译学院，培养专业同传人才。

同声传译与交替传译相比，孰难孰易呢？一般说来，同声传译要求译员有更敏锐的听力和更快的反应能力，以及具备边听边译的能力，应当说比交替传译的门槛更高一些。但不能说交替传译各方面都比同传容易。比如交替传译对记忆和笔记的要求比同传高，对口译产出质量的要求也比同传高，听众期望值高，对译员出现的失误不大宽容理解。而且译员与听众面对面地接触，提高了对译员举止、表情等形象方面的要求。所以的确有一些习惯于做同声传译的译员不愿意做交替传译。

二、同声传译需要具备的素质

第一，同声传译译员需要具备扎实的英汉基础和熟练的运用能力，特别是听说能力。对英语的掌握上，译员必须做到发音准确，口齿清晰，思维迅速敏捷，听到源语后能够迅速准确地理解，并几乎同时用目标语流畅地表达出来，确保无误解、无误译，并且不遗漏任何细节。对汉语掌握也同样重要，译员如果汉语水平不够到位，就无法准确理解和翻译，更无法在两个语言系统之间自如地转换。因此，译员要注意提高英汉两种语言的能力。

第二，同声传译人员应掌握丰富的百科知识，具有丰富的人文科学以及自然科学知识。国际会议议题广泛，内容多样，涉及领域广泛。因此，译员要广泛阅读，不断更新和拓展自己的知识结构。为了应对各种可能的议题，他们必须具备宽泛的知识面和相应的词汇储备。同时，随着社会的进步和科技的发展，译员还要不断学习新的主题，跟上时代的步伐。

第三，同声传译是一项高度紧张的工作，对译员的脑力要求非常高，要求译员时刻保持全神贯注，不容有丝毫分心或放松。因此，同声传译人员必须具备出色的心理素质，能够承受巨大的工作压力和精神压力。

第四，同声传译不仅是一种脑力劳动，也是一种体力劳动。口译人员往往要较长时间保持高度紧张的工作状态，几乎没有休息的时间。因此，译员要拥有旺盛的精力和充沛的体力，甚至要具备良好的肌肉协调能力，以适应这种高强度的工作。①

---

① 王逢鑫. 高级汉英口译教程[M]. 北京：外文出版社，2004：412.

三、同声传译的要领与技巧

要想做好同声传译,译员必须懂得一些要领和技巧,并通过大量练习和实践,掌握及运用这些要领和技巧。

(一)意译为主

首先必须明确同声传译的任务是传达原讲话的内容与精神而不是再现原话的语言形式。译员绝不能把精力集中在讲话人所用的具体词句上。这样一方面影响理解原话,另一方面影响记忆。记住一句话的内容比记住其具体词句容易得多。一篇十多页的文章我们听一遍大致可以复述其主要精神和内容。但如果从一本词典中任选几页给我们读一遍,一般人恐怕记不住几个词条。同传译员是在高度紧张的情况下一边译刚听过的话一边听发言人正在讲的话,这决定了译员绝不能对词句斤斤计较,不能以代码转换为主进行翻译,而只能以意译为主,把直译限制在专有名词和专业术语及其他两种语言基本对等的词的翻译上。而且译员开始口译与讲话间的时间差(ear-voice-span,简称 EVS)越大就越要采用意译。

(二)根据不同的口译任务和译员的具体条件科学地分配用于听与说的精力

同传译员要同时进行听与说两件事,嘴巴和耳朵要协调配合。既不能全神贯注地听,又不能全神贯注地说,必须一心二用,合理地分配对听与说的注意力。两种注意力如何得到合理分配,只能因人而定,因事而定。"因人而定"主要是指依译员的特点而定。听力理解能力强、口头表达能力相对略弱的译员应该在"说"上多投入一些注意力;反之,则应该在"听"上多投入一些注意力。此外,讲话人的特点也会影响译员注意力的分配。如果讲话节奏分明、清楚易懂,译员则可以在"说"上多投入些精力;反之,如果发言人口音较重、节奏含糊,那就需要在"听"上多投入一些精力。译员应当切记:无论做什么口译,"听懂"都是第一位的基本要求。听不清楚讲话,不明白讲话人在说什么,表达能力再强也无从发挥作用。可以说,在"听"上分配多少精力决定译员在"说"上投入的精力,而在"听"上具体投入多少精力应以听懂为原则。而"因事而定"指的是以工作的特点而定。前面已经分析过英译汉主要难在听力理解方面,译员只要听明白了讲话的内容,就不难用母语表达出来。一般说来译员应把主要精力放在听上。而汉译英主要难在英语口头表达,译员一般应将注意力放在说上。

(三)同声传译一般不记笔记

同声传译时,译员译的是讲话人刚刚说过的一两个意群,至多是一句不太长的话。现场一般只要求译员有较好的瞬间记忆能力,对译员的记忆压力不大,不会造成太大的记忆困难,所以一般不记笔记。译员如果记笔记就等于是在做"听"和"说"两件事的同时又增加了一件事,只会增加工作难度。但这并不是说同传译员什么也不记,实际上同传室内常常备有纸和铅笔。译员可根据自己的特点,在必要时略作记录,比如记录较大的数字和列举的人名、地名等，切记记录越少越有利于集中精力听和说。一般来说只记点数字就可以了，译列举的人名、地名等专用名词时，最好的办法是紧跟讲话——译出，一时来不及译，重复原名也可在一定程度上达到交流目的。因为除日语等少数外语外，将其他主要外语的专用名词译作汉语时可采用音译的方式。

（四）做好同传的关键——断句、处理语序、合理拿捏EVS

可以说，英汉之间进行同声传译的关键在于断句和处理语序。而断句和处理语序的具体方式又和译员与讲话人之间的EVS密切相关。同声传译不同于交替传译，一般说来，不等讲话人说完一句话就要开口翻译。为了使所译的话比较符合目标语的习惯，译员要灵活地采取各种手段，随时调整自己的语序，而不像接续口译的译员听完了一句话或更多的话，可以比较从容地安排语序。断句和调整语序的能力在很大程度上能体现同传译员的水平。调整语序的实质是要求译员采取手段尽量使译文的语序贴近原话以减少听与记的压力，最大限度地减少干扰。视译是训练断句和语序调整能力的重要方法。如果译员在视译工作场景下能够做到熟练断句、灵活调整，经过一定的适应性训练，这些能力可以转移到同声传译工作场景。

英语与汉语语序最大的差别体现在定语与状语位置上。汉语中定语与状语一般放在中心词之前。而英语重形合（hypotaxis），大量使用关联词来连接句子的各种成分，定语与状语位置比汉语灵活，后置的情况较多。而且英语定语从句使用频率大大超过汉语。定语从句与中心词之间又有各种不同的意义关系，所以定语与状语会给同传造成一定的困难。在同传过程中，处理英汉在定语和状语上的差别，尤其考验译员的断句和语序调整的能力。本部分仅举两例，对同传译员的应对策略作简要说明。

例1[①]：英译汉

On the contrary,
  相反
continued economic growth in the developing countries
  发展中国家经济继续增长
has an important part to play in supporting the healthy development of the world.
  可发挥重要作用   促进了世界经济健康发展。

从例1可以看出，由于英语定语 in the developing countries 和状语 in supporting the healthy development of the world 均后置，给同传造成了不便。本例中译员解决定语语序靠的是缩短EVS，将后置变成了前置。状语语序的解决实际利用了汉语意合（parataxis）的特点，在译完"可发挥重要作用"后，直接说"促进……发展"，让听众意会前后的意义关系，而不照原话译成"在促进世界经济健康发展方面发挥重要作用"（这样译使译员

---

① 齐涛云. 商务英语翻译教程（口译）（第三版）[M]. 北京：中国水利水电出版社，2022.

与讲话人之间的时间差显得太大，使汉语句子中断时间显得过长）。不可否认，例句中的处理办法与原话有一点差距，但在同传时不失为一种办法。当然本句还有其他处理办法。译员先说出"可以发挥重要作用"，听到后面状语短语的意思后可再补充"在促进世界……方面发挥重要作用"，通过重复"发挥重要作用"一方面译全了句子，另一方面也在一定程度上弥补了汉语句子中断过长的缺陷。

例2①：汉译英
中国如期举办这一全球贸易盛会，
  China is hosting this global trade event as scheduled
体现了中国同世界
  showing that China is willing to
分享市场机遇、
  share with the world market opportunities
推动世界经济复苏的真诚愿望。
  and promote the world economic recovery.

  从例2可以看出，中文"真诚愿望"的定语很长，为"中国同世界分享市场机遇、推动世界经济复苏的"。按照笔译处理方式，这个长定语翻译成英语时应该后置：sincere desire to share its market opportunities with the world and contribute to global economic recovery. 如果同传也采用这种处理方式，译员就要等听到中心词"真诚愿望"后才能开口翻译。这样做 EVS 拉得很长，会产生两个不好的后果：①等待时间过长引起译文中出现过长的停顿，会给听众带来译文不流畅的感觉；②译员在等待过程中的记忆负荷过重，等开口翻译完"真诚愿望"时，很可能会遗忘一部分长定语信息。本例中译员采用了"适度预测"的技巧，在听到"中国同世界"后，就预测演讲者会表达中国"愿意"的态度，基于此开口翻译，使用了 is willing to 把后面信息串联起来。有经验的译员经常能预测出与演讲人讲话内容基本相同的结果。但是如果预测内容与真实内容出现较大偏差时，译员还要在后续的译文中进行必要的修正。

  合理把握 EVS 对同声传译至关重要。译员应根据自身的条件与习惯选择最适合自己的 EVS 长度。EVS 太长了，虽然译员掌握好语序了，但上下句极易相互干扰，往往容易顾此失彼，自乱阵脚；时间差小了，听与说的干扰小一些，但要求译员熟练地掌握各种灵活手段理顺句中的词序。一般来说，译员落后讲话一个小意群到半句（两三个小意群）为宜，这样原句讲完时已可译出大半句。这时意思都明朗了，译员便可利用句子间的自然停顿以较快的速度译完全句，等下句开始一两个意群后便可再开口翻译。这一两个意群所占用的时间便也构成了译员所译句子间的自然停顿。

  值得注意的是，有些句子不听完很难判断其意思是肯定还是否定。这时不要把前半

---

① 齐涛云. 商务英语翻译教程（口译）（第三版）[M]. 北京：中国水利水电出版社，2022.

句译得太明确，可先把前半部分的内容摆出来，听完后再用"关于这问题"或"关于这一点"把结论性的内容引出来。

(五) 处理失误的原则与技巧

同传是高度紧张的工作，出现这样或那样的失误是在所难免的。而且即使译员知道自己出现了失误，也不可能让讲话人停下来等自己纠正，所以同传译员应该掌握处理失误的原则和技巧。首先，译员要有冷静的头脑、机敏的反应力，不能一出差错就紧张慌乱，从而影响接下来的翻译。译员应判断失误(一般多是错译或遗漏)的性质。如果失误不太关键一般不要纠正，译员的同伴尤其不要越俎代庖。个别地方未听清、未听懂可以跳过去，不必耿耿于怀，要集中精力翻译后面的话，否则会因小失大。与交替传译的情况相同，译员精益求精的精神应该体现在平时的学习与训练中，临场时应该顺其自然。谨小慎微只会影响大局，追求完美可能会造成更多的失误。如果是重大的关键失误则必须纠正，以免造成实质性的负面影响。最好能在同传过程中就用比较自然的办法纠正过来。例如发言人说"奥地利政府中出现了极右势力掌权的现象"。译员若把奥地利译成了 Australia，这种失误是必须纠正的，否则会造成严重的政治影响。译员可以在说出 Australia 后很自然地补充一句"I mean Austria"，既纠正了错误又不显山露水。此外还可以用 sorry it should be，or rather 等话纠错。如果译时来不及纠正而又是非纠不可的错误也可以先用笔记下来，等发言中有较长停顿时纠正，甚至等到发言结束后纠正，但这种情况要严格控制。如果译员发现发言人的明显口误，那么应该直接译成正确的，而不必先照错的译再纠正解释。对不属口误类的错误，译员应该照译，不要加任何说明。译员遇到自己不懂的专业术语或新词，可以重复原文。这样做，听众中的内行人可能懂，同时也可以引起其他听众的注意。

(六) 临场时的某些技术问题

同声传译的译前准备与交替传译基本一致，但是在同传现场却可能会遇到与交传不一样的挑战。有时发言人事先没有把稿子交给译员，临场时却又念稿，这会给译员造成很大困难，因为稿子一般都是书面语言，用词比较讲究，句子结构往往复杂，信息量大。遇到这种情况译员也不必慌乱，可以请搭档去要稿子，然后一边听，一边看稿视译。在实在要不到稿子的情况下，译员首先保证把讲话的要点翻译出来，在此基础上尽量多地译出细节性内容。

为了提高同声传译的效果，还应该注意一些具体技术问题。译员要熟悉会场的同传设备，要能恰当地掌握自己说话的声音，掌握与话筒的距离。一般来说，离话筒要近一点，说话声音要轻一点。这样既可减少自己的声音对自己的干扰，又不影响听众听清译出的话。与话筒的距离要相对稳定，不然听众所接收的译员的声音会忽大忽小。使用耳机的方式因人而异。有的译员把两个耳机紧紧扣在耳朵上，觉得这样有利于集中听，但有的译员感到这样会增加禁锢感和封闭感，更容易疲劳，所以把一个耳机扣在耳朵上，一个耳机只戴一半。还有人干脆只戴一个耳机。这样做头脑固然会清醒一些，但加大了自己声音的干扰。总之，同传是劳动强度很大的工作，其工作特点和工作环境条件极易使译员感到疲劳。通常两三个译员在同一个口译箱轮流工作，一般不超过半个小时就要轮换。两个译员交替时要处理好关机与开机。译员自己要说话或要咳嗽时一定要关掉话筒或者按 cough 键。口译时不能用手摸话筒，那样会对听众造成噪声刺激。译箱内空间小，很容易缺氧，使译员感到头昏，所以最好不要把门关得太严。

第四单元　糖尿病与血糖管理

第一节　糖尿病与血糖管理口译知识点

一、糖尿病知识概述

糖尿病（diabetes mellitus，缩写为 DM，国外专家在口语表达中也经常称之为 diabetes）是一种代谢性疾病（metabolic disease），它的特征是（it is characterized by）患者（patient）的血糖（blood glucose）长期高于标准值。高血糖（hyperglycemia，high blood sugar）会造成俗称"三多一少"的症状（symptom）：多食、多饮、多尿及体重下降。

糖尿病分为 1 型糖尿病（Type 1 diabetes mellitus，T1DM）和 2 型糖尿病（Type 2 diabetes mellitus，T2DM）。无论是哪一种糖尿病，如果不进行治疗，可能会引发诸多并发症（complication）。急性并发症包括糖尿病酮症酸中毒（diabetic ketoacidosis，DKA）与高渗性非酮症糖尿病昏迷（Hyperosmolar nonketotic diabetic coma，HNDC）；严重的长期并发症则包括心血管疾病（cardiovascular disease）、卒中（stroke）、慢性肾脏病变（nephropathy）、糖尿病足以及视网膜病变（retinopathy）等。

根据世界卫生组织（World Health Organization，WHO）统计数据，糖尿病患者人群从 1980 年的 1.08 亿上升至 2014 年的 4.22 亿。低收入国家和中等收入国家的患病率上升速度高于高收入国家。

据国际糖尿病联盟（International Diabetes Federation，IDF）统计，2021 年全球成年糖尿病患者人数达 5.37 亿人，其中中国成年糖尿病患者人数达 1.41 亿人，占比超过 26%。

糖尿病是失明（blindness）、肾衰竭（renal/kidney failure）、心脏病发作（heart attack）、卒中和下肢截肢（lower extremity amputation）的主要病因。2000 年至 2019 年，糖尿病导致的死亡率增加了 3%。2019 年，糖尿病以及糖尿病引起的肾脏疾病估计导致 200 万人死亡。健康饮食、保持一定频率的锻炼活动、维持正常体重及避免使用烟草有助于预防 2 型糖尿病或推迟其发病。

患者通过注意饮食、身体活动、服药以及定期筛查和诊治并发症，可以治疗糖尿病，并避免或延缓其后果。

糖耐量受损（impaired glucose tolerance，IGT）和空腹血糖受损（impaired fasting glucose，IFG）是指介于正常与糖尿病之间的一种过渡状态。糖耐量受损患者或空腹血糖受损患者发展为2型糖尿病的风险较高，不过这一情况并非不可避免。

T1DM的病因为身体无法生产足够的胰岛素(insulin)或根本无法生产胰岛素，病理上也被叫作胰岛素依赖型糖尿病(insulin-dependent diabetes mellitus, IDDM)或是青少年糖尿病(属于先天性疾病，大多数是在婴儿时期至青少年时期发病，故得此名)，病因不明。1型糖尿病与2型糖尿病的发病机理完全不同，1型属于自身免疫性疾病，可能是由基因或由自体免疫系统破坏了产生胰岛素的胰腺胰岛β细胞所引起的，因此患者必须注射胰岛素治疗，目前世界上没有治愈此病的方法。

T2DM始于胰岛素阻抗作用异常(细胞对于胰岛素的反应不正常、不灵敏)或细胞对胰岛素没有反应，而胰脏本身并没有任何病理问题。随着病情发展，胰岛素的分泌亦可能渐渐变得不足。2型糖尿病最为常见，占全世界糖尿病患者的80%~90%。

糖尿病的诊断标准包括几个重要指标：餐后两小时血糖(2-hour postprandial blood glucose level, 2hPBG)、空腹血糖(fasting plasma glucose, FPG; fasting blood glucose, FBG)，以及糖化血红蛋白(glycated hemoglobin, HbA1c, or A1c)。

二、血糖知识概述

血糖或血浆葡萄糖(plasma glucose)，指血浆中的葡萄糖浓度，是静脉血(venous blood)经抗凝和离心后测得的血糖，又称静脉血浆葡萄糖。近年来在相关会议中，部分美国顶级医生讲课时也会使用"blood sugar"而不讲"blood glucose"，因此口译时译员也不一定要严格将"血糖"译作"blood glucose"。

毛糖(capillary glucose)，即毛细血管血糖。常见的指尖采血(fingerstick)即为毛细血管血糖，国内医生经常将其简称为"毛糖"。

三、糖尿病相关检查与监测

口服葡萄糖耐量试验(oral glucose challenge test)，为检查葡萄糖代谢功能的一项检查，用于诊断血糖升高不明显的可疑糖尿病。受检者服用一定量的葡萄糖后，在特定时间点(0.5小时、1小时、2小时、3小时)进行血糖测定，用于评估受检者的自身血糖调节能力(regulation)。

糖化血红蛋白为血液中葡萄糖与红细胞中血红蛋白相结合的物质。糖化血红蛋白随血糖的变化而变化，能反映出患者在抽血检验前四周到前八周之间的平均血糖水平。

在糖尿病的管理(diabetic management)中，血糖监测(blood glucose monitoring, BGM)起着至关重要的作用。传统的血糖监测方法经常是通过间断性测量血糖来获取血糖数据，简单而言，就是依赖指尖血糖监测(fingerstick testing/finger stick blood sugar/finger-stick glucose monitoring)，此过程由护士或由患者自己进行，即自我血糖监测(self-monitoring of blood glucose, SMBG)；也无论监测频率如何，无论一天七次、四次还是两次；抑或近年来国外医生提出的随机血糖监测，即每天在不固定的时间点进行指尖血糖监测，十指连心，每次监测都会给患者带来一定的痛苦。

近年来，连续性血糖监测系统(continuous glucose monitoring system, CGMS)技术日

渐成熟，各个相关会议中相应的内容和讨论也时有提及。CGMS 是通过连续记录血糖的变化，提供更加全面和准确的血糖数据，从而帮助医生和糖友（diabetes patient）更好地了解血糖波动情况。连续性血糖监测（continuous glucose monitoring，CGM）是通过埋植于皮下组织的微电极（microelectrode），记录组织间液葡萄糖氧化反应产生的电信号，间接反映测量血糖的新型微创血糖监测技术。

CGM 可在 1 型糖尿病（T1DM）、2 型糖尿病（T2DM）、妊娠糖尿病（gestational diabetes）患者的血糖控制和生活方式管理中进行广泛应用，同时在新生儿、ICU 危重症患者的血糖管理、减重、运动锻炼指导和饮食营养调整优化等领域也有诸多潜在应用场景。随着技术的进步和产品的成熟，CGM 的应用场景也在不断拓大。

在 T1DM 和 T2DM 患者中，大量的临床试验（clinical trial）已证实应用 CGM 能显著提高血糖控制达标率、减少低血糖事件（hypoglycemia event）和高血糖事件，并能提高生活质量（quality of life，QoL）。对于仍保持活跃运动的糖尿病患者，CGM 对于及时补充热量，保证运动中能量提供，防止低血糖具有重要意义。在妊娠糖尿病或糖尿病合并妊娠患者管理中，CGM 具有较高的准确性和安全性。

对于处在 ICU 或在围手术期（peri-operative period）的危重患者，CGM 可以实现精准个体化的血糖控制，降低医源性低血糖（iatrogenic hypoglycemia）的风险和术后不良事件。

在运动和保健方面，CGM 的应用也得到更多的关注。CGM 最早应用于保持活跃运动的 1 型糖尿病患者，后来人们发现将其用于长跑运动员可以合理规划赛程中的饮食和能量摄入。此外，CGM 指导下的生物反馈减肥、锻炼方案优化及健康生活方式培养也成为了在欧美保健领域的时尚，帮助使用者进行膳食选择调整，帮助其远离高糖而低饱腹感的食物，通过加强运动来调节血糖。

CGMS 是一种微创血糖监测方式，通过监测皮下组织间液内的葡萄糖浓度而反映血糖水平，可连续监测佩戴者 24 小时内每时每刻的血糖值。CGMS 设备体积较小，为可穿戴设备，可固定于上臂或腹部。其机理是把一根无菌、细软的传感器植于皮下，24 小时连续监测患者的血糖水平，可实时传输血糖数据，可供 CGMS 使用者及医生查看。

CGMS 应用的主要限制是成本，但其毕竟能够减少疼痛体验，并提供连续的间接血糖数据，这对于临床研究意义重大。而近年来，数字医疗、精准医疗（precision medicine）、互联网医疗、人工智能（artificial intelligence，AI）、大数据（big data）在临床医学中越来越多被提及，而 CGM 与这些概念都能完美融合，将个体患者（individual patient）、患者群体（patient population）、特定医学社区、医生和医院联系起来，这将有助于在糖尿病防控和血糖达标方面发挥更重要的作用。

四、糖尿病治疗

国内对糖尿病的管理，有所谓的"五驾马车"（five pillars）一说，即饮食控制、运动、糖尿病教育、自我血糖检测、药物治疗。其英文对应为：dietary control, physical activity, diabetes education, self-monitoring of blood sugar, and regular medication, 不同的讲者、出版物可能在具体细节上稍有差异。

糖尿病药物分为两大类，一类是口服药物(oral drugs)，另一类是注射药物(injectable drugs)，主要为胰岛素。口服药物简单介绍如下：

1. 双胍类(biguanides)：主要是二甲双胍(metformin)，主要通过抑制肝脏葡萄糖输出起到降糖作用。

2. 格列奈类(glinides)：如瑞格列奈(repaglinide)、那格列奈(nateglinide)。

3. 磺脲类(sulfonylureas)：如格列齐特(gliclazide)、格列吡嗪(glipizide)、格列美脲(glimepiride)等。

4. 噻唑烷二酮类(thiazolidinediones)：如罗格列酮(rosiglitazone)、吡格列酮(pioglitazone)，主要是在增加靶组织对胰岛素的敏感性上起作用。

5. α葡萄糖苷酶抑制剂(alpha-glucosidase inhibitors，AGI)：如阿卡波糖(acarbose)、伏格列波糖(voglibose)，通过抑制α葡萄糖苷酶从而延缓对碳水化合物的吸收，降低餐后血糖。

6. 二肽基肽酶-Ⅳ抑制剂(Dipeptidyl peptidase-Ⅳ inhibitors，DPP-4i)：如沙格列汀(saxagliptin)、西格列汀(sitagliptin)等，主要是对提高内源性GLP-1水平起作用。

7. 钠-葡萄糖共转运体2抑制剂(sodium-glucose cotransporter 2 inhibitors，SGLT-2i)：如达格列净(dapagliflozin)、恩格列净(empagliflozin)，主要是通过促进肾脏排泄葡萄糖起作用。

糖尿病注射类药物，主要是胰岛素，根据其作用时间不同，可分为超短效胰岛素、短效胰岛素、中效胰岛素、长效胰岛素及预混胰岛素五类。胰岛素的用药方式为皮下注射(subcutaneous injection)。

此处说明，以下所列的具体起效时间、作用高峰时间及持续时间等数字，因研究结果及患者人群不同，不同出版物及演讲时所述之具体时间各不相同，读者应以了解口译相关信息为主，而无须刻意比较不同出版物间对于具体细节描述的细微差异。

1. 超短效胰岛素(rapid-acting insulin)

皮下注射后一般10~20分钟起效(it begins to affect blood glucose)，作用高峰(it peaks in)1~2小时，持续时间(it continues to work for)3~5小时，须在餐前立即皮下注射，也可用于临时高血糖的降糖治疗。代表药物有门冬胰岛素(诺和锐)、赖脯胰岛素(优泌乐、速秀霖)等。

2. 短效胰岛素(short-acting insulin)

起效时间30~60分钟，作用高峰2~4小时，持续时间6~8小时，须在餐前30分钟进行皮下注射。代表药物有普通胰岛素、生物合成人胰岛素(诺和灵R)、精蛋白锌重组人胰岛素(优泌林R)、重组人胰岛素(甘舒霖R、优思灵R)等。

3. 中效胰岛素(intermediate-acting insulin)

起效时间2~4小时，作用高峰4~10小时，持续时间10~16小时，可单独使用或作为基础胰岛素与超短效或短效胰岛素混合餐前使用。代表药物有精蛋白生物合成人胰岛素(诺和灵N)、精蛋白锌重组人胰岛素(优泌林R)、精蛋白重组人胰岛素(重和林N、优思灵N)、低精蛋白重组人胰岛素(甘舒霖N)等。

4. 长效胰岛素（long-acting insulin）

起效时间 2~4 小时，注射后体内药物浓度相对稳定，无明显高峰（pronounced peak），持续时间 24~36 小时，作为基础胰岛素使用，每日注射 1~2 次。代表药物有甘精胰岛素（来得时）、地特胰岛素（诺和平）等。

5. 预混胰岛素（premixed/combination insulin）

将两种不同的胰岛素，如超短效或短效胰岛素与中效胰岛素按一定比例预先混合而成（a mix of rapid- or short-acting insulin combined with an intermediate-acting insulin），短效成分可快速降低餐后血糖，中效成分缓慢持续释放，起到代替基础胰岛素的作用。药品上的数字代表了短效和中效胰岛素各种所占的比例，30 代表短效 30%，中效 70%；25 代表短效 25%，中效 75%；50 则代表短效和中效各占 50%。代表药物有门冬胰岛素 30（诺和锐 30R）、精蛋白生物合成人胰岛素（诺和灵 30R、诺和灵 50R）、精蛋白锌重组赖脯胰岛素混合注射液（优泌乐 25R、优泌乐 50R）、精蛋白锌重组人胰岛素混合注射液（优泌林 70/30）等。

除降低血糖的药物外，糖尿病患者通常还需要降压药（hypotensive drugs/hypotensor）和他汀类药物（statins）来降低并发症风险。

糖尿病治疗中，值得关注的一点就是避免低血糖事件的发生。低血糖是指血糖水平低于标准范围，其发生原因众多，但通常与糖尿病治疗相关，在糖尿病治疗中应努力预防并避免低血糖事件。如果血糖水平过低，可能会出现以下体征（vital signs）和症状（symptoms）：脸色苍白（pale face）、颤抖（tremor）、出汗（sweating）、头痛（headache）、饥饿感或恶心（nausea）、心律不齐（arrhythmia）或心动过速（tachycardia）、疲劳（fatigue）、易怒或焦虑（irritability/anxiety）、难以集中注意力（inattentiveness）、头晕（dizziness）、嘴唇、舌头或脸颊出现刺痛感（tingling）或麻木感（numbness）等。

随着低血糖情况进一步加剧，可能会出现下列体征和症状：意识混乱（clouding of consciousness）、行为异常（abnormal behavior）、丧失协调性、言语不清、视力模糊（blurred vision）、梦魇等。

而重度低血糖症可能导致意识丧失（loss of consciousness）与癫痫发作（epileptic seizure）。

低血糖需要立即治疗。治疗方案包括摄入高糖饮食或应用药物，以便快速将血糖恢复至正常范围。

第二节　真实世界口译情境

一、主题会议

如前文所述，现代社会，无论国内外，无论是在发展中国家或是在发达国家，糖尿病发病率高，国内患病人数更是以亿计，故医学会议中涉及糖尿病/血糖管理概念的较多，以下主题的医学会议可能涉及糖尿病/血糖管理：

糖尿病诊疗相关会议；各个外科手术主题的会议，鉴于 DM 患者的血糖控制会影响手术结果，大多数会议中都会提到 DM 手术患者的围手术期血糖管理（perioperative blood glucose management），因为良好的血糖控制有助于提高手术成功率并加快康复，以及减少术后并发症；各个内科会议，只要讲到病例讨论，就一定会提到患者是否有糖尿病，以及相应的糖尿病管理措施；代谢减重外科的相关会议也会提到糖尿病与血糖管理；DM 治疗的新药研发；持续血糖监测技术与设备；无创式血糖监测与可穿戴设备；因为 DM 的诸多慢性并发症，眼科、神经内科、肾内科、心内科等相关会议中也时有提及 DM、血糖管理、DM 并发症的治疗与控制等相关内容。

二、行业特点

对于糖尿病主题，中外演讲者口语中都会使用一些缩略语或部分缩略语的表达方式，例如国内医生习惯将"糖化血红蛋白"简称为"糖化"，将"毛细血管血糖"简称为"毛糖"等，而英语讲者喜欢将"HbA1c"简称为"A1c"。

三、口译难点

糖尿病口服用药类型较多，药品有通用名（generic name）和商品名（brand name）之分（上列药品名均为通用名）。而对于糖尿病口服药物的口译听辨，译员可能会面临以下一些难点：

1. 国外讲者英文发言时对同一药名发音可能略有差别，如日本、法国、意大利和北欧讲者与英美讲者比，发音差异明显，且各有特点，而国内讲者在用中文发言时也可能会略带口音。

2. 国内讲者在中文发言时，时有讲到英文缩略语，举例，如：钠-葡萄糖共转运体 2 抑制剂（sodium-glucose cotransporter 2 inhibitors, SGLT2i），中文讲者发言时，大概率不会用"钠-葡萄糖共转运体 2 抑制剂"这样的表达，很可能讲到的是"SGLT2 类药物"或"SGLT2 抑制剂"，而"2"的读音因人而异，有些讲者会按照中文读为"二"，而有些讲者可能会按照英文读为"two"，此类汉语中夹英文缩略语，而英文缩略语中继续夹汉语的情况并不少见，这一现象在肿瘤治疗方面较为明显。

3. 药品通用名难度尚可，但在国内讲者讲到药品商品名时，可能因为药物比较新，尚未确定最终的中文商品名；也可能因医生个人选择，国内讲者在提及时，会直接讲英文，而不同讲者因为口音及英语水平不同，发音略有差异，而有些时候会议主办方以及部分与会者会相对关注具体的药名，这对译员提出较高的要求。

4. 部分药物的中文翻译不止一个，例如：sodium-glucose cotransporter 2 inhibitors, SGLT2i，能查到的中文译名就有"钠-葡萄糖共转运体 2 抑制剂""钠-葡萄糖共转运蛋白 2 抑制剂""钠-葡萄糖协同转运体抑制剂""钠-葡萄糖协同转运蛋白 2 抑制剂"，这些中文译名虽然仅存在细节的差异，但也增加了听辨时的难度，译员应能够快速反应，将听到的内容与自己的知识储备或会前准备内容快速配对处理后译出。

第四单元　糖尿病与血糖管理

第三节　中英对照篇章及分析

一、英译中

It has been heard already diabetes is a worldwide problem and certainly in China you do have a lot of patients who need to be taken care of very well in order to help them control their diabetes and related comorbidities. As you well know, the main goal in diabetes is to be sure that people do not develop complications from the disease and they have a good quality of life, not just extended life but also good quality of life and that has to do with helping them control their blood sugars as well as other conditions very well. And certainly, the introduction of technologies like glucose monitoring has definitely helped in the better appreciating the blood sugar levels that people have, so that we can make better decisions with them. So with that, let me then start in what I want to cover today is, first of all, how do we know in a patient either diabetes is well controlled or not? The historical value of glycohemoglobin A1c. The introduction of home blood glucose monitoring and monitoring in the hospital, the availability of now continuous glucose monitoring. The relationship of all these measures with complications. What the targets are in clinical practice, and then some practical recommendations.（本段内容选自2022年一位美国糖尿病诊疗专家的学术演讲，有删改调整。）

◎ **参考译文**：大家已经听到了，糖尿病是全世界的问题，而当然在中国，你们也确实有很多的患者，他们需要良好的诊疗，这样才能帮助他们控制糖尿病以及相关疾病。你们也都很了解，糖尿病的主要目标就是要确保人们不会出现疾病所致的并发症，以及他们能有不错的生活质量，而不仅仅是寿命的延长，也要好的生活质量，这就要帮助他们控制血糖以及其他疾病，要控制得好。当然，技术的引入，例如血糖监测，确实帮助到了更好地理解患者的血糖，所以我们就能够据此作出更好的决策。接下来，让我们，我今天想讲的是，首先，我们如何知晓一位患者的糖尿病是否控制良好？糖化血红蛋白的历史价值。引入居家血糖监测以及医院内监测，现在连续血糖监测的可及性。所有这些指标与并发症的关系。临床实践中的目标，以及后面的一些实用建议。

◎ **分析**：

1. 这位讲者没有口音，语速适中，但从句和连接词的使用导致句子比较长，同传时译员应注意断句；

2. "patient"近年来多译作"患者"而非"病人"（恐有歧视之嫌）；

3. "develop"意为"人开始出现疾病的症状"，故译作"出现"；

4. 按照顺句驱动的技巧，"更好地理解患者的血糖"和"能够据此作出更好的决策"两处中"患者的"和"据此"均为预测先说，其中"据此"无误，而"患者的"并不准确，但并非关键表述，不影响听众理解；

5. "appreciate"一词近年来在医学会议中出现的频率越来越高,意思为"看到、理解";

6. "home blood glucose monitoring"中的"home",口译时译作"居家",相比"在家"或"家庭"等表述更符合国内医生的表述习惯;

7. "measures"一词,除"措施"之外,更常见的意思就是"指标"。

Excellent. Great. Thank you very much, professors. Thank you for the introduction and for having me today with all of you. It has been heard already, diabetes is a worldwide problem. And certainly, in China, you do have a lot of patients who need to be taken care of very well in order to help them control their diabetes and related co-morbidities. As you will know, the main goal in diabetes is to be sure that people do not develop complications from the disease. So that they have a good quality of life, not just extended life, but also good quality of life. And that has to do with helping them control their blood sugars, as well as other conditions, very well. And certainly the introduction of technologies like glucose monitoring has definitely helped in the better appreciating the blood sugar levels that people have so that we can make better decisions with them. With that, let me then start. What I want to cover today is, first of all, how do we know in a patient, either diabetes is well controlled or not. The historical value of hemoglobin A1c, the introduction of home blood glucose monitoring, monitoring in the hospital, the availability of now continuous glucose monitoring, the relationship of all these measures with complications, what the targets are in clinical practice and then some practical recommendations.

◎ **参考译文**:非常好,非常感谢,教授,感谢您的介绍,感谢邀请我来到这里,很开心今天和大家见面。糖尿病已经是一个全世界范围内的问题了,尤其是在中国,中国有很多的患者,他们需要接受非常仔细的护理,才能够控制糖尿病和相关的合并症。糖尿病主要的目标就是要确保不要发展出疾病的并发症,这样能获得良好的生活质量,不只是延长生命,而且还要保证好的生活质量,这就要帮助他们控制血糖,还有一些其他的情况也要控制得很好。还有随着技术的进步,比如说血糖监控,能够很好地帮助监测人们的血糖,这样我们就能够作出更好的决策。讲到这里,我来开始我今天的演讲,我想提到的,首先,我们如何了解一个患者的血糖控制得好,还是不好,糖化血红蛋白的既往数值,居家血糖监测的引入,以及院内血糖监测的引入,现在连续性血糖检测的可及性,以及这些方法与并发症之间的关系,临床实践的目标,以及一些实用建议。

◎ **分析**:

1. "It has been heard already"未译出,并无影响;

2. "to be taken care of"译作"护理",这是常见的错误,可译作"诊疗"或"处理";

3. 将"develop"译作"发展出",可处理为"出现,进展为";

4. "quality of life"译为生活质量,近年来的医学会议口译中,这一表达的出现频率越来越高,有时也缩写为QoL;

5. "the introduction of technologies"译作"随着技术的进步",其实是随着技术的引入,"引入"与"进步"意义明显不同,但并不影响听众的整体理解;

6. "cover"译作"提到",此处理不妥,可译作"讲到、包括"。

So it's a busy agenda, but I will go relatively quickly in some of these points just to illustrate the importance of all these different aspects in diabetes care. The first question that we have with some of our patients is how do we know if their diabetes is well controlled? Now, I don't know about your patients, but many of my patients say, I think my diabetes is well controlled because I feel well. So, the first education point is to tell them that people may feel well, but that doesn't mean that their diabetes is well controlled. We do need to measure their blood sugars. And, of course, the introduction of hemoglobin A1c was one of the main drivers of success in the past, and even in the present time, because we do have good information of how high the blood sugars have been in the last 90 days in our patients, but also the introduction of glucose monitors was very important in diabetes care. Because with this devices and by patients breaking their fingers in obtaining capillary glucose levels, we have a good sense of what their blood sugars are at different points in time during the day. This has become important in clinical care, both in the outpatient, but also in the inpatient setting so that we know what the blood sugars are in established patterns of blood sugars in patients and make the right decisions about adjusting their treatments.

◎ **参考译文**:有些内容我讲得相对快一点,就是说明所有这些不同方面在糖尿病诊疗中的重要性。第一个问题,我们要问到部分患者的是,就是怎么知道患者的血糖控制良好?我不知道你们的患者如何,但是我很多的患者,他们会说"我觉得我血糖控制得挺好的,因为我感觉挺好的"。所以首先第一个教育要点在于,要告诉他们,他们可能感觉不错,但不代表他们的血糖控制得就很好,我们确实需要去测量他们的血糖。还有糖化血红蛋白的引入,是成功的因素之一,过去如此,甚至现在也是一样,因为我们确实有了很好的信息,了解了在过去90天当中,在患者体内的血糖有多高。还有一些血糖监测设备的引入也非常重要,因为有了这些器械,患者扎一下手指,就能获知他们的毛糖水平,我们就有很好的了解,了解到他们的血糖在每天不同时间点的情况。这在临床上已经变得非常重要,门诊如此,在住院情况下也是一样,这样我们就可以知道他们的血糖情况如何,就能知道患者血糖的特定情况,然后作出正确决定,调整其治疗方案。

◎ **分析**:

1. "So it's a busy agenda"意思是"日程安排内容很多",类似的表达还有"This slide is quite informative";

2. "to illustrate the importance of all these different aspects in"此处可以预测先说,在"XX"中的重要性,此处无非就是说糖尿病诊疗/管理;

3. "了解了在过去90天当中,在患者体内的血糖有多高",这一部分的同传,要么拉长 EVS，要么对"糖化血红蛋白"的意义有一定了解，可以做到预测先说；

4. "breaking their fingers"译作"扎一下手指"，此处讲者很可能讲的是"pricking"，译员可能听作了"breaking"，两个单词发音十分相近。但译员如果做过译前准备，就应该了解扎指尖测血糖是很长一段时间以来临床上和患者自我监测血糖最常用的方式，译员应该能够译出"扎一下手指"。此处若被译作"弄破手指"，听众虽然不会形成任何误解，但可能会对译员的专业程度产生怀疑；

5. "capillary glucose levels"译作"毛细血管葡萄糖水平"，如果译员熟悉相关领域，可以简化处理为"毛糖"，更加贴合临床实际情况。

But the most recent introduction of continuous glucose monitors has really come to modify a lot of the approaches that we have in diabetes care, because we have now more information. We can have a reading of blood sugars basically every minute, if we want to, and assess the blood sugars and with that truly build patterns over the 24 hour period, for as many days as people wear the continuous glucose monitors. And that gives us a very good idea of when the blood sugars are elevated, when the blood sugars are low, whether people are in the right range or not. And this allows us to make better decisions. Again, both in the outpatient and sometimes in the inpatient setting. Also, although I have to say that in the hospital, CGM continues glucose monitors are not used that frequently yet, but my prediction is that they will continue to grow and be used more and more. We do know that glycol hemoglobin A1c is related to the risk of complications. These are data from the diabetes control and complications trial, the DCCT, very important study in type 1 diabetes that demonstrated that A1c levels are related to retinopathy, nephropathy, neuropathy, so that people with the highest A1c levels are the ones with the highest risk. This is one of the reasons why we emphasize controlling blood sugars effectively in patients with diabetes.

◎ **参考译文**：最近兴起的连续血糖监测，这个也越来越改变了我们应对糖尿病的方式，因为现在我们能获取更多的信息。我们几乎每分钟都能得到血糖读数，如果你想的话，然后去评估血糖，这样我们才能真正地建立24小时的血糖模式，因为人们可以佩戴连续血糖监测很多天。这能让我们非常好地理解，理解何时血糖会升高，何时血糖会降低，我们还能知道他们有没有控制在合理的范围内。这些能让我们作出更好的决定。再次强调，它既可以用于门诊患者，也可以有时用于住院患者。但我也要说，在医院内，CGM，连续血糖监测，其实用得不那么频繁，但是我的预测是他们在未来会越来越多地得到使用。我们都知道糖化血红蛋白与并发症风险相关，这些数据是来自糖尿病控制和并发症试验，DCCT试验，这个试验非常重要，是针对1型糖尿病的，结果显示糖化的水平与视网膜病、肾病、神经病等这些并发症都相关。所以糖化水平最高的人，他的风险就最高。这也是为什么我们强调有效的血糖控制，对糖尿病患者的血糖控制。

◎ **分析**：

1. 关于"But"的处理，有时候有些讲者的口头禅就是"but"，有时候"but"也并非真正意义上的转折，有些讲者在讲完"but"之后，稍一停顿，改变了原有思路，"but"之后的内容在语义上并无转折。此处译员并未译出，效果反而比直接译作"但是"要好。此处更好的处理是将"but"译作"而"，在不明确语义是否有转折且对较长一句话进行同传的情况下，"而"的表达更加灵活，它既可表示连接，也能表示一定意义的语义转折；

2. "if we want to"译作"如果你想的话"，此处译员作了人称调整，这一操作对于听众理解并无太大影响，可能是下意识所为，但应尽量避免，如果讲者讲到"in our hospital"，译员也习惯性地进行人称转换的话，就可能造成部分误解；

3. "continue to grow and be used more and more"译作"未来会越来越多地得到使用"，并未译出 grow。在同传的模式下，这样处理并不影响听众理解；

4. "A1c"译作"糖化"，在同传语速较快的情况下，专科医生也可以接受这样处理，这也是医生常用的表达，并不影响听众理解；

5. "等这些并发症都相关"的表达，是同传译员的过度翻译。虽然中文中经常会出现此类表达，但英译中同传时译员不应随口添加，否则可能会导致不必要的误解。

But we should also remember that glycol hemoglobin A1c levels may be affected by different factors. And you see here in the screen, different elements that may affect blood sugars, either increase or decrease, their levels. Notably, anemia, for example, can affect A1c level. So the first thing, to also assess in our patients, is their hemoglobin level, if it is really low? And what I mean by really low is perhaps less than ten grams, then the value of the hemoglobin A1c may not be very accurate. Of course, it will depend on other aspects as well. As you can see there, the type of anemia, the use of different medications, etc. It's something to keep in mind as you continue to evaluate A1c levels in your patients. But there is no question that we have really evolved in diabetes care, because there was a time. And some of you may remember, we only had urine testing for diabetes management and that helped to reduce marked hyperglycemia, but the intermittent finger-stick glucose monitoring, the monitors that we continue to use in clinical practice, help us intensify treatment. But now, of course, the benefit of continuous glucose monitors is the possibility of intensifying glucose management without increasing the risk of hypoglycemia, which is on its own an important target in diabetes care.

◎ **参考译文**：但是我们还要记得一件事儿，糖化血红蛋白水平会受到一些因素的影响。在屏幕上你可以看到，不同的因素都会影响血糖，无论使其增高还是降低。比如说贫血能够影响糖化的水平。所以，首先，要去评估我们的患者，评估他们的血红蛋白水平，看看它是否特别低。我说得特别低，也许是不到 10 克，这时糖化血红蛋白的值可能就不是很准确了。当然了，这还取决于其他的一些方面，你可以看到，贫血的类型、不同的药物使用等。所以大家要考虑到，你在评估糖化血红蛋白的时候要考虑到患者的这些方面。但毫无疑问，我们在糖尿病护理方面进展很大。因为曾经一度，在座的各位有些人可能还记得，我们只有尿检用于糖尿病管理，这帮助我们减少明显的高血糖。但是正是这种间歇式手指血糖监测，这种监测我们一直在临床实践当中使用，能帮我们加强治疗。但是现在，当然了，连续血糖监测的优点是它能够加强血糖管理，而不增加低血糖的风险，而这本身也是我们在糖尿病控制当中很重要的一个目标。

◎ 分析：

1. "increase"译作"增高"，其实此处译作"升高"更符合汉语表达习惯，但不影响听众理解；

2. "diabetes care"译作"糖尿病护理"，此处是典型的错译，应该译作"糖尿病诊疗"。将"care"译作"护理"是医学口译中常见的错误；

3. "reduce"译作"减少"，此处译作"减低"或"降低"更符合汉语表达习惯，此处可能会让听众产生一点误解；

4. "finger-stick glucose monitoring"译作"手指血糖监测"，此处可译作"指尖针刺血糖监测"最为准确，但用得更多的表达是"指尖血糖监测"，不一定非要译出"针刺"；

5. "intensify treatment"译作"加强治疗"，但应译作"强化治疗"，这一处理并不影响听众的理解，但能反映出译员对糖尿病主题的熟悉程度；

6. "hypoglycemia"正确译作"低血糖"，但很多时候不少讲者对"hypoglycemia"和"hyperglycemia"的发音非常相似，此时译员最好能够理解上下文的逻辑关系，这样才能够保证翻译正确，而如果不了解讲者逻辑，纯靠听力，就有译错的可能，会让听众觉得莫名其妙。

But let's also remember that when we use glucose monitors in the outpatient or in the inpatient setting, the monitors need to be very accurate. And I know that we're gonna be hearing more about this later on. And monitors need to go through a process to evaluate their quality, so that the readings that we obtained with our patients are appropriate. One very practical way to know whether the blood sugars that we are obtaining with our meters are accurate is to test the blood sugars, basically, at the same time in the laboratory. And with a glucose meter, they should be close to each other. The values are probably not gonna be exactly the same, but as long as they are within a 10% to 15% range, I think that's considered appropriate in most cases. But this is important in terms of hospitals establishing a quality control program to be sure that the meters that are used are adequate. And of course there are specific recommendations. These are the recommendations from the Association of Diabetes Care and Education Specialist in the United States, where the use of monitors is, of course, encouraged in patients with diabetes are both in the outpatient and inpatient settings, but again, to looking at, but looking at the accuracy of all these devices is extremely important to be sure that what we're doing with our patients is correct.

◎ **参考译文**：但是我们也要记住，我们在使用血糖检测仪的时候，在门诊或者住

第四单元 糖尿病与血糖管理

院的条件下，检测仪要非常准确。我知道在这一点上我们后面会听到很多。检测仪需要经过一个流程以评估其质量，从而我们获得的读数，仪表读数是准确的。有一个非常实用的方法，可以知道我们获得的血糖，仪表的读数是否准确，就是检测血糖，基本同时在检验科也检测一下血糖。两个值很可能并不完全一样，但只要它们控制在10%~15%的范围内，我想就可以认为是合适的，大部分情况都是如此。很重要的是，医院要建立一个质量控制计划，以确保医院所用的血糖仪是准确的。当然还有一些具体的推荐。这是ADCES的指南，是美国的，鼓励使用血糖仪，鼓励糖尿病患者使用，无论是在门诊还是住院，而且看这些设备的准确度是非常重要的，从而确保我们为患者所做的都是正确的。

◎ 分析：

1. 此处的"glucose monitors"指的是"血糖检测仪"，注意与前文的"血糖监测"相区别；

2. "laboratory"译作"检验科"，非常贴合国内医疗现状，国外医院没有所谓的"检验科"，只有"laboratory"。而"laboratory"的词义就是实验室，因此在翻译时，译员容易将"laboratory"译作"实验室"，但随着中外交流越来越频繁，此语境下"实验室"的表达也越来越多地被接受；

3. "The values"译作"两个值"，也可以译作"两者"，但要表达出复数对比的感觉，如果只译作"值"，中文表达也没有问题，但需要听众多理解一层，如果译作"两个值"，则听众更能直观地理解；

4. "quality control program"译作"质量控制计划"，也可以译作"方案"或"项目"，但如果将其译作"体系"就稍有过度解读之嫌；

5. "adequate"译作"准确的"，此处难度较大，"adequate"有一个释义是"质量达标"，用在此处才是最为合适。但在同传的形式下，译员如果对于质量体系没有深刻的理解，将其译作"准确的"也未尝不可；

6. "looking at"连续两次出现，译作"看"，但如果能处理为"看、检查"，就能完美反映出讲者语气与重点的改变。

Avoiding hypoglycemia is important. Now, for older individuals, we may be less strict, and not 70%, but let's say more than 50% of the time is okay. But because of the risk of hypoglycemia, we want older individuals to be in really less than 1% …with hypoglycemia. And you can see here in pregnancy, in gestational diabetes, in type one diabetes and pregnancy, it's very hard to be avoiding all these fluctuations. So it's very similar targets. But for people who have type two diabetes or gestational diabetes. We want the blood sugars to be almost perfect, because we know the impact on the mother and the baby of having high blood sugars. So you see here now this table that gives you an idea of how these measures of timing range and A1c compare. For example, if someone has an A1c of 10.6%, most likely it means that only 20% of the time, this person is in an adequate range. If we have a patient with an A1c of 6.7%, which is usually the goal that we establish less than 7% in many of our patients. And that corresponds exactly to what I already said, 70% of the time the blood sugar is in a good range. These are studies in type one and type two diabetes. This one on the right is only on type one diabetes with very similar results.

◎ 参考译文：避免低血糖很重要。对于较年长的患者，不用那么严格，不用70%了，但要超过50%。当然低血糖也会有风险，所以我们也希望老年患者一定要小于1%，低血糖的时间不到1%。还有在妊娠期，妊娠期糖尿病，在1型糖尿病和妊娠期，很难避免这些波动，所以目标也很相似。但是如果有2型糖尿病或者是妊娠期糖尿病，我们希望血糖控制接近完美，因为母亲和孩子都会受到高血糖的影响。在这个表格当中看到时间范围指标和糖化的比较。比如，如果某人的糖化是10.6%，很可能就意味着只有20%的时间，这个人是控制在合适范围内的。如果我们有个患者，糖化是6.7%，也就是我们设立的低于7%的目标，大多数的患者也都是如此，它就对应着我之前已经说过的70%的时间，血糖是在好的范围内的。这主要是对1型和2型糖尿病的研究。右边的这个仅研究1型糖尿病，但结果相似。

◎ 分析：

1. "But because of the risk of hypoglycemia"在翻译时，应更贴近原文的逻辑，即强调低血糖的风险，此处的处理稍偏离了讲者的逻辑。翻译为"当然低血糖也会有风险"可能让听众感觉低血糖的风险是理所当然的，而原文意在强调这是一个需要考虑的重要因素。更合适的翻译可能是"但由于低血糖的风险"，这样的表述更加直接和明确；

2. "… with hypoglycemia"，此处为了让中文表达通顺，同传时译者作了适当的重复，译作"低血糖的时间不到1%"，虽然是无意之举，但在事实上却是通过语言重复强调了部分内容，因此语音语气上不应再有加重；

3. "gives you an idea"此处并未译出，考虑到中文的通顺，不译出完全可以；

4. "This one on the right is only on type one diabetes with very similar results"处理为"这主要是1型和2型糖尿病的研究"，这里的"主要"一词可能会误导听众，让人误以为研究只关注1型和2型糖尿病，而实际上研究可能也涉及其他类型的糖尿病，"主要"一词应予以避免，口译时也应避免随口弱化语气或改变所指范围。

Here we see a table from a recent paper which shows how just even small differences can result in differential clinical decisions. For instance, just this change between the venous and the point of care measurement, a small change of about 10~20 mg/dL would result in a change of insulin dosing by two units. So it depends on what the treatment is. Not just the magnitude of the inaccuracy, but where the inaccuracy falls. So the last thing that I would point to is here we see a difference of 10~15 mg/dL, resulting in a two-unit difference. But here at a little bit lower decision a measurement range, the decision threshold is the same, right. We see an almost 50 mg/dL difference between the measurements and it still results in only a two-unit insulin dose. So it depends on where the measurement takes place, the magnitude of the difference and the decision threshold. So knowing that the measurement will influence the insulin dose, we want to think about what causes inaccuracy in the measurement. And so here is a diagram showing how glucose biosensors are constructed. We here we have an outer membrane and enzyme layer, typically glucose oxidase or glucose dehydrogenates. We will then have an inner membrane to screen out some interferences and the electrode at which the electrochemical sensor where the measurement is made.

◎ **参考译文**：这里有一张表格，来自最近的一篇文章，显示仅仅是很小的差别就能带来不同的临床决策。比如说，静脉血糖和POC检测的一点小小的区别，10~20mg/dL就会改变胰岛素剂量，两个单位。所以它取决于治疗方式是什么，不仅仅是误差的大小，而是误差在哪里出现。最后我想说的是，在这里我们可以看到10~15mg/dL会带来两个单位的差别。这里还有更低一点的指标范围，它的决策阈值是一样的，这里几乎是50mg/dL的误差，它同样带来的是两个单位的胰岛素变化，所以这取决于在哪里测量、差异程度和决策阈值。所以我们知道测量会影响到胰岛素的剂量，那我们就要想测量中的误差是什么原因导致的。这张图展示的是葡萄糖生物传感器的结构，有一个外膜、酶层，主要是葡萄糖氧化酶或者葡萄糖脱氢酶。然后有内膜能够去除干扰，还有电极，上面的电化学传感器就是测量的位置。

◎ **分析**：

1. "differences"译作"差别"，此处译作"差异"为好，相比而言，"差异"的"专业感"更强一些；

2. "point of care test"是指在标本采样现场进行即刻分析，免去了标本在实验室内的复杂处理程序，可译作"POCT检测"或"即时检测"，近年来"床旁检测"的说法使用得越来越少；

3. "inaccuracy"译作"误差"，此处准确译法为"不准确度"，此为检验医学中的专业术语，有着明确的定义，但对于非检验医学专业人士，想准确区分"不准确度""精密度"和"误差"有一定难度。

二、中译英

那么大家都知道这个血糖监测，其实方法是有很多的。到目前为止，各种版本的指南，还是认为毛细血管的血糖监测，还是比较重要且基础的。中国血糖监测的临床应用指南，从11版开始，至今已经发展到第三版，在这期间，也就差不多五到六年修订一次。他这个制定的背景是大家都知道的。中国在医学的各个方面，相对来说要落后于其他国家的。所以，在糖尿病的管理方面，尤其在血糖的监测方面，就比较落后一点。这个管理的状态的话，现状也不是那么乐观，那么当然近几年的话，我们有了长足的进步。像我们沿海地区，最近这几年的话，这个糖尿病管理也非常地好啊。（本段内容选自2024年一位国内专家的学术演讲，有删改调整。）

◎ **参考译文**：We all know that there are many ways of glucose monitoring. And it is believed that the capillary blood glucose is very important and basic, glucose monitoring method. In China, the clinical guidance of glucose monitoring, from 2021 version, we have three versions till now, from 2011 version to 2021 version, so it will be revised every five or six years. At the very beginning, the background of the guideline was that we all know that in the past, China, in terms of medicine, modern medicine was not that advanced compared to other countries, especially western countries. And in diabetes management, especially the glucose monitoring, the methods were left behind. The management status quo is not that optimistic. But in recent years, we've made huge progress, for example, coastal areas in recent years, at local level, we actually manage diabetes well.

◎ 分析：

1. 此处中文为部分演讲实录，对语气词进行了细微处理，此类演讲风格非常普遍且真实，面对语气词运用较多且发言较零碎的讲者，同传时其演讲内容的信息密度也许不是很高，但在表达逻辑上可能会让译员面对一定压力。面对此类讲者，译员可跟随讲者发言，多用连接词、短句、同位语、插入语、从句结构等进行同传；译员也可适度拉长 EVS，使译入语的英文句子听起来更为完整；

2. "临床指南"译作"clinical guideline"；

3. "差不多五到六年这么修订一次"口译时译员用了将来时，此处应使用过去时；正确的翻译应为"it was revised every five or six years"，以反映过去的修订周期；

4. "这个管理的状态的话"可直接处理为"management"，使用"management status quo"可能会显得过于正式或冗长，除非在特定的学术或专业语境中要强调现状，否则范畴词无须译出；

5. "基层"译作"local level"，也可根据具体语境处理为"grassroot level"或"community level"。

大家其实在这个方面，还是有很多疑问的。就是我们这个毛糖测定到底能不能算是一种比较好的方法？能不能运用到我们的一些更精，要求更精细的方面？比如说诊断方面。现在这种情况，我们应该做到一个什么样的程度呢？其实呢，21版的这个指南里面，把15版原来要求的"准确性要求"跟"精确性"的这个要求改为了"准确度"跟"精密度"。那这个字面上的更改，实际上它反映的是什么呢？是我们对毛糖的测定有了一个更精细的要求。这个要求从原来的定性的要求，转变为一个定量的要求。这个也是对毛糖测定仪器的一个要求。这个要求其实是跟 ISO，国际认证标准 15197 的这个标准是匹配的。因为我们临床医生可能对这个血糖仪，背后的一些包括计量方面的要求，可能并不是很了解。

◎ 参考译文：In terms of this, we still have a lot of questions, for example, the capillary blood glucose monitoring, whether it is a good method. Can it be applied to things that require higher accuracy, for example, diagnosis. Currently, how can we do it? To what extent? So in 2021 version, it changes some phrases in 2015, for example, changing "accurate requirement" and "precise requirement" to "requirement of accuracy" and "precision". So literally, it changed like this, but it reflects that we have more precise requirements on capillary measurement. The requirement changed from qualitative to quantitative, so this is the requirement of the capillary devices. And the requirement, with ISO, ISO 15197, they are consistent. So for clinical practitioners, we don't know the underlying specific measurement requirements, we lack knowledge on this.

◎ 分析：

1. "Can it be applied to things that"此处"things"的处理不是最佳，此处可以考虑预测先说，毛糖测定大多用于诊断和管理；

2. "准确度"为"accuracy"，精确度为"precision"；

3. "ISO 15197"的读音为"ISO one five one nine seven"；

4. "临床医生"也可以简单处理为"clinicians"。

那么毛糖的监测，其实在国内、在国外都是差不多。关键都是建议还是以个体化的治疗方案为主，就是我们这个频率不是固定的，是要根据具体的患者情况，方案的治疗情况等来进行。这个 21 版的指南的要点 3，更改的这个要点 3，那么这里面的话呢，也谈到了糖化血红蛋白，由于目前我们国内的糖化监测的标准化程度越来越高了，所以在这个 21 版的血糖监测指南里，也把它列入到了这个糖化，作为糖尿病的诊断标准之一，作为诊断标准之一，那么可能应该是说跟我们的最近版的，就是 21 版的中国 2 型糖尿病管理指南是一致的。那么当然，我们知道这个糖化血红蛋白，它的影响因素比较多。15 版的时候，没有对它的影响因素进行归类。而新一版的指南里，把糖化血红蛋白影响因素，进行了一个比较详细的分类，这样的话呢，也有利于我们在临床上进行糖化，这个质控的进行。

◎ 参考译文：The monitoring of capillary blood glucose, both in home and abroad are similar. The key point is to recommend personalized treatment, so the frequency is not fixed, but it should be based on patient's condition and treatment regimen or other factors. In 2021 version, the key point three was revised, and it mentioned HbA1c. Because, currently in China, the monitoring of HbA1c is more standardized. So in 2021 version of Glucose Monitoring Guideline, it was listed, HbA1c was listed as the diagnosis criteria, one of the criteria. So, the latest version, 2021 Type Two Diabetes Management Guideline. It is in line with it. HbA1c has many different influencing factors, so for the 15 version, it didn't categorize the influencing factors, but in the latest version, the influencing factors are categorized in detail. So it is beneficial for, HbA1c, the quality control of it, clinically.

◎ 分析：

1. "个体化治疗"可译作"personalized treatment"，有时候也被称作"个性化治疗"；

2. "影响因素"译作"influence factor"；

3. 国内医生喜欢讲"临床上"或"在临床上"，可处理为"in clinical practice"。

我们可以看到糖尿病、肾病在病理上和它的这个临床上是对应的，早期就是高滤过状态，肾小球肥大，那么后面呢，逐渐地开始出现KW结节。这个时期呢，继续保持一个高滤过状态，同时有微量蛋白尿，有高血压的形成。到糖尿病肾病的进一步发展，就是差不多到了一半的肾小球都出现KW结节的时候呢，这时候病人就会出现大量的蛋白尿，同时肾功能也开始逐渐有异常。这时候，10到20年的这个时间，糖尿病肾病进展的一个基本过程。那我们非常希望对糖肾患者的治疗，最好你就在它高滤过期就开始给干预。其次，就是在微量白蛋白尿期，也要给干预。这时候，因为病人在多数情况下在内分泌科医生的手里，我们是非常倡导他们早期使用SGLT-2抑制剂去进行很好的干预。但是，即便是病人到了临床蛋白尿期，出现了大量蛋白尿，依然不晚。这个时期还是要给病人进行一个非常好的干预，不要轻易地把这部分病人放弃掉。

◎ 参考译文：We can see diabetic nephropathy, pathologically and clinically, are consistent. In the early stage, it's high GFR stage and glomerular hypertrophy, and it gradually progresses to KW nodules, at this time, keep high GFR level, and there is microalbuminuria, hypertension. With further progression, around half of glomerulus develop KW nodules, at this time patients have massive albuminuria, and the kidney functions also become abnormal. In 10 to 20 years, the diabetic nephropathy progresses, this is the basic progress. We hope that for the treatment we should intervene at the high GFR stage and for the microalbuminuria stage, intervention is also needed. During these stages, patients are mostly seen by the endocrinologists. And we highly recommend that they use SGLT-2 inhibitor for better intervention. Even when they get to clinical proteinuria stage and has massive albuminuria, it's still not late, so at this time we can do better intervention for patients, we shouldn't give them up.

◎ 分析：

1. "病理上和它的这个临床上是对应的"中的"对应"译作了"consistent"，此处可以处理为"corresponding"，"consistent"的处理稍微有点过度；

2. "糖肾"这类的不规则表达，也是国内讲者常用的表达方式，意思是"糖尿病肾病"，译员需要快速理解和反应；

3. "高滤过状态"译作"high GFR"，要比"high filtration"更易理解；

4. "干预"译作"intervention"。

但是2型糖尿病人，病情比较快。你看青少年早发2型糖尿病人和普通的2型糖尿病人，那么他的胰岛功能的下降速度是非常快的。而且对各种药物的失效，它比较容易失效。所以他有遗传背景，再加上早发2型糖尿病，那他的病情，很容易就发展到多种药物进行治疗。另外还有，和你看早发2型糖尿病人和青少年1型比的话，那么这些病人，发生蛋白尿还高啊，比这个1型糖尿病早发的，不，比1型糖尿病人，就发生蛋白尿的机会还要多。而且呢，终末期肾病也比较多。所以这个早发2型的还是挺麻烦的。

与成年 2 型糖尿病比的话，他同样这个早发 2 型糖尿病的蛋白尿也比较多。而且，发生的肾病是老年糖尿病的 5 倍，死亡风险增加 2 倍，所以早发 2 型这个是不太好的一个事情。而且和成人 2 型糖尿病比，早发 2 型糖尿病的心血管风险也会高很多。和 1 型比，你看这个心血管死亡，这个累计风险都要高。

◎ **参考译文**：But for the type two diabetes patients, the disease develops fast. The juvenile early-onset T2DM patients, compared to normal T2DM patients, the pancreas islet function declines fast. And the failure of drugs is very likely to happen. It's very likely to fail. So with genetic factors and early-onset type 2 diabetes, it's very likely to develop to multiple drug treatment. And early-onset T2DM, compared with youth type one, it has more albuminuria, and has more albuminuria compared with T1DM patients, and with more terminal kidney diseases. So the early-onset type 2 is complicated. And compared with adult T2DM, it has higher albuminuria and kidney disease, is five times more than elderly T2DM and the mortality is two times more, so it's not very promising. And compared with adult type 2 diabetes, the cardiovascular risk is way higher than type one. For example, regarding the cardiovascular death, the cumulative risk is higher.

◎ **分析**：

1. "青少年"此处译作"youth"，正确的是"juvenile"，但"youth"的翻译不影响英语听众的理解，同传时想不到"juvenile"，处理为"youth"也可勉强接受；

2. "再加上"此处译作"and"，但近些年的会议中，直接处理为"plus"也是可以的；

3. "蛋白尿"译作"albuminuria"，也可译作"proteinuria"，这是糖尿病肾病主题的高频词汇，译者应提前作好准备，目前最好不要译作"protein urine"，虽然"protein urine"的发音和"proteinuria"有些类似，但只是巧合而已；

4. "累计风险"为"cumulative risk"。

长期高血糖的一个状态可以造成一个下肢和周围血管的病变，造成足部和溃疡，足部发生感染，溃疡以及深部组织的坏死，就形成糖尿病足。所以说大家知道糖尿病足的治疗是非常艰难的，它的病程长、治愈难、心理负担高、经济负担高、致残率高和致死率高。那这么艰难的疾病，我们怎么去治疗呢？还有它的消耗是非常大的。不是说就咱们中国治疗糖足，因为在座各位老师都知道说病人的换药费用很高，不光是在中国，你在美国，在哪儿它的治疗费用都高。除非他放弃治疗，只要想治疗，它治疗费用就是高。那尽管糖尿病足治疗起来非常困难，还有它的预防其实是非常有效的，我们的医务人员可以抽出几分钟的时间去检查他的脚，就说把健康教育要前移，来筛查这些病人。所以说咱们糖尿病足还是可防可治的。现在咱们缺乏什么，缺乏咱们糖尿病足的多学科的合作，不是说我做伤口，单纯做伤口，对于我的糖尿病病人，我就控制他的血糖，其实它是相关很多问题的。

◎ **参考译文**：The long-term hyperglycemia may lead to severe lower limbs and peripheral vessel lesions, causing foot ulcer, infection and deep necrosis, forming diabetic foot. So we all know that the treatment for diabetic foot is very hard because it has long disease course, difficult to cure, high mental pressure and financial burden, high disability rate and mortality rate. So how we can treat it, because it's so difficult and the fee is very high in China, we all know that my colleague, for example, the fee for a patient is very high for changing dressing, not only in China but also in the U.S., the fee is really high, only if stop receiving treatment. Though, it's very difficult to treat, the prevention is very effective. So the medical practitioners can take a few minutes to check the patient's feet and do the education in advance to screen the patient. So the diabetic foot is preventable and treatable. So what we lack now? We lack the MDT of diabetes. It doesn't mean that we only do wound care or control the blood sugar separately, but there are also many related issues.

◎ 分析：
1. 现在有些讲者会用"老师"来称呼与会者、医务人员等，可灵活对应处理；
2. "换药"指更换伤口处的敷料；
3. "做伤口"可处理为"do wound care"。

当伤口局部病原微生物的繁殖发生了感染，以及感染的播散，这个我们要开始局部伤口感染，我们就要使用局部的抗菌剂。咱们现在银离子敷料是广谱杀菌，又不产生耐药，应用是非常广的。那当它往感染周围播散和全身感染的时候，不光局部要使用抗菌剂，还要配合全身的一个抗感染治疗。对于伤口湿性愈合，XX专家说了，伤口湿性愈合越湿越好。其实不是越湿越好，一定要保持它的一个平衡状态。像原来似的，咱们就伤口干性愈合，因为现在这个30分钟的讲课时间，讲不了那么全面。干性愈合，我就说，比如说晾腊肉，这个肉晾成干干的，像木乃伊，干干的，它的组织是没有活性的。但如果说，比如说在战争年代，把这个人打得遍体鳞伤，给他扔到水里，身上有大量的伤口，大量的感染的伤口，扔到水牢里头，马上细菌在水里头有繁殖。到你的伤口里不断地繁殖造成感染，最终人死于全身的感染中毒。

◎ 参考译文：When the wound pathogen reproduces and causes infection, and with the spread of the infection, we have to use local antibacterial agent, for example, silver ion dressing is broad-spectrum bactericidal and non-resistant, which is widely used. So when the infection spreads to the peripheral, to the whole body, not only treat locally but also the full body. You may think that somebody said, the moister the better, but it is not like that. We have to keep a balance just like before, the dry healing. Because we only have 30 minutes and we cannot go through comprehensively. Dry healing, in my opinion, for example, the cured meat gets dry, like mummy, very dry, so its tissue is not active at all. But in wartime, if one has a lot of wounds and is put in the water, with a lot of wounds, infected wounds. In the water, the bacteria would reproduce and then the wounds would be infected. And the person will die because of the systemic infection.

◎ 分析：

1. "这个我们要开始局部伤口感染"属于口误，对于此类讲者，EVS 可以适当放长，从而去除明显口误同时组织语言；

2. "杀菌"为"bactericidal"；

3. "全身感染中毒"此处译作"full body infection"，其实可以处理为"systemic infection"。

第四节　补充练习

一、中译英

连续性血糖监测是通过植于皮下组织内的微电极，记录组织间液葡萄糖氧化反应产生的电信号，从而间接测量血糖的新型微创血糖监测技术。CGMS 是微创的血糖监测系统，通过检测皮下组织间液的葡萄糖浓度而反映血糖水平，它可不间断地监测使用者一天中每时每刻的血糖值。CGM 的佩戴设备体积较小，为可穿戴式设备，可固定于上臂或腹部，该设备内有芯片，有一根细微软管连接仪器与探测头，探测头插入皮下组织。葡萄糖传感器则是 CGM 技术的关键部分，大多数传感器是基于电化学理论设计的酶传感器。传感器可连续使用 14 天，每 5 分钟记录 1 次血糖值，并储存形成连续的血糖图谱，方便患者真实精准地记录日常生活。简单而言，就是把一条无菌、纤细且柔软的传感器植入皮下，从而实现 24 小时持续监测佩戴者的血糖水平，通过蓝牙传输血糖数据，还可以把实时的血糖值发送到手机上供佩戴者查看。

CGM 有以下功能：连续监测，CGM 设备能连续、动态地监测全天人体血糖值的变化；记录功能，CGM 可记录并储存每个时间段的血糖值以及其他相关事件，如进餐、运动及用药等；数据分析，通过上传监测数据并进行数据处理，可以得到连续的血糖图谱，以便医生对患者的血糖控制情况进行总体把控；发现隐匿性高血糖和低血糖事件，CGM 能够发现不易被传统血糖监测方法监测到的隐匿性高血糖及低血糖事件；个性化血糖管理，CGM 技术可提供海量的血糖信息，有望使糖尿病管理方案的制定更具针对性，真正做到精准控糖。

如今，在部分国家和地区，对于 2 型糖尿病（T2DM）、1 型糖尿病（T1DM）、妊娠糖尿病（GDM）患者，CGM 在血糖控制和生活方式管理中得到广泛应用，同时在新生儿、ICU 危重症患者的血糖管理，减重、运动指导和饮食营养优化等领域也已成为热点。随着技术进步及产品成熟，CGM 的应用场景将不断拓宽。

在 T1DM 和 T2DM 患者中，CGM 的应用已经被大量临床试验所证实，其能显著提升血糖控制达标率、减少低血糖及高血糖事件并提高生活质量。对于希望运动的糖尿病患者，CGM 对于及时补充热量、保证能量供给、防止低血糖等都具有重要指导价值。在妊娠糖尿病或糖尿病合并妊娠患者管理中，CGM 具有可靠的准确性和安全性。

在非糖尿病领域，CGM 在 ICU 危重症患者或围手术期的使用有助于精准地个性化血糖控制，降低医源性低血糖风险及术后不良事件。在新生儿低血糖症应用中，CGM 有利于及时发现、早期处理低血糖，从而改善患儿预后。

此外，CGM 在运动领域和健康保健领域的应用也日益受到关注。CGM 最早应用于希望坚持运动的 1 型糖尿病患者，后来发现应用于正常健康的长跑运动员可以合理规划赛程中的饮食和能量摄入。近年来，CGM 指导下的生物反馈减肥、优化锻炼方案和健康生活方式管理在部分国家的保健领域成为时尚，旨在引导使用者的食物选择，远离高糖、低饱腹感的食物，并鼓励通过加强运动来调节血糖。

◎ **参考译文**：Continuous glucose monitoring (CGM) is a new minimally invasive blood glucose monitoring technology that indirectly measures blood glucose by recording the electrical signals generated by the oxidation reaction of glucose in the interstitial fluid through microelectrodes implanted in the subcutaneous tissue. CGMS is a minimally invasive blood glucose monitoring system that reflects blood glucose levels by detecting the glucose concentration in the interstitial fluid of the subcutaneous tissue. It can continuously monitor the user's blood glucose level at all times of the day. The CGM wearable device is small in size and can be fixed on the upper arm or abdomen. The device contains a chip and a fine hose connecting the instrument and the probe, which is inserted into the subcutaneous tissue. Glucose sensors are the key part of CGM technology. Most sensors are enzyme sensors designed based on electrochemical theory. The sensor can be used continuously for 14 days, recording blood glucose values once every 5 minutes, and storing them to form a continuous blood glucose map, which is convenient for patients to record their daily lives accurately. In simple terms, a sterile, thin and soft sensor is implanted under the skin to continuously monitor the wearer's blood glucose level for 24 hours, transmit blood glucose data via Bluetooth, and send real-time blood glucose values to the mobile phone for the wearer to view.

CGM has the following functions: continuous monitoring, CGM equipment can continuously and dynamically monitor the changes in human blood sugar levels throughout the day; recording function, CGM can record and store blood sugar levels in each time period and other related events, such as meals, exercise and medication; data analysis, by uploading monitoring data and processing data, a continuous blood sugar map can be obtained so that doctors can have an overall control of the patient's blood sugar control; discover hidden hyperglycemia and hypoglycemia events, CGM can discover hidden hyperglycemia and hypoglycemia events that are not easily monitored by traditional blood sugar monitoring methods; personalized blood sugar management, CGM technology can provide a large amount of blood sugar information, which is expected to make the formulation of diabetes management plans more targeted and truly achieve accurate blood sugar control.

Nowadays, in some countries and regions, CGM is widely used in blood sugar control and lifestyle management for patients with type 2 diabetes (T2DM), type 1 diabetes (T1DM), and gestational diabetes (GDM). At the same time, it has also become a hot topic in the fields of blood sugar management, weight loss, exercise guidance, and diet nutrition optimization for newborns and critically ill patients in the ICU. With technological progress and product maturity, the application scenarios of CGM will continue to expand.

In patients with T1DM and T2DM, the application of CGM has been confirmed by a large number of clinical trials, which can significantly improve the blood sugar control rate, reduce hypoglycemia and hyperglycemia events and improve the quality of life. For diabetic patients who want to exercise, CGM has important guiding value for timely replenishment of calories, ensuring energy supply, and preventing hypoglycemia. In the management of patients with gestational diabetes or diabetes combined with pregnancy, CGM has reliable accuracy and safety.

In the non-diabetic field, the use of CGM in critically ill patients in the ICU or perioperative period helps to accurately personalize blood sugar control, reduce the risk of iatrogenic hypoglycemia and postoperative adverse events. In the application of neonatal hypoglycemia, CGM is conducive to timely detection and early treatment of hypoglycemia, thereby improving the prognosis of children.

In addition, the application of CGM in the fields of sports and health care is also receiving increasing attention. CGM was first used in patients with type 1 diabetes who wanted to stick to exercise, and later it was found that it could be used in normal and healthy long-distance runners to reasonably plan their diet and energy intake during the race. In recent years, biofeedback weight loss, optimized exercise programs and healthy lifestyle management guided by CGM have become fashionable in the health care field of some countries. They aim to guide users' food choices, stay away from high-sugar, low-satiety foods, and encourage blood sugar regulation through increased exercise.

二、英译中

The disease burden related to diabetes is very high and rising in every country, fueled by the global rise in the prevalence of obesity and unhealthy lifestyles. The recent estimates show a global prevalence of 382 million people with diabetes in 2013, expected to rise to 592 million by the year of 2035. The etiology classification of diabetes has now been widely accepted. Type 1 and type 2 diabetes are the two main types, with type 2 diabetes accounting for the majority ($>85\%$) of total diabetes prevalence. Both forms of diabetes can lead to multisystem complications of microvascular endpoints, including nephropathy, retinopathy, neuropathy, and macrovascular endpoints including ischemic heart condition, stroke and peripheral vascular disease. The premature morbidity, mortality, reduced life expectancy and financial and other costs of diabetes make it an important public health issue.

The slow onset of type 2 diabetes, and its usual presentation without the acute metabolic disturbance seen in type 1 diabetes, means that the true time of onset is difficult to be determined. There is also a long pre-detection period, and up to 50% of cases in the population may be undiagnosed.

Because the ratio of detected/undetected cases may vary over time and between locations, epidemiology research aimed at defining the true prevalence of type 2 diabetes has relied on special studies in which the presence and absence of disease are defined by the oral glucose tolerance test (OGTT). The WHO recommends the use of the 75g OGTT, with diabetes defined by fasting glucose 7.0 mmol/L or more and/or 2-hour post-challenge glucose 11.1 mmol/L or more. Recently, the American Diabetes Association (ADA), the WHO and other authoritative bodies have approved the use of HbA1c for the diagnosis of diabetes with a cut-off of 48 mmol/mol (>6.5%) in a standardized laboratory.

As in type 1, there is marked geographical variation, but the pattern is different. The prevalence is lowest in rural areas of developing countries, generally intermediate in developed countries, and highest in certain ethnic groups, particularly those that have adopted Western lifestyles. Populations with the highest prevalence have a high prevalence of obesity. The hypothesis is that genetic susceptibility to obesity would be disadvantageous in times of food abundance, but advantageous when food is scarce, driving its persistence by natural selection. This 'thrifty genotype' hypothesis is supported by evidence of gene-environment interaction; individuals who migrate from low-prevalence areas to the West are at increased risk of type 2 diabetes. Diabetes is up to four to six times more prevalent in South Asians and African-Caribbeans in the UK compared with European white populations. There is only a small gender difference in the global numbers of people with diabetes, with about 14 million more men than women estimated to have diabetes in 2013. The prevalence increases sharply with age in both sexes.

◎ 参考译文：由于全球肥胖和不健康生活方式的流行，与糖尿病相关的疾病负担在每个国家都很高且呈上升趋势。最近的估计显示，2013年全球糖尿病患病人数为3.82亿，预计到2035年将上升至5.92亿。糖尿病的病因分类现已被广泛接受。1型和2型糖尿病是两种主要类型，其中2型糖尿病占糖尿病总患病人数的大多数(>85%)。两种类型的糖尿病都可导致多系统并发症，包括微血管并发症，包括肾病、视网膜病变、神经病变；以及大血管并发症，包括缺血性心脏病、卒中和外周血管疾病。糖尿病的过早发病、死亡、预期寿命缩短以及经济和其他成本使其成为重要的公共卫生问题。

2型糖尿病发病缓慢，且通常没有1型糖尿病那样的急性代谢紊乱，这意味着很难确定其真正的发病时间。此外，2型糖尿病的诊断前期较长，高达50%的病例可能未被诊断出来。

由于发现/未发现病例的比例可能随时间和地点而改变，旨在确定2型糖尿病真实患病率的流行病学研究须依赖专门的研究，这些研究通过口服葡萄糖耐量试验（OGTT）来定义疾病的存在与否。WHO 建议使用 75g 的 OGTT，糖尿病定义为空腹血糖 7.0 mmol/L 或以上和/或餐后 2 小时血糖 11.1 mmol/L 或以上。最近，美国糖尿病协会（ADA）和 WHO 等权威机构已批准在标准化实验室中使用 HbA1c 诊断糖尿病，临界值为 48 mmol/mol（>6.5%）。

与 1 型一样，2 型糖尿病也存在明显的地域差异，但模式有所不同。发展中国家农村地区的糖尿病患病率最低，发达国家的患病率一般中等，某些族群的患病率最高，尤其是那些采用西方生活方式的族群。患病率最高的人群肥胖患病率也很高。假设是，肥胖的遗传易感性在食物充足时不利，但在食物匮乏时有利，这种特性通过自然选择推动其持续存在。这种"节俭基因型"假设得到了基因与环境相互作用的证据支持；从患病率低的地区迁移到西方的人患 2 型糖尿病的风险增加。与欧洲白人相比，在英国的南亚人和非洲裔加勒比人患糖尿病的概率会高 4 至 6 倍。全球糖尿病患者人数的性别差异很小，2013 年估计男性糖尿病患者比女性多 1400 万左右。男女两性糖尿病患病率随年龄增长而急剧上升。

第五单元　心脏介入

第一节　心脏介入口译知识点

　　介入治疗（interventional/intervention treatment）有别于大多数人对于临床医学的常规理解，即"内科就是吃药，外科就是开刀"的概念。介入治疗，既不属于内科治疗（medical treatment），也不属于外科治疗（surgical treatment），是随着近年来材料学、工程学以及医学技术的不断进步，尤其是影像学水平的快速发展，而形成的一种独特的治疗方式。简单理解，就是一种微创操作（minimally-invasive procedure），在其过程中操作者通过特殊的影像方法，能够在屏幕上实时"看到"人体内部器械及操作的全过程。简而言之，操作医生在血管内用导管（catheter）和微导管（microcatheter）将特殊的器械（device）送到人体内的病变部位（lesion），通过物理、化学的手段直接消除或减轻病变，从而达到治疗目的。

　　心脏介入治疗包括：冠状动脉造影术（coronary arteriography，CAG）、经皮冠状动脉腔内成形术及支架术（percutaneous transluminal coronary angioplasty，PTCA，and stent）、二尖瓣球囊扩张术、射频消融术（radiofrequency ablation）、起搏器植入术（pacemaker implantation）、先天性心脏病介入治疗、冠状动脉腔内溶栓术、左心耳封堵术（left atrial appendage occlusion，LAAO）等。

　　冠状动脉造影是一种侵入性/有创性检查（invasive examination），旨在显示向心肌供血的冠状动脉的影像。检查时，患者接受局麻（local anesthesia），使用血管造影机，通过人手腕处的桡动脉（radial artery）或腹股沟处（groin）的股动脉插入心导管，沿动脉逆行至升主动脉根部，然后送至冠状动脉开口处，注入一种特殊的造影剂（contrast medium/contrast），使冠状动脉显影。此操作可清晰显示整个左冠或右冠的主干（trunk）及其分支（branch）的血管腔，可以判断血管有无狭窄病灶，可以明确诊断病变部位、范围严重程度等信息，为决定后续治疗方案（内科治疗、手术治疗或介入治疗）奠定基础，也用于随访监测疗效。

　　此处简单介绍一下冠状动脉及其重要血管分支：

　　左冠状动脉主干（left main artery，LM），分为左前降支（left anterior descending，LAD），其又分为对角支（diagonal branches，D1，D2）以及间隔支（septal branches，S1，S2），以及左回旋支（left circumflex，LCX），其有分出钝缘支（obtuse marginal branches，OM1，OM2）。

右冠状动脉（right coronary artery，RCA），分为锐缘支（acute marginal branch，AM）、后降支（posterior descending artery，PDA）以及左室后支（posterior lateral artery，PLA）。

自1977年世界首例经皮冠状动脉腔内成形术成功完成后，以PTCA为基础的经皮冠状动脉介入治疗（percutaneous coronary intervention，PCI）技术和器械就得到了快速发展，至今已经成为治疗冠心病的重要方法之一。我国从1984年开始开展PTCA技术，20世纪90年代开展冠状动脉内支架植入术，从裸金属支架（bare metal stent，BMS）、药物洗脱支架（drug-eluting stent，DES），到生物可吸收支架（bioresorbable scaffold，BRS），经过一代又一代的不断探索进步，冠心病介入技术、治疗策略、新器械研发方面，都已经取得了巨大成就，目前我国已经成为全球开展PCI数量最多的国家，部分相关技术已经位居世界前列。

冠状动脉球囊成形术（coronary balloon angioplasty），是将球囊扩张导管沿导丝（guidewire）轨道送达冠状动脉的靶病变（target lesion）处，利用球囊加压充盈（inflation）后产生膨胀力而使冠状动脉狭窄（stenosis）得到扩张，是所有冠心病介入治疗技术的基础。球囊扩张导管（简称球囊）（balloon）在PCI中的作用已从最初的单纯球囊血管成形术（plain old balloon angioplasty，POBA）逐步扩展，现在的功能包括：病变预扩张（pre-dilation）、辅助支架的输送释放和后扩张（post-dilation）以及载药（药物涂层球囊，drug coated balloon，DCB）治疗等。球囊根据设计特性可分为顺应性、半顺应性和非顺应性球囊；根据操作特点可分为快速交换和整体交换球囊（over-the-wire，OTW）；根据特殊功能，可分为最初的灌注球囊以及目前临床上的切割球囊、棘突球囊、双导丝球囊和DCB等新型球囊。

冠状动脉球囊成形术的并发症包括：

冠状动脉痉挛（coronary artery spasm）、冠状动脉夹层及壁内血肿（coronary artery dissection and intramural hematoma）、分支闭塞（branch occlusion）、冠状动脉破裂或穿孔（rupture or perforation）等。

单纯PTCA可能会有血管急性闭塞（acute vascular occlusion）和再狭窄（re-stenosis），而冠状动脉支架能有效地处理夹层（dissection），提供机械支撑并减轻弹性回缩。

冠状动脉支架包括：

裸金属支架：这是最早投入临床使用的支架，相较于单纯球囊扩张，BMS的优势在于更大的即刻管腔获得以及较小的弹性回缩，但内膜增生所致的晚期管腔丢失，或称为支架再狭窄（stent re-stenosis）是其主要缺陷，因此已经基本被DES取代。目前仅少量用于有介入指征的抗栓治疗禁忌或高出血风险患者。

药物洗脱支架：第一代DES携带的雷帕霉素（rapamycin）或者紫杉醇，在血管局部抑制血管平滑肌细胞迁移和增殖（migration and proliferation），一定程度上解决了支架再狭窄的问题。然而，第一代DES的晚期支架血栓或获得性贴壁不良（malapposition）的风险有所增加。第二代DES药物通常采用脂溶性（lipid solubility）更好的佐他莫司（Zotarolimus）、依维莫司（Everolimus）或其他雷帕霉素衍生物，其聚合物涂层的生物相容性更好。第二代 DES 的支架血栓的发生率更低。目前流行的新一代 DES 采用了更先进的聚合物涂层技术(coating technology)，包括单面涂层技术、可降解(degradable)聚合物涂层技术、无聚合物涂层技术以及采用纳米工程改良的涂层技术等。

生物可吸收支架：为避免异物永久留存于患者体内，BRS 的理念应运而生。自从 2006 年第一代 BRS 进入大规模临床验证以来，全球已有很多款 BRS 进入临床研究。

心脏射频消融术(catheter radiofrequency ablation，经常为 RF)，是将电极导管(electrode catheter)经静脉或动脉血管送入心脏内腔预定部位，释放射频电流，从而导致局部心内膜及心内膜下心肌凝固性坏死，以达到阻断快速心律失常(arrhythmia)异常传导束和起源点的介入性技术。射频消融术目前已成为根治阵发性心动过速最有效的方法。

心律失常是指心脏的正常节律发生了异常改变。心律失常包括房室折返性心动过速(预激综合征)、房室结折返性心动过速、心房扑动/房扑(atrial flutter)、房性心动过速/房速、室性期前收缩/早搏、室性心动过速/室速、心房颤动/房颤(atrial fibrillation，A-fib/AF/Afib)。临床表现以心慌、心悸(palpitation)、胸闷(chest distress)、乏力(fatigue)、头晕(dizziness)等为主要表现，严重者可能出现胸痛(chest pain)、呼吸困难(difficult breathing)、肢冷汗出、意识丧失、抽搐等表现。

电生理检查和射频消融术，要在一间有特殊设备的手术间进行，称为导管室(catheter room/lab)。导管室人员包括电生理医生、助手、护士和技师。

首先进行导管插入部位(腹股沟、手臂、肩膀或颈部)的皮肤消毒，使用局麻药进行局部麻醉；然后用穿刺针穿刺静脉/动脉血管，电生理检查导管通过血管插入心腔；心脏电生理检查所用的电极导管长而可弯的导管，能将电信号传入和传出心脏。电极导管记录心脏不同部位的电活动，并发放微弱的电刺激来刺激心脏，以便诱发心律失常，明确心动过速诊断；然后医生通过导管找到心脏异常电活动的确切部位[此过程被称为"标测"(mapping)]，再通过消融仪发送射频电流消融治疗，从而根治心动过速。

心房颤动，简称房颤，是最常见的心律失常之一。房颤患者最大的风险在于容易出现栓塞事件(embolic event)，如急性脑梗死(acute cerebral infarction)、急性心肌梗死(acute myocardial infarction，AMI)，房颤高危栓塞患者须积极抗凝治疗(anticoagulant/anticoagulation therapy)，而药物抗凝治疗有导致包括脑出血在内的出血风险，左心耳封堵术通过介入手术的方式应用国产或进口封堵器堵塞左心耳，预防房颤时左心耳(LAA)血栓的形成，可达到药物抗凝的治疗效果，降低房颤患者由血栓栓塞引发长期残疾或死亡的风险，而出血风险大大降低。因此，左心耳封堵术可消除患者对长期口服抗凝治疗的依赖性，为不能长期接受抗凝治疗、不愿药物抗凝治疗以及出血高风险的患者提供新的治疗选择。

经导管左心耳封堵术(transcatheter left atrial appendage occlusion，LAAO)是一种通过在心房颤动患者左心耳内置入封堵器，以达到预防 AF 相关的栓塞性事件的治疗方法。经典式 LAAO 要求采用全身麻醉、经食管超声心动图(transesophageal echocardiography，TEE)引导，且需要心外科及体外循环医师后备支持，以随时应对各种突发情况。但是，随着经验累积、器械迭代发展，LAAO 的手术风险不断降低，全身麻醉、TEE 检测等措施在一些情况下反而可能会增加患者的相关风险，增加手术及康复的时间和费用。已有临床研究表明，X 线透视下引导 LAAO 也是安全和有效的。截至 2021 年底，我国 LAAO 总数已突破 3 万例，可实施 LAAO 的中心数量超过 500 家，国内外的部分术者已积累了丰富的经典式和简化式的 LAAO 经验。

简化式 LAAO 一般采用局部麻醉，术中主要在 X 线透视、经胸超声心动图 (transthoracic echocardiography, TTE) 引导评估下完成。这种操作流程一般不需要全身麻醉和 TEE 的全程引导，简化了经典式 LAAO 的流程。术后患者可直接被转运至普通病房，无手术相关并发症的情况下，可在术后 6~12 小时下床活动，缩短康复过程和住院时间。

但简化式 LAAO 也并不排斥 TEE 或心腔内超声 (intracardiac echocardiography, ICE) 的引导及监测，若术前影像学评估提示手术难度较大和/或手术风险高的患者，可视具体情形转为镇静或全身麻醉，给予 TEE 或 ICE 辅助引导及进一步评估封堵效果。

第二节　真实世界口译情境

一、主题会议

随着医学技术的发展，越来越多的医院提供"不开刀的心脏病治疗"。相较于冠心病的搭桥手术以及心脏瓣膜疾病的开胸换瓣手术，心脏介入治疗，因其确切的疗效、微创性及便捷性，更受患者的青睐。近年来，随着人口老龄化的加剧及经济水平的提升，国内心脏介入的操作量连年上升，而随着各家介入器械公司的产品引进和迭代，现在医学会议中涉及心脏介入的会议不在少数，以下主题的医学会议可能涉及心脏介入：

介入器械公司与国家监管机构间的咨询会议、国家监管机构对器械生产公司的 GMP 核查、大医院心脏介入操作的在线直播会议、国外介入专家在国内的学术路演、先天性心脏病专题会议、心脏电生理专题会议、介入器械临床应用的国内外医生交流会议、各类心脏主题的医学会议以及其他主题医学会议进行病例讨论时，在回顾患者病史时，如患者之前接受过心脏介入治疗，一定会提及，而且介入后的持续用药很可能会影响到患者的治疗计划。

二、行业特点

为了构建最基础的心脏介入知识体系，前文介绍了各种心脏介入操作，包括：冠脉造影(CAG)、冠脉成形术(PTCA)、射频消融术、左心耳封堵等。

冠脉造影(CAG)，是相对基础的介入操作，也是大多数其他介入治疗的基础，现在基本无专门以此为主题的医学口译会议；冠脉成形术，如前文所述，我国在操作量、操作技术和操作经验方面，都处于领先地位，因此也少有专门以此为主题的医学口译会议，偶尔有些此主题的医学口译会议，会议主题也是针对 PTCA 中尚有治疗争议或难度较大的具体内容，例如主题为"分叉处病变"（bifurcation lesion）的专门会议。

射频消融术也被相应领域的医生称为"电生理"（electrophysiology），此主题的医学口译会议也常被称为"电生理会议"，行业内部分公司会定期召开此主题会议；与二尖瓣球囊扩张术、起搏器植入术、冠脉腔内溶栓这三个主题相关的医学口译会议较少；先心病介入治疗，偶尔在心内科或儿科会议中会有提及；左心耳封堵术，相关公司会定期召开此主题会议。

介入治疗一般被称为"介入操作"（interventional procedure），以区别于外科手术（surgery operation），但近年来"介入手术"的说法也会被提及。而对于介入操作前的准备，不少医生习惯称之为"术前准备"（Pre-op preparation），对于介入操作后的随访观察（follow-up and observation），不少医生称之为"术后随访"（post-op follow-up），口译时译员可灵活处理。

介入操作相较于开胸手术，虽然风险及术者压力相对较小，但近年来很多会议会进行介入操作的远程实时直播，对于介入操作直播会议，操作者仍然有相当的操作压力以及会议的直播压力，故此类会议操作时术者往往更关注介入操作本身，发言往往简单快速，而同时可能会有多位点评嘉宾（panelist）在进行同时发言/讨论/点评，有时会给同传带来一定困难。

三、口译难点

心脏介入口译的难点有四：

（一）相对复杂的心脏解剖及电生理基础

普通译员一般应具备常规的知识储备，例如绝大多数人的心脏居左，人的心脏分为左右心房及左右心室，心脏的血液循环方向为右心房—右心室—肺动脉—肺静脉—左心房—左心室—主动脉，心脏的供血动脉为冠状动脉等。此等水平的知识储备对于现在主题越来越细致且不断更新的心脏介入会议完全不够，因此译员要在会前进行充足的学习与准备。

心脏的解剖更加注重三维立体结构，尤其是心脏电生理主题和左心耳封堵主题，以及瓣膜介入的主题（下一章节详述），译员需要对心脏解剖有相对的了解，并且具备一定的立体空间想象能力。对于重要的冠状动脉名称及缩略语表达，译员要烂熟于心，同传时能做到随口译出。心脏内部亦有众多重要的解剖结构，会议举办方在会前不一定能够提供会议当中所要用到的课件，而就算会前提供了讲者的演讲课件，课件中大概率也不会提及这些细微而重要的解剖结构。而在讲课讨论时，医生往往会随口说出这些结构，且医生语速往往较快，译员临时查单词表或查询网络资源根本来不及，这就造成了此类内容同传时难度较大，译员如果没有与此主题相关的足够经验，或没有良好的会前准备，很可能对中文表达的理解都有困难。

而心脏电生理相较于心脏解剖，更是难上加难。心脏解剖结构，无论是壁、隔、环、瓣还是心肌、血管等，都是实际看得见的实体结构，译员通过经验的积累，以及有效的会前内容准备，花一定时间，达到熟悉的水准并不难。而心脏电生理看不见摸不着，就算对于非心内科的医生而言也是难点，对于没有医学背景的译员，想要做到心中有数，难度较大。

(二) 中文表达中英文的使用

在会议交流时，不少临床上使用的介入器械及耗材在中文中仍然沿用英文的商品名，这就需要译员对相关产品有一定的熟悉度，在英译中时能迅速判断出哪些内容"无须翻译，跟读即可"；而在中译英时，对于不同中文讲者的发言，能够快速判断出讲者讲的是哪一款器械，有时因为中文讲者的口音与英语发音问题，在无辅助材料进行纯口语交流时，译员要对产品器械非常熟悉，才能够瞬间作出判断。当然，绝大多数会议的主题发言部分，都会主要围绕某一款具体的产品器械展开。但在讨论与问答环节时，与会者时常会提及数种产品及器械，此时译员的压力较大。因为在讨论及问答环节，无论同传还是交传，问答双方随时停顿，对信息的准确度要求极高，容错率相较于主题演讲低得多，一旦译员漏译或错译，势必影响交流。另外，现今不少国内医生都有国外交流培训经验，有些医生出于各种原因，会在中文表达中夹杂一些英语，有时是几个单词，有时可能是几句话，而往往又毫无规律可循，有时医生讲出关键英文词，会对译员有所帮助，但有时这样反复切换的语言表达方式也会对译员造成一定压力。

(三) 英文缩略语、中文的省略以及特色表达

心脏介入主题的会议会出现大量缩略语，如果不理解这些缩略语，译员对内容的理解就会有困难，但想要及时处理好这些缩略语，译员需经验积累或会前有针对性地准备。在此主题下，除了标准缩略语外，国内外医生又"创造"了大量缩略语，口语中经常随意讲出，译员只能依靠知识储备和经验来应对此类情况。

举个例子，心脏电生理主题会议中会提及一个缩略语"SNO"，发音同"snow"，SNO 是 slow or no 的缩略语，意思是"缓慢传导或传导阻滞"，而电生理主题会议的一大特色就是课件画面色彩绚丽，各类颜色及形状丰富，如译员提前并不了解这一缩略语，此时极易被误导，是按照"snow"的形态理解再翻译，是跳过或是跟读，这一决策往往需要在瞬间作出，难度极大。又或讲者说到"ICE"，发音就是"ice"，但实际是 intracardiac echocardiography 的缩略语，意思是"心脏内超声"，译员如果不提前作了解，耳中听到的是"snow"和"ice"，眼中看到的是五彩斑斓的幻灯片，多少会受到一定影响。再或演讲时的幻灯片上使用缩略语，而讲者却使用完整表达，或反其道而行之，此时译员如果同时听发言、看课件、做同传，加之部分译员 EVS 较长，此时译员很可能无法将前几秒听到的完整表达与幻灯片上看到的缩略语进行正确匹配，此时就可能产生混乱，最常见的情况就是译员跳过不译，导致信息遗漏。英文缩略语还有一种现象，就是同一个中文表达存在两个英文缩略语的情况，例如"左上肺静脉"，其英文表达实际存在两个缩略语，分别是"LSPV"和"LUPV"，虽然两者仅相差了一个字母，但译员在经验不足的情况下，口译时也可能会产生一定困惑。

英文缩略语主要存在于解剖、操作方法、术式、产品等方面，而中文讲者在发言时

所用到的省略无处不在，这对不熟悉此领域的译员会造成极大的挑战。英文缩略语需要译员进行充分的会前准备；而中文的省略则需要译员对于会议主题和相关知识有较好的理解或在此领域有一定的经验。

在中文中，医学术语也存在大量省略。例如，绝大多数医生习惯讲"左室"而非"左心室"，而且不同医生对于"室"的发音也不同，既有三声也有四声，译员需要对其口音极为熟悉，能够做到"肌肉记忆"。而且在进行中译英时，如果中文讲者不使用英文缩略语，译员就不应使用缩略语，而"左室"译作"LV"不妥，应译作"left ventricle"，这个词的中文有两个音节，而其英文对应单词的音节翻了一番还多，而这一表达使用频率极高，故而译员在保持发音清晰的同时还要提高语速。再比如不少医生会将"左下肺"作为"左下肺静脉"的省略表达，其实这是错误的表达方式，沟通时能不产生歧义是严格局限于当前的语境内，以及讲者与听众间的默契。此时如果译员将其译作 left lower lung，只是译对了字面意思，但译错了其意义，此时最好译作"left inferior pulmonary vein"，译员如果译作"left inferior pulmonary"，则不符合此情境下英语的表达习惯，而且因为中国医生未使用英文缩略语，译员最好也不使用，而且就算想用，也不一定能瞬间反应出"LIPV"的表达。此类例子不胜枚举。

此主题的中文发言中还存在一种特殊的情况，就是讲者用一个与医学无关且非常具象化的生动表达，甚至成语，来描述某一具体操作方法或步骤。例如电生理会议中，讲者用"回头望月"来表示一个器械的具体操作步骤，此时想要完美译出，首先要理解讲者所表达的具体步骤，将其译出后快速补充译出中文表达的意象。但在同传过程中，译员如果之前没有遇到过这种情况，想在两秒内完成这一过程，难度较大。再比如讲者用"孙悟空""牛魔王"来形容介入过程中某款器械操作与周围解剖结构的关系，同时还有一丝传统式的幽默。同传时译员能够跟上讲者思路，理解该器械与周围结构的关系，并能准确译出，已属不易，而想要瞬间找到英语文化中对应"孙悟空"与"牛魔王"关系的文学或神话人物形象，还要尽可能保证听众能够理解，因为并非所有听众均为英语母语者，这对于译员是极大的挑战；而如果译者选择直译，绝大多数的听众只会是一头雾水，极可能会认为同传出了问题。此时讲者又很可能希望英语听众能够理解并欣赏他的表达，甚至会提问，所以此时译员的临时决断能力就显得尤为重要，译员首先应着重将器械操作与周围解剖关系译出，如果想得过多，很可能顾此失彼，导致听众不知所云。

（四）客户的某些具体要求

客户会对具体表达提出明确的口译要求。比如在某些具体主题的医学口译会议中，部分客户会明确要求将"leak"（意思是"漏"）译作"分流"而非"漏"，而"leak"以及"leakage"在医学口译中又常规译作"漏"。此主题医学口译会议中，译员如果不特别注意，很容易陷入惯性思维；又或者先译作"漏"，然后"猛然觉察"，再改口说"分流"，但前面话已出口，无法收回，以上两种情况都会达不到客户的要求。

再比如某些客户对于自己的医学会议口译质量要求极高，简单而言就是要求译员同传时做到"纤毫毕现"，每一个专业术语、每一个操作的详细描述，都要求100%准确译出,有些客户还会专门安排监听人员,建立微信群,同传过程中随时与译员沟通。在这样的要求下,客户唯一不会在意的只有单复数表达的偶尔出错,其他任何漏译、错译、译出语模糊、专业表达含糊等情况都不接受。这样的要求对于该主题经验丰富的译员都有一定挑战,对于第一次接触这一主题的译员更是严苛。译员如果没有丰富的经验或开展大量的会前准备,客户很容易在会后给出负面评价,进而要求下次会议换译员。

第三节 中英对照篇章及分析

一、英译中

What is a coronary angioplasty? Coronary angioplasty is a technique for dealing with narrowings in coronary arteries, and these narrowings can typically cause angina, chest pain or breathlessness. And the way that they're dealt with is a small tube placed into the artery. The wire is passed down the artery, and over that wire, balloon is positioned in the area of narrowing and inflated. When that's been done, one can also place stent, which is a metal scaffold which will keep the artery open and resolve that narrowing and hopefully remove or reduce the symptoms of chest pain and breathlessness. (本段内容选自2023年一位英国医生的采访,有删改调整。)

◎ **参考译文**:什么是冠状动脉成形术?冠状动脉成形术是一种技术,用于治疗冠状动脉的狭窄,这种狭窄通常会导致心绞痛、胸痛或呼吸困难。处理的方法是将一根小管子放入动脉。导丝向下穿过动脉,通过导丝,将球囊置于狭窄的区域并充气。完成之后,还可以放支架,支架是一种金属的架子,其会保持动脉畅通并解决狭窄的问题,并有望去除或减轻胸痛和呼吸困难的症状。

◎ **分析**:

1. "coronary angioplasty"译作"冠状动脉成形术",译员在初次完整表述之后可以将其简化为"冠脉成形";

2. "narrowing"译作"狭窄",容易理解,专业的表达是"stenosis";

3. "tube"指的是"catheter",意为"导管";

4. "wire"指的是"guidewire",意为"导丝";

5. "balloon"译作"球囊"。

Is coronary angioplasty a safe procedure? What are the risks? So the coronary angioplasty is an extremely safe procedure. It's generally carried out through a small artery in the wrist or the leg. And the small risks include damaging the artery, causing a small heart attack or occasionally causing a stroke. The risk of any of these complications runs at less than one in a hundred for a standard procedure, and in most cases, this can be carried out as a day case, with the patient being discharged home either the same day or overnight. So an extremely safe procedure.

◎ **参考译文**：冠状动脉成形术是一种安全的操作吗？有哪些风险？冠脉成形是一种特别安全的手术。它通常通过手腕或腿部的小动脉进行。一些小风险包括动脉损伤、引起轻微心脏病发作或偶尔导致卒中。任何这些并发症的发生风险不到百分之一，只要进行标准操作，而且在大多数病例中，这一操作可以作为日间手术进行，患者可以当天或过一夜就出院回家。所以是一个极安全的手术。

◎ **分析**：

1. 严格意义上说，"procedure"应被译作"操作"，但现在将其翻译为"手术"也不算错，不少专业人士会同时使用这两种表达，现在会议中"介入操作"与"介入手术"的界限越来越模糊；

2. "stroke"译作"卒中"，此处不应译作"中风"，中风是非专业人士的表达方式。当然在中医会议中，"中风"是中医学里的一个专业概念；

3. "day case"译作"日间手术"，译员如果对这一概念熟悉的话，后面的"with the patient being discharged home either the same day or overnight/患者可以当天或过一夜就出院回家"可以做到预测先说。

What is the difference between coronary angioplasty and bypass surgery? So the major difference between a coronary artery bypass operation and angioplasty is that the former is a surgical procedure where the patient is anesthetized, the heart is exposed, and an incision in the chest and the narrowings in the artery are bypassed using other blood vessels. This can either be a vein from the leg or can be an artery from inside the chest wall, and that's placed across the area of narrowing. A coronary angioplasty, in contrast, is a technique where the narrowing itself is dealt with a balloon or stent, and the narrowing is stretched open. And that's a much less invasive procedure, as mentioned, usually carried out in the arm or a leg, carrying a risk about one in a hundred, so a smaller procedure with a much more rapid recovery.

◎ **参考译文**：冠状动脉血管成形术和搭桥手术有什么区别？冠状动脉搭桥手术和血管成形术的主要区别在于，前者是一种外科手术，患者接受麻醉，心脏暴露，胸部做切口，动脉狭窄处用其他血管绕过。这要么可以是腿部的静脉，也可以是胸壁内的动脉，将其置于狭窄的区域。冠状动脉血管成形术，相比而言，对狭窄的处理是使用球囊或支架，并将狭窄处撑开。这是一种有创性小得多的手术，正如前面所提到的，通常在手臂或腿部进行，其风险约为百分之一，因此手术规模较小，恢复速度更快。

◎ **分析**：

1. "bypass surgery"为"旁路手术"，但更常见的说法是"搭桥手术"；

2. "So the major difference between a coronary artery bypass operation and angioplasty"译作"冠状动脉搭桥手术和血管成形术的主要区别在于"。前文表达非常明确，此处就是预测先说；

3. "stent"为"支架"，是介入操作中最基础的概念。

第五单元　心脏介入

　　Is coronary angioplasty a major surgical procedure? Coronary angioplasty is not a major surgical procedure. It's a minor interventional procedure, does not involve an incision, does not involve general anesthesia, does not involve a long period of recovery. So typically, one will recover within a few hours after the procedure, and will back up as normal within a few days. How many days should I rest after coronary angioplasty? So this largely depends on how complex the procedure is, but in a standard angioplasty procedure, it would rest for approximately 48 hours and mobilize normally following that. You can easily return to driving within a few days, and work within a few days.

　　◎ **参考译文**：冠状动脉成形术是一项大型外科操作吗？冠状动脉成形术不是一种大型外科手术。它是一种小型的介入操作，不涉及切口，不涉及全身麻醉，也不涉及长时间的恢复。因此在通常情况下，患者会在手术后几小时内恢复，并在几天内恢复正常。冠状动脉成形术后我应该休息几天？这在很大程度上取决于操作有多复杂，但在标准的血管成形术中，要休息大约48小时，这之后就可以正常活动了。患者可以在几天内轻松恢复驾驶，并在几天内进行工作。

　　◎ **分析**：

　　1. "general anesthesia" 译作 "全身麻醉"，更常用的说法是 "全麻"；

　　2. "mobilize" 有时在口译中表示 "动员"，但此处表示 "移动、活动"；

　　3. "You can easily return to driving"，此处灵活处理成 "患者可以在几天内轻松恢复驾驶"。

　　The best way to understand this is probably a clinical vignette. This will kind of put this into crystal clear focus on what I'm talking about. This is an actual patient of mine. He's a 55-year-old male. He was an avid runner who presented with a three month decline in exercise tolerance. He has a history of hyperlipidemia and was on a statin already. There is a strong family history of premature CAD. He had a pretty unremarkable exam. His ECG showed a left bundle, and he went for a SPECT scan. And you can see on the SPECT scan that there is pretty significant ischemia involving the infra lateral wall with preserved LVEF. This is what you want to see in the cath lab. This is an angiogram of the right coronary artery with a very discrete focal lesion involving the distal right coronary artery. This is something that anybody would treat without question and feel very good about that they've done a good job for this patient. So there's nothing controversial here, and there's nothing really to discuss. This would be pretty straightforward.（本段内容选自2020年一位美国医生的演讲，有删改调整。）

　　◎ **参考译文**：理解这一点的最佳的方法可能就是临床案例。这会使我所讲的内容愈加清晰。这是我的一位真实患者。55岁，男性。他热衷于跑步，三个月来运动耐量下降。他有高脂血症病史，并且已经在服用他汀类药物。其家族史中有很多早发性CAD。他的检查结果非常正常。他的心电图显示左束支，他做了SPECT扫描。可以在SPECT扫描中看到，有相当严重的缺血，涉及下侧壁，但LVEF保留。这就是大家希望在导管室看到的结果。这是右冠状动脉的血管造影，有一个非常不连续的局灶性病变，涉及远端右冠。这种情况下任何人都会毫无疑问地接受治疗，并且会为自己为这位患者所做的出色治疗感到非常高兴。这里没什么争议，也没什么可讨论的。这里很简单。

◎ **分析：**

1. "vignette"来源于法语，使用频率较低，此处可灵活处理为"临床病例"或"病例介绍"；

2. "He's a 55-year-old male"译作"55 岁，男性"，这样的表述比起直接译作"他是一位 55 岁的男性"更符合中文病例报告的语言习惯；

3. "He was an avid runner"经过词性转换，处理为"他热衷于跑步"，中文中倒不一定非要加上"之前"来反映时态，也不符合中文病例报告的习惯；

4. "left bundle"译作"左束支"，但此处是讲者省略的表达方式，完整的表达是"left bundle branch block, LBBB"，即"左束支传导阻滞"，译作左束支并不影响专业人士的理解，但听起来感觉差一些，如译员医学素养良好，此处可以补充译出；

5. "This is what you want to see in the cath lab"处理为"这就是大家希望在导管室看到的结果"。其中"cath lab"常规译作"导管室"，"you"可以灵活处理。

The more challenging situation would be as if the angiogram showed this. So more diffuse disease involving the ostium of the PDA, some diffuse disease involving one of the circumplex marginal branches. So we said that the patient had infra lateral ischemia. And when you have these borderline lesions, the ideal way to assess this in the cath lab is to do some sort of hemodynamic assessment with an FFR protocol or a resting grading protocol. And from this, we know that the this, the PDA, probably doesn't need to be fixed, whereas the circumflex should be fixed. And so you can feel very good that you've used evidence based medicine to manage this patient appropriately and manage their symptoms, and this is borne out in the FAME trial. I'm not going to go through all this in detail, but we know that from FAME and trials like FAME, that hemodynamic assessment of borderline lesions is superior to an angiographic assessment in terms of late events, and that PCI and hemodynamically significant lesions is superior to medical therapy when there is a hemodynamically significant lesion proven by pressure wire.

◎ **参考译文：** 更具挑战性的情况是，如果血管造影显示这种情况。PDA 开口处有更多弥漫性病变，部分弥漫性病变涉及回旋支边缘分支之一。我们说患者有下侧壁缺血。遇到这些临界病变时，在导管室评估的理想方法是用 FFR 方案或静息分级方案进行血流动力学评估。由此，我们知道，PDA 可能不需要处理，而回旋支应予处理。这是可以感觉非常好，因为我们已经在用循证医学对患者进行合适的管理了，并且控制了他们的症状，这在 FAME 试验中得到了证实。我就不过这些细节了，但是从 FAME 以及类 FAME 的试验当中我们知道，就晚期事件而言，PCI 对于血流动力学显著病变优于内科治疗，只要压力导丝证实存在血流动力学显著病变。

◎ **分析**：

1. "So more diffuse disease involving the ostium of the PDA"中"so"为部分英语讲者的口头禅，一般不必翻译，"PDA"直接跟读即可，"disease"可以译作"病变"，直接翻译为"疾病"的话，稍显突兀；

2. "borderline lesion"意为"临界病变"，指冠状动脉造影显示的冠状动脉病变的狭窄程度为40%~70%；

3. "fix"作为动词意思颇多，医学口译中译员也不时会遇到，可表示"固定""修复""解决"等，此处译作"处理"为佳；

4. "bear out"意为"证实、验证"。

But this is the angiogram that my patient has. So this is a patient that I took care of a few years ago who has a total occlusion of proximal right coronary artery with robust collaterals from the left system. And you know, this is where things kind of fall apart. I mean, what do we do with this patient? It kind of depends on which hospital you show up in terms of what the recommendations are. I mean, he doesn't really have a lot of left coronary disease. There's nothing to justify bypass surgery for him. He is truly symptomatic and doesn't have a lot of room for medication because his heart rate and blood pressure are already pretty low. So what do you do with him? And that's really what I want to talk about.

◎ **参考译文**：这是我的患者的血管造影。这是我几年前治疗的一位患者，他的右冠状动脉近端完全闭塞，但有稳定的侧支循环来自左冠脉系统。大家也知道，这就是事情出问题的地方。我的意思是，我们该怎么处理这个患者？这有点取决于你去哪家医院，要看医院给的建议是什么。我的意思是，他的左冠问题并不严重。没有任何理由为他做搭桥手术。他确实有症状，没有太多药物治疗的空间，因为他的心率和血压已经很低了。那么对他该怎么办呢？这才是我真正想谈的。

◎ **分析**：

1. "But this is the angiogram that my patient has. So this is a patient that I took care of a few years ago…"此段内容虽有调整，但尽量保留了讲者的语言风格，此处的"But"和"So"都是非常典型的无意义连接词，无须处理；

2. "he doesn't really have a lot of left coronary disease"处理为"他的左冠问题并不严重"，非常符合国内医生的表达，此处可以比较此句与"他的左冠状动脉疾病并不严重"之间的效果差异。

So CTOs are pretty common. The definition that we use for academic purposes is TIMI 0 flow for greater than three months on a coronary angiogram. We see this in up to a third of coronary angiograms done around the world. CTO PCI attempt rates have been low historically, and they continue to remain quite low. If you look at this box at the bottom, this sort of explains why the overall success rate of CTO PCI nationally is only around 59% and that compares with the 96% success rate if the artery still has some flow in it. And it comes at a price, the risk of complication is 1.6% versus 0.8% for an artery that's patent, so less likely to succeed, much higher risk of a complication, so not as appetizing a lesion to treat. But that doesn't mean that these people are not suffering from symptoms and don't have ischemia.

◎ **参考译文**：CTO 很常见。我们用于学术目的的定义是，TIMI 0 级血流，持续超过三个月，经冠状动脉造影判断。我们在多达三分之一的冠状动脉造影中都看到这种情况，全球都是如此。CTO PCI 的尝试率历来很低，而且现在仍然很低。你如果去看底下的这个框，这可以解释为什么全国 CTO PCI 的总体成功率仅是 59% 左右，而如果动脉中仍有血流，成功率就是 96%。这也是有代价的，并发症的风险是 1.6%，对比动脉通畅的风险是 0.8%，所以不大可能成功，而并发症的风险要高得多，所以这一病灶治疗起来没那么有吸引力。但这并不意味着这些人没有症状，也没有缺血。

◎ **分析**：

1. TIMI 是 Thrombolysis In Myocardial Infarction 的缩写，冠脉血流等级（TIMI 分级）是心脏病学中一个关键的评估工具，用于判断冠状动脉的血流状况。TIMI 分级系统分为 0 级到 3 级共四个等级。TIMI 0 级：无血流；TIMI 1 级：微弱血流；TIMI 2 级：部分血流；TIMI 3 级：完全血流。TIMI 分级系统提供了一个标准化的方法来评估和比较不同患者的血流状况；

2. "attempt rate" 译作"尝试率"，此种表达不多见；

3. "so not as appetizing a lesion to treat" 译作"所以这一病灶治疗起来没那么有吸引力"，"appetizing" 在这里是一个比喻用法，意指某些病变或病例对于医生来说不那么"诱人"或"有吸引力"，因为它们治疗起来风险较高且成功率较低。翻译为"所以这一病灶治疗起来没那么有吸引力"是合适的，它传达了原文的意思，即治疗这类病变的吸引力较低；

4. "suffer" 并未译出，减弱了语气。"suffer" 在医学语境中通常指的是患者经历症状或疾病的困扰。在翻译中，这个词应该被译出，以保持原文的语气和信息的完整性。例如，可以翻译为"但这并不意味着这些患者没有症状，也没有缺血的困扰"。

So the big barriers are obviously the lack of clinical evidence, the observational data that we have is just that it's observational, and it has its own inherent biases, and the randomized clinical trial data that we have today has been somewhat controversial and quite limited in terms of its implementation and how to interpret it. What we do know is that symptomatic relief is achievable in CTO PCI, we can improve LV function, we can expect better tolerance of a future acute coronary syndrome if that were to occur. And we also know that failed CTO PCI is associated with a higher future adverse cardiac event rate. The ongoing controversy really is about the relative value. It remains a ⅡA indication in AHA/ACC guidelines, and the biggest challenge here is the variable expertise. So, you know, look at a system like ours, where we have multiple community hospitals and a large referral center hospital. You know, we do a great job here of taking care of patients out in the community and identifying patients who need more advanced care and referring them to providers that have expertise.

◎ **参考译文**：因此，最大的障碍显然是缺乏临床证据，我们拥有的观察性数据只是观察性而已，它有其固有偏倚，而我们今天的随机临床试验数据在实施和解读方面存在一些争议，而且非常有局限性。我们确实知道的是，CTO PCI 可以缓解症状，我们可以改善左室功能，我们可以预期对未来急性冠状动脉综合征的耐受性会更好，如果出现这种情况的话。我们也知道，CTO PCI 失败与较高的未来不良心脏事件发生率相关。持续的争议实际上是在于相对值。它仍然是 AHA/ACC 指南中的 ⅡA 指征，这里最大的挑战是不同的专家意见。大家知道，看看我们这样的系统，我们有多家社区医院和一家大型转诊中心医院。大家也知道，我们在这里做得很好，照顾社区里的患者，确定需要更高级别诊疗的患者，并将他们转给有专业知识的医生。

◎ **分析**：

1. "bias" 译作"偏倚"，偏倚指的是由系统性而非随机性导致的测量值与真值的偏离，会削弱研究的真实性。所有的观察性研究都有其固有偏倚。此处常见的错误是下意识地译作"偏见"；

2. "interpret" 译作"解读"；

3. "we can improve LV function" 译作"我们可以改善左室功能"，优于"我们可以改善 LV 功能"；

4. "expertise" 可表示"专长""专业知识"以及"专家意见"；

5. "more advanced care" 译作"更高级别诊疗"，此处常见的错误是将"care"译作"护理"；

6. "providers" 此处处理为"医生"，要优于"提供者"，此处的 provider 指的是提供专业医疗服务的人员，译作"提供者/供应者"虽然准确，但不符合中文语境。此外注意以 er 结尾的名词可能是人也可能是机构，要根据具体语境带入。

And so we have a system in place, but that may not always be the case in outlying areas where there isn't a coordinate system to manage these patients, and that leads to variable care. Let's get into the nuts and bolts of some of the physiology. So we know that patients who have collateralization of the CTO artery are ischemic, and this is irrespective of the size and robustness of the collaterals. If you are able to cross the CTO and measure the FFR, it's always less than 0.8, which is what we think is significant. This chart shows that it doesn't matter how big the collaterals are, how robust the collaterals are. If you cross a CTO that's collateralized, it is going to have an ischemic FFR. And we already talked about how important FFR is in the assessment of borderline lesions.

◎ **参考译文**：我们是有一个体系，但情况可能并非如此，对于偏远地区，在那里没有一个协调的系统来管理这些患者，而这会导致不一致的诊疗。让我们来深入了解一些生理学的细节。我们知道，CTO 动脉侧支循环的患者是缺血的，而这与侧支循环的大小和强度无关。如果你能够穿过 CTO 并测量 FFR，它总是小于 0.8，我们认为这是有意义的。这张图显示，侧支循环有多大、侧支循环有多强都并不重要。如果你穿过有侧支循环的 CTO，它会出现缺血性 FFR。我们已经讲过 FFR 在评估临界病变方面有多重要。

◎ 分析：

1. "variable"有多重含义，此处处理为"不一致的"，同传时译员在未听到下文时，这样处理比较合适，优于"时好时坏的""可变的""多变的"等处理方式；

2. "collateralization"或"collateral circulation"意为"侧支循环"，指的是血管主干近侧分支和远侧分支之间形成血管网，在主干血管发生阻塞时，这一血管网能实现部分血流循环，以补充主干血供的不足，有时甚至可以完全代替，这就能保证组织的血供。

That what I'm saying here is that all CTOs, no matter how well collateralized they are, they're just ischemic. They're ischemic by the modern interpretation of what ischemia is and what would warrant treatment? You know, the ischemic burden that that would warrant PCI has been identified in historical literature, anything more than 10% ischemia on a SPECT scan is determined to be associated with adverse cardiac events and potentially benefit from revascularization. This is even seen in the COURAGE trial. So I mean, we think about the COURAGE trial as encouraging the medical management of CAD but in the nuclear sub study, the COURAGE trial, they did identify a subset of patients who did benefit from revascularization with PCI, and those are the patients that had at least 10% ischemia on a SPECT scan. So based on some of this historic data, we use a cutoff, it's a little arbitrary, but a cut off of around 12.5 percent on a nuclear study of myocardial ischemia, where we think patients would have some clinical benefit from CTO PCI.

◎ 参考译文：我在这里要说的是，所有的 CTO，无论其侧支循环有多好，都是缺血的。根据现代对缺血的解释，它们是缺血性的，那什么情况需要治疗？大家知道，需要进行 PCI 的缺血负荷已在过去的文献中得到确认，SPECT 扫描中任何超过 10% 的缺血都被认为与不良心脏事件有关，并可能从血运重建中获益。这甚至在 COURAGE 试验中也能看到。所以我的意思是，我们认为 COURAGE 试验鼓励对 CAD 进行内科管理，但在核医学亚组研究中，COURAGE 试验，他们确实确定了一个患者亚组，确实从 PCI 血运重建中获益，这些患者在 SPECT 扫描中至少有 10% 的缺血。因此，根据一些历史数据，我们设定了一个截止值，有些随意，但截止值大约为 12.5%，在对心肌缺血的核医学研究中，我们认为患者会从 CTO PCI 中收获一些临床获益。

◎ 分析：

1. "ischemic burden"译作"缺血负荷"；

2. "anything more than 10% ischemia on a SPECT scan is determined to be associated with adverse cardiac events"译作"SPECT 扫描中任何超过 10% 的缺血都被认为与不良心

脏事件有关",此处的"被"字翻译腔过重,"SPECT扫描中任何超过10%的缺血都确定与不良心脏事件相关"的处理更好些;

3. "nuclear"处理为"核医学",在此补充"医学"二字更合适些。

This is also borne out in some level in larger trials, like the SYNTAX trial. There's a CTO subset analysis of the SYNTAX trial where they looked at the impact of incomplete revascularization on four-year event rates, and they show an association between incomplete revascularization on four-year mortality, revascularization need and future MACE. And the biggest predictor of incomplete revascularization and STNTAX was CTO. And you can see that in the PCI arm, nearly half of patients with CTO ended up with incomplete revascularization whereas about a third in the CABG arm. So even in the CABG arm, CTO patients were not being revascularized. One thing that needs to be added is that the CTO PCI attempt rate and SYNTAX is pretty low by modern standards, but it just shows how important this concept of incomplete revascularization is on long term outcomes.

◎ **参考译文**:这也在某种程度上得到了更大规模试验的证实,像SYNTAX试验。SYNTAX试验中有一项CTO亚组分析,他们研究了不完全血运重建对四年事件发生率的影响,结果显示不完全血运重建与四年死亡率、血运重建需求和未来MACE之间存在关联。不完全血运重建和SYNTAX的最大预测因素是CTO。可以看到,在PCI组中,近一半的CTO患者最终血运重建不完全,而在CABG组中,这一比例约为三分之一。因此,即使在CABG组中,CTO患者也没有血运重建。需要补充的一点是,CTO PCI尝试率和SYNTAX相当低,按照现代标准是如此,但这只显示了不完全血运重建这一概念对长期结果有多重要。

◎ **分析**:

1. 国外医学试验一般会从试验全名中挑选部分字母,组成一个全大写字母的首字母缩略词,以此来命名试验,例如本篇中提到的"COURAGE"和"SYNTAX"即是如此,译员遇到时应及时分辨,跟读即可,切记不可直接意译。例如"COURAGE"试验的全称为"the Clinical Outcomes Utilizing Revascularization and Aggressive Drug Evaluation trial",译员跟读即可,切记不可译作"勇气"试验,而"SYNTAX"试验的全称为"the Synergy between PCI with Taxus and Cardiac Surgery trial",听到"SYNTAX"时,译员也不可将其译作"语法/句法"试验,否则只会让听众不知所云;

2. "CABG"有些国外讲者的发音是"cabbage",此时译员应结合上下文内容以及幻灯片内容,作出及时准确判断,切记不可仅根据听到的信息强行翻译;

3. "arm"意为"组",同"group",尽量译作"组",近些年有些医生直接译作"臂",例如"单臂研究""臂中",这是语言入侵现象,如同近些年来其他一些毫无中文美感且奇葩的"硬核翻译"一样,口译时译员应尽量予以纠正。

Now this is also seen prospectively, so this is data from the SCAR registry. So in

Sweden, anybody who has a cardiac catheterization in Sweden is followed in this database, and you can see the long term outcomes of patients who present for catheterization for any indication. So you look at the six year outcome data and how much higher the cumulative mortalities in patients who had a CTO at the time with their index coronary angiogram. And you can also see on the panel on the right that there is a clinical benefit of successfully opening the chronic total occlusion, although the attempt rates were pretty low and the success rates were pretty low in the SCAR registry, but there is a beneficial, beneficial impact, and it seemed to be strongest among younger patients who presented with an acute coronary syndrome. And that sort of supports this prospective data, which looks at patients who presented with STEMI and had a concomitant CTO in a non, you know, in a non-infarct artery, you look at the dramatic impact that having a CTO at the time of STEMI has, both acutely and in the long term, on mortality. So it's not a benign entity to have the CTO. Now, whether or not treating this CTO is going to improve that outcome is obviously debatable, but we're identifying a patient who's at a much higher risk of an event in the future.

◎ **参考译文**：前瞻性研究中也可看到，这是来自 SCAR 登记的数据。在瑞典，任何接受过心脏介入的人都会放在这个数据库中，大家可以看到患者的长期结果，这些患者因为各种指征而进行介入。看看六年结果的数据，以及当时有 CTO 且进行冠脉造影患者的累积死亡率有多高。还可以在右侧看到，成功打开慢性完全闭塞具有临床获益，尽管 SCAR 登记的尝试率很低，成功率也很低，但确实存在获益的影响，而且似乎在急性冠状动脉综合征的年轻患者中最为明显。这在某种程度上支持了这一前瞻性数据，该数据研究了患有 STEMI 且在非梗塞动脉中同时有 CTO 的患者，可以看到在 STEMI 时患有 CTO 对死亡率的显著影响，无论是急性影响还是长期影响。因此，患有 CTO 并非良性。现在，治疗 CTO 是否会改善这一结果显然是有争议的，但我们正在识别未来发生事件风险更高的患者。

◎ **分析**：

1. "see the long term outcomes of patients who present for catheterization for any indication."按照顺句驱动的方式被处理为"可以看到患者的长期结果，这些患者因为各种指征而进行介入"。其中"catheterization"被处理为"介入"，而非"导管插入术"，更符合中文的语言表达习惯；

2. "STEMI"意为"ST 段抬高型心肌梗死"，口译时译员无须将其展开翻译，跟读即可。

二、中译英

血栓栓塞，尤其是脑卒中，是房颤患者最常见的并发症。口服抗凝药物治疗是房颤患者的基础治疗策略，但抗凝治疗在降低栓塞风险的同时也会带来出血风险的升高。大规模真实世界研究显示，90%以上的心源性栓子来自左心耳，通过左心耳封堵来预防脑卒中的发生有极大的获益。我国为房颤大国，左心耳封堵的应用和推广可为我国房颤患者带来极大获益。（本段内容选自2023年一位国内医生的采访，有删改调整。）

◎ **参考译文**：Thromboembolism, especially stroke, is the most common complication in patients with atrial fibrillation. Oral anticoagulant therapy, for patients with atrial fibrillation, is the basic treatment strategy, but anticoagulant therapy reduces the risk of embolism while also increasing the risk of bleeding. Large-scale real-world studies have shown that more than 90% of cardiogenic emboli come from the left atrial appendage, and there is great benefit in preventing stroke by occluding the left atrial appendage. As a country with a high incidence of atrial fibrillation, the application and promotion of left atrial appendage occlusion can bring great benefits to patients with atrial fibrillation in our country.

◎ **分析**：

1. "房颤"指"心房颤动"，国内绝大多数医生都选择用其简称，可被译作"atrial fibrillation"，英文中有时也简称为A-Fib；

2. "口服抗凝药物治疗是房颤患者的基础治疗策略"按照顺句驱动的方法可处理为"Oral anticoagulant therapy, for patients with atrial fibrillation, is the basic treatment strategy"，"治疗策略"译作"treatment strategy"；

3. "真实世界研究"译作"Real world study"，这一概念在最近几年越来越热门。

心房颤动，简称房颤，是一种严重的慢性疾病，房颤患者的卒中风险升高，生活质量下降，心衰发生率，甚至死亡率均会增加。其中，卒中是房颤患者最为重要的并发症。研究显示，90%以上的非瓣膜性房颤脑卒中是由左心耳内的血栓脱落造成的。血栓脱落后随血液进入脑部导致患者发生卒中。LAAC是将左心耳进行封堵的一种非常好的手术方式，这样左心耳就不会形成血栓，即使形成了血栓也不会掉出来。对于LAAC，目前已经进行了很多项的探究，随着循证证据的累积，其安全性和有效性已得到证实，适应证也逐渐增宽。

◎ **参考译文**：Atrial fibrillation, abbreviated as AF, is a serious chronic disease. Patients with AF have an increased risk of stroke, decreased quality of life, increased incidence of heart failure, and even increased mortality. Among them, stroke is the most important complication for patients with AF. Studies have shown that more than 90% of non-valvular atrial fibrillation strokes are caused by the detachment of blood clots in the left atrial appendage. After the blood clot detaches, it enters the brain with the blood and causes a stroke in the patient. LAAC is a very good surgical method to block the left atrial appendage, so that the left atrial appendage will not form a blood clot, and even if a blood clot is formed, it will not fall out. Many studies have been conducted on LAAC. With the accumulation of evidence-based evidence, its safety and effectiveness have been confirmed, and its indications have gradually expanded.

◎ 分析：

1. 房颤译作 atrial fibrillation，其英文简写并不单一，有 AF、Afib 及 A-fib 等；

2. "卒中"的正确中文读音为"促众"（音），但不少医生将其读为"族忠"（音），口译时译员了解即可。

总体而言，目前 LAAC 主要用于以下几类人群：有高出血风险、高卒中风险的患者；有抗凝药物禁忌证或不能长期使用的患者；虽然进行了最佳抗凝药物治疗，但仍发生栓塞事件的患者；因发生过出血事件而不能使用抗凝药物的患者；因生活习惯、工作性质或认知障碍不适合进行长期抗凝治疗的患者；房颤消融产生左心耳电隔离的患者。这些患者进行 LAAC 后，可以减低抗凝药物的剂量，甚至不用抗凝药物，药物不良反应的发生率降低，生活质量也相应提高。

◎ 参考译文：In general, LAAC is currently mainly used in the following populations: patients with high risk of bleeding and stroke; patients with contraindications to anticoagulants or patients who cannot use them for a long time; patients who still have embolic events despite optimal anticoagulant treatment; patients who cannot use anticoagulants because of previous bleeding events; patients who are not suitable for long-term anticoagulant treatment due to lifestyle, work nature or cognitive impairment; patients with left atrial appendage electrical isolation caused by atrial fibrillation ablation. After LAAC, these patients can reduce the dose of anticoagulants or even not use anticoagulants, reduce the incidence of adverse drug reactions, and improve their quality of life accordingly.

◎ 分析：

1. "患者人群"译作"patient population"，医学口译中"人群"译作"population"；

2. "认知障碍"译作"cognitive impairment"；

3. "药物不良反应的发生率降低，生活质量也相应提高"中的"药物不良反应的发生率降低"译作"reduce the incidence of adverse drug reactions"是准确的，这里常将"reduce"处理为"降低"而非"减少"。"生活质量也相应提高"译作"and improve their quality of life accordingly"，这里的"accordingly"表明了生活质量的提高是与药物不良反应减少相一致的。

自 2002 年 PILOT 研究首例器械植入至今，左心耳封堵已经历了 20 多年的循证发展，在国内也有 10 年的使用经验。自 2014 年，LAAC 在国内进入临床应用开始，最近几年 LAAC 经历了高速发展。虽然 LAAC 在我国起步较晚，但有相当多的相关研究和探索。最初我们探索这项术式的可行性、安全性及有效性，尤其是短期，并进行了相关研究。之前在国际上有两个里程碑式的研究——PROTECT-AF 和 PREVAIL 随机对照试验。这两项研究均显示，与传统口服抗凝药物华法林相比，W 封堵器可持续降低患者的心脑血管事件发生率，甚至在出血风险方面也低于华法林，证实了 LAAC 的安全性和有效性。

◎ **参考译文**：Since the first device implantation in the PILOT study in 2002, left atrial appendage occlusion has undergone more than 20 years of evidence-based development, and has 10 years of experience in use in China. Since LAAC entered clinical application in China in 2014, LAAC has experienced rapid development in recent years. Although LAAC started late in our country, there have been quite a lot of related research and exploration. Initially, we explored the feasibility, safety and effectiveness of this procedure, especially in the short term, and conducted relevant research. Previously, there were two landmark studies internationally—the PROTECT-AF and PREVAIL randomized controlled trials. Both studies showed that compared with the traditional oral anticoagulant warfarin, the W occluder can sustainably reduce the incidence of cardiovascular and cerebrovascular events in patients, and even has a lower risk of bleeding than warfarin, confirming the safety and effectiveness of LAAC.

◎ **分析**：

1. "研究"此处译作"study"，医学口译中，涉及实验室的研究更多译作"research"，其他类的可译作"study"，"trial"意为"试验"；

2. 在此主题的医学口译实践中，中文发言中经常会夹杂大量英文，译员需要在同传时能够及时识别，缩短 EVS，快速跟读出相应内容；

3. "封堵器"可用"occluder"来表达。

由于传统口服抗凝药物华法林可以与多种药物/食物产生相互作用，在使用时需要定期查血，因此会降低患者的用药依从性。新型口服抗凝药物 NOACs 的出现解决了这些问题，但仍有出血的风险。在 NOACs 时代，LAAC 还有优势吗？PRAGUE-17 多中心、随机、非劣效性试验，在非瓣膜性房颤患者中比较了 LAAC 与 NOACs 在预防卒中方面的安全性和有效性。3.5 年的随访显示，在高卒中、高出血风险的患者中，LAAC 在预防房颤相关心血管、神经系统和出血事件方面不劣于 NOACs。

◎ **参考译文**：Since the traditional oral anticoagulant warfarin can interact with a variety of drugs/foods, regular blood tests are required when using it, which will reduce patients' medication compliance. The emergence of new oral anticoagulants, NOACs, has solved these problems, but there is still a risk of bleeding. In the era of NOACs, does LAAC still have advantages? The PRAGUE-17 multicenter, randomized, non-inferiority trial compared the safety and effectiveness of LAAC and NOACs in preventing stroke in patients with non-valvular atrial fibrillation. 3.5 years of follow-up showed that in patients with high stroke and high bleeding risk, LAAC, in terms of preventing atrial fibrillation-related cardiovascular, neurological, and bleeding events, is not inferior to NOACs.

◎ **分析**：

1. "查血"此处译作"blood tests"，不少国外讲者也会使用"blood works"的表达；

2. "NOAC"的读音同"no arc"，全称是"novel oral anticoagulants"，而非"new oral

anticoagulants";

3."LAAC 在预防房颤相关心血管、神经系统和出血事件方面不劣于 NOACs",按照顺句驱动的方法,处理为了"LAAC, in terms of preventing atrial fibrillation-related cardiovascular, neurological, and bleeding events, is not inferior to NOACs."这样的处理虽然不是最佳,但能极大地减轻译员的同传压力。

此外,国内相关试验也证实了 LAAC 的安全性和有效性均较好。虽然大多为观察性研究,但国内患者数量大,能反映中国真实的临床情况。在封堵器类型方面,目前我国已经有了十多种不同类型的封堵器。多数器械的安全性和有效性都得到了一定的验证,长期随访结果也在积累当中。在术式探索方面,我们不但探索了单纯的左心耳封堵术,还探索了房颤消融联合左心耳封堵一站式手术,相关研究也提示患者预后较好。其次,包括我们科室在内的多个中心都在探索 LAAC 的简化术式,这种术式不需要进行全身麻醉和食管超声,仅在局麻下便可进行。

◎ 参考译文:In addition, relevant domestic trials have also confirmed that LAAC is safe and effective. Although most of them are observational studies, the number of domestic patients is large, which can reflect the real clinical situation in China. In terms of occluder types, there are currently more than ten different types of occluders in our country. The safety and effectiveness of most devices have been verified to a certain extent, and long-term follow-up results are also being accumulated. In terms of surgical exploration, we have not only explored simple left atrial appendage occlusion, but also explored a one-stop surgery of atrial fibrillation ablation combined with left atrial appendage occlusion. Related studies also suggest that patients have a good prognosis. Secondly, many centers, including our department, are exploring simplified LAAC procedures, which do not require general anesthesia and esophageal ultrasound, and can be performed only under local anesthesia.

◎ 分析:

1."一站式手术"译作"one-stop surgery",同样"一站式服务"译作"one-stop service";

2."简化术式"译作"simplified procedures","改良术式"译作"modified procedures";

3."食管超声"此处译作"esophageal ultrasound",但并非最佳,在心脏介入主题中,应译为"transesophageal Echocardiography"或可简化为"TEE",两者均可为听众所接受。

此外,其他团队和中心也进行了一些相关的探索,包括术中进行影像学指导是否对患者有益?是否可以做到零射线?这些研究对于稳步推动临床实践都是非常有益的尝试。LAAC 在临床上的应用并非一蹴而就,不能着急,应该稳步推进。总体而言,我们目前的道路正确,很多研究正在进行中。对于好的方法、术式及器械,我们都应该持续推进。目前,我们主要面临着患者、医生和我们中国人群自己数据的三方面问题。患者方面,目前仍有很多患者并不知晓 LAAC 术式。由于 LAAC 术式的安全性和有效性已经得到了验证,因此未来还需要进一步做好患者宣教工作。首先,让患者了解房颤的卒中风险和危害。

◎ **参考译文**:In addition, other teams and centers have also conducted some related explorations, including whether imaging guidance during surgery is beneficial to patients? Is it possible to achieve zero radiation? These studies are very useful attempts to steadily promote clinical practice. The clinical application of LAAC is not achieved overnight, so we should not be impatient and should advance steadily. Overall, we are on the right path and many studies are ongoing. We should continue to advance good methods, procedures and equipment. At present, we are mainly facing three problems: patients, doctors and our own data of the Chinese population. On the patient side, there are still many patients who are not aware of the LAAC procedure. Since the safety and effectiveness of the LAAC procedure have been verified, further patient education will be needed in the future. First of all, let patients understand the stroke risks and hazards of atrial fibrillation.

◎ **分析**:
1. "零射线"此处其实指代的是"零辐射",所以处理为"zero radiation";
2. "一蹴而就"有"轻而易举、一次成功"之意,此处译作"overnight",译员如果临时反应不过来,也可将其简单处理为"is not easy",同传时听众也可接受;
3. "危害"一般处理为"hazard"。

其次,使患者明确了解传统口服抗凝药物和NOACs均可降低房颤患者的卒中风险,NOACs更优一些,但患者的出血风险和药物不良反应也有不少。而LAAC既可降低患者的卒中风险,又可降低出血和药物不良反应风险。适宜的患者可以考虑选择LAAC。从医生角度而言,目前仅心内科医生和房颤专业医生比较了解LAAC这一术式,其他医生可能并不十分了解。因此,我们需要对医生进行培训,多加交流,让更多的医护人员了解LAAC这一术式及其价值。对于LAAC相关人员,应该对这项技术本身、相关器械、心脏结构、影像知识等进行培训。进行LAAC操作时,一步一个脚印,掌握好手术指证,规范操作,提高成功率,降低并发症的发生。这样就能使得LAAC有良性、规范发展,从而使更多患者获益。

◎ **参考译文**:Secondly, patients should be made aware that both traditional oral anticoagulants and NOACs can reduce the risk of stroke in patients with atrial fibrillation. NOACs are better, but patients also have a lot of bleeding risks and adverse drug reactions. LAAC can reduce the risk of stroke in patients, as well as the risk of bleeding and adverse drug reactions. Suitable patients can consider choosing LAAC. From a doctor's perspective, only cardiologists and doctors specializing in atrial fibrillation are relatively familiar with the LAAC procedure, and other doctors may not be very familiar with it. Therefore, we need to train doctors and communicate more so that more medical staff can understand the LAAC procedure and its value. For LAAC-related personnel, training should be provided on the technology itself, related equipment, heart structure, imaging knowledge, etc. When performing LAAC operations, take one step at a time, master the surgical indications, standardize the operation, improve the success rate, and reduce complications. This will enable LAAC to develop in a benign and standardized manner, so that more patients can benefit.

◎ **分析**：

1. "适宜的患者"译作"suitable patients"，其实"appropriate"一词在此处更合适些；
2. "一步一个脚印"相类似的表达可以直译；
3. "降低并发症的发生"，此类表达中的"发生""情况""局面"等，可以不必译出。

除此之外，我们还应该有我们中国人群自己的数据和高质量的研究。对国产封堵器设计、实施一系列研究，尤其是RCT研究，即随机、多中心试验。在指南中这类研究的推荐级别更高，更有利于规范推动LAAC的发展。此外，我们还应探究一些更加简便的术式，探究相关新器械的可行性、安全性和长期结局。对于一站式手术，我们也进行了很多年的探索。最开始的时候，对进行一站式手术，我们也有诸多顾虑。因为我们长期做房颤的导管消融，包括射频消融、冷冻消融等。之后，随着LAAC的出现，这两种术式我们都掌握得比较好了。由于这两种术式都需要静脉穿刺、房间隔穿刺，术中也都会用到一些鞘管、导管。于是我们就考虑一次进行这两种术式，这样既可以减少耗材应用，也可以减低患者的痛苦，还可以降低总费用。

◎ **参考译文**：In addition, we should also have our own data and high-quality research of the Chinese population. A series of studies have been designed and implemented on domestic occluders, especially RCT studies, i.e. randomized, multicenter trials. In the guidelines, such studies have a higher recommendation level and are more conducive to standardizing and promoting the development of LAAC. In addition, we should also explore some simpler procedures and explore the feasibility, safety and long-term outcomes of related new devices. We have also explored one-stop surgery for many years. At the very beginning, we also had many concerns about performing one-stop surgery. Because we have been doing catheter ablation for atrial fibrillation for a long time, including radiofrequency ablation, cryoablation, etc. Later, with the emergence of LAAC, we have mastered these two procedures better. Since both procedures require venous puncture and atrial septal puncture, some sheaths and catheters will be used during the operation. So we considered performing these two procedures at one time, which can not only reduce the use of consumables, but also reduce the pain of patients and reduce the total cost.

◎ **分析**：

1. "冷冻消融"译作"cryoablation"；
2. "射频消融"译作"radiofrequency ablation"，这是心脏电生理学中常用的术语。
3. "耗材"此处译作"consumables"，国外讲者有时也会用"supplies"表示耗材。

第五单元 心脏介入

之后我们进行的相关研究也证实了一站式手术的安全性和有效性。同时，我们还在不同患者中进行研究。例如脑梗后患者，这类患者多有跛行，精神状态也欠佳，他们是否可以进行一站式手术？之后我们研究结果证实，脑梗后患者进行一站式手术的结果较非脑梗后患者更好，患者的获益更多。目前相关研究也已发表，并得到了广大同道的认可。此外，我们还对心衰、肥厚型心肌病等患者进行了探究，相关结果也很好。截至目前，我们已经进行了超过千例的一站式手术，并对前期的 900 例患者进行了总结，并在去年进行了发表。

◎ **参考译文**：The related studies we conducted later also confirmed the safety and effectiveness of one-stop surgery. At the same time, we also conducted studies on different patients. For example, patients after cerebral infarction, most of these patients have claudication and poor mental state. Can they undergo one-stop surgery? Later, our research results confirmed that the results of one-stop surgery for patients after cerebral infarction are better than those for patients without cerebral infarction, and patients benefit more. At present, relevant studies have also been published and recognized by the majority of colleagues. In addition, we have also explored patients with heart failure, hypertrophic cardiomyopathy, etc., and the relevant results are also very good. So far, we have performed more than a thousand one-stop surgeries, and summarized the results of 900 patients in the early stage and published them last year.

◎ **分析**：

1. "跛行"最好译作"claudication"，而不要处理为"limp"或"cripple"，后两者较口语化；

2. "精神状态也欠佳"译作"poor mental state"，医学口译中，"poor"经常用来表达"不佳"或"欠佳"之意。

研究结果显示，一站式手术可使预期栓塞事件发生率降低 76%，出血事件发生率降低 80%，且并发症较少。同时研究也证实了大部分手术患者可以停用抗凝药物，证实了一站式手术的长期安全性和有效性。未来我们应该进一步推广这一术式，从而使更多患者获益。与此同时，我们还进行了其他研究，包括围手术期抗凝药物的使用，6 个月之后对一级预防的患者是否还应该使用阿司匹林等。目前，这些研究正在进行中，期待未来可以为临床实践提供一定的借鉴。

◎ **参考译文**：The results of the study showed that one-stop surgery can reduce the expected incidence of embolic events by 76%, the incidence of bleeding events by 80%, and there are fewer complications. At the same time, the study also confirmed that most surgical patients can stop taking anticoagulants, confirming the long-term safety and effectiveness of one-stop surgery. In the future, we should further promote this procedure so that more patients can benefit. At the same time, we have also conducted other studies, including the use of perioperative anticoagulants, whether aspirin should still be used for primary prevention patients after 6 months, etc. At present, these studies are in progress, and we hope that they can provide some reference for clinical practice in the future.

◎ 分析：

1. "围手术期"译作"perioperative"，指术前、术中及术后三个阶段，这是一个十多年前从国外引入的概念，相对于以往外科更加注重手术而相对忽视术前准备和术后康复及管理的情况，这一概念更注重手术患者在治疗过程中的全程管理，而这一概念也逐渐从外科推广到涉及介入操作的其他专科；

2. "一级预防"译作"primary prevention"，指在问题出现前采取措施，防止疾病或伤害的出现，从而减少人群的患病或受伤的风险。

第四节 补充练习

一、中译英

心脏电生理检查使用数根带电极的心导管，置入右心房及右心室的不同部位，冠状静脉窦内（相当于左心室后壁），以及接触房室束，其中一根置于右心房或右心室作临时起搏之用。同步记录体表、右心房上部和下部、右心室流入道或心尖部或流出道的心电图，以及房室束电图。然后按不同的程序以电刺激起搏心脏，再作记录。本检查有助于了解窦房结功能、房室传导功能、旁道传导束的定位、室上性和室性心动过速的发病机制和病灶的定位、预测或评价药物或电起搏治疗的疗效。可为消融、手术切除异常病灶或切断异常折返通道提供参考，成为心律失常患者消融、植入电子装置或外科手术治疗前必须施行的检查。

PTCA 为在瑞士工作的德国医生 Gruentzig 于 1977 年率先创立的首个介入治疗冠心病的方法。本法用带球囊的导管置入狭窄的冠状动脉处向球囊注入含对比剂的液体，使球囊扩张撑开狭窄部位而使血流重建。至 1992 年，美国施行此手术的例数已超过外科冠状动脉旁路移植术。1997 年国内 PTCA 例数已达到 8725 例，为此前 12 年的总和，成功率达到 95.9%。PTCA 适应证从单支血管病变引起的稳定型心绞痛发展到治疗多支病变、急性心肌梗死（直接 PTCA 治疗）和慢性完全闭塞性病变（CTO）。由于 PTCA 不能有效清除血管内的粥样物质，手术本身足以损伤血管内膜和中膜，再狭窄的发生率较高，尤其术后血管弹性回缩、内膜撕裂引起的急性闭塞，后果严重。为解决这些问题，应用过激光成形术、超声成形术、腔内斑块旋切术、斑块旋磨术、切割球囊术、血栓抽吸术等，但效果仍不尽如人意。1992 年中国引入裸金属支架（BMS）置入术，在 PTCA 后将支架置入已被扩张的冠状动脉腔狭窄部位，防止血管的回缩和形成夹层，21 世纪初，BMS 的置入率达到 80.6%，但因仍有 20%~30% 的支架内狭窄率，现已被药物洗脱支架（DES）所取代。2002 年我国与国外几乎同步应用雷帕霉素或紫杉醇涂层的 DES。

这些药物可延迟支架的内皮化，配合术后用双联抗血小板药物至少1年，虽然1年后仍可能有支架内血栓形成，但已使支架内狭窄率降至5%～10%。近年这种支架得到广泛应用，占到置入支架总数的95%以上，其中中国产品占到70%以上。新一代的支架是既有药物涂层又能完全降解的生物可降解支架(BVS)，此种支架在完成机械性支撑血管防止其回缩后，逐渐自行降解而代谢掉，血管内不残留异物，其再狭窄率将会更低，前景乐观。由于冠心病介入治疗早已不单是经皮冠状动脉腔内成形术，故现已统称为经皮冠状动脉介入治疗(PCI)。21世纪以来，我国冠心病介入治疗例数每年以20%～40%的速度增加，2009年例数已超过日本和其他欧洲国家，2013年例数已近45万，仅次于美国，居世界第二位。

◎ **参考译文**：Cardiac electrophysiology examination uses several cardiac catheters with electrodes, which are placed in different parts of the right atrium and right ventricle, in the coronary sinus (equivalent to the posterior wall of the left ventricle), and in contact with the atrioventricular bundle. One of them is placed in the right atrium or right ventricle for temporary pacing. The electrocardiogram of the body surface, the upper and lower parts of the right atrium, the inflow tract or apex or outflow tract of the right ventricle, and the atrioventricular bundle electrogram are recorded simultaneously. Then the heart is paced with electrical stimulation according to different procedures, and then recorded again. This examination helps to understand the function of the sinus node, the atrioventricular conduction function, the location of the bypass conduction bundle, the pathogenesis of supraventricular and ventricular tachycardia and the location of the lesions, and predict or evaluate the efficacy of drug or electrical pacing therapy. It can provide a reference for ablation or surgical removal of abnormal lesions or cutting off abnormal reentry channels, and become a necessary examination for patients with arrhythmias before ablation, implantation of electronic devices or surgical treatment.

PTCA is the first interventional treatment for coronary heart disease pioneered by German doctor Gruentzig working in Switzerland in 1977. This method uses a balloon-carrying catheter to be inserted into the narrowed coronary artery and a liquid containing a contrast agent is injected into the balloon, causing the balloon to expand and open the narrowed area to restore blood flow. By 1992, the number of cases of this operation in the United States had exceeded that of surgical coronary artery bypass grafting. In 1997, the number of PTCA cases in China reached 8,725, which was the sum of the previous 12 years, with a success rate of 95.9%. The indications for PTCA have evolved from stable angina pectoris caused by single-vessel lesions to the treatment of multiple-vessel lesions, acute myocardial infarction (direct PTCA treatment) and chronic total occlusion (CTO). Since PTCA cannot effectively remove atherosclerotic material in the blood vessels, the operation itself is enough to damage the vascular intima and media, and the incidence of restenosis is high, especially acute occlusion caused by postoperative vascular elastic retraction and intimal tearing, which has serious consequences. To solve these problems, laser angioplasty, ultrasound angioplasty, intraluminal plaque atherectomy, plaque atherectomy, cutting balloon surgery, thrombus aspiration, etc. have been used, but the effect is still unsatisfactory. In 1992, China introduced the bare metal stent (BMS) implantation. After PTCA, the stent was placed in the narrowed part of the dilated coronary artery cavity to prevent the retraction of the blood vessel and the formation of dissection. At the beginning of the 21st century, the implantation rate of BMS reached 80.6%, but because there was still a 20% to 30% in-stent stenosis rate, it has now been replaced by drug-eluting stents (DES). In 2002, my country and foreign countries almost simultaneously applied DES coated with rapamycin or paclitaxel. These drugs can delay the endothelialization of the stent. Combined with the use of dual antiplatelet drugs for at least 1 year after surgery, although in-stent thrombosis may still occur after 1 year, the in-stent stenosis rate has been reduced to 5% to 10%. In recent years, this type of stent has been widely used, accounting for more than 95% of the total number of implanted stents, and Chinese products account for more than 70%. The new generation of stents is a biodegradable stent (BVS) that is both drug-coated and fully degradable. After completing the mechanical support of the blood vessel to prevent it from retracting, this stent gradually degrades and metabolizes by itself, leaving no foreign matter in the blood vessel. The restenosis rate will be lower, and the prospect is optimistic. Since coronary intervention is no longer just percutaneous coronary angioplasty, it is now generally referred to as percutaneous coronary intervention (PCI). Since the 21st century, the number of coronary interventions in my country has increased by 20% to 40% each year. Since 2009, the number of cases has exceeded that of Japan and other European countries. In 2013, the number of cases was nearly 450,000, second only to the United States, ranking second in the world.

二、英译中

Invasive cardiac interventions can reduce mortality and morbidity in selected patients with acute coronary syndromes, severe valvular disease, heart failure, and ventricular arrhythmias. However, randomized trials demonstrating improved cardiac outcomes have excluded patients with advanced malignancies, such as advanced solid organ cancers receiving ongoing treatment and incurable hematologic neoplasms with guarded prognosis. There is a paucity of direct clinical trial evidence to inform the risks and benefits of invasive cardiovascular interventions in these individuals.

In parallel with various seminal cardiovascular trials, there have been paradigm-changing developments in cancer therapies, including targeted biologic therapies and immunologic treatments. These have led to important improvements in survival in many patients with advanced cancers. As targeted cancer therapies continue to evolve, event-free and overall survival has increased, placing individuals at increased risk of experiencing cancer therapy-related cardiovascular toxicity and also unrelated adverse cardiovascular outcomes as competing risks. Health care providers have been reluctant to refer patients with advanced cancer for invasive cardiac procedures because of the likelihood of succumbing to death from cancer before any benefit from the invasive cardiac intervention can be realized. However, longer life expectancy among many patients challenges this notion.

Given the limited clinical trial data on invasive cardiac interventions in patients with advanced cancer, an evidence-based approach to decision making in these individuals requires an understanding of the patient's expected cancer-specific survival. If the anticipated survival exceeds the length of time needed to derive benefit from an invasive cardiac intervention, then one might extrapolate that an individual is likely to benefit from the cardiac intervention. Our aim is to summarize the current data to guide decision making in patients with common metastatic cancers or malignancies with poor prognosis eligible for cancer-specific treatments (referred to as advanced cancer) who also have severe cardiovascular disease. To achieve this aim, we describe the evidence supporting invasive cardiac interventions in the general population, and we integrate the literature that exists for these interventions in cancer populations. A key consideration in patients with advanced cancer is the competing risk of cancer death, which may influence the patient's likelihood of benefitting from an invasive cardiac intervention. Thus, we describe the survival expectations for several of the most common cancers. We conclude by describing a conceptual framework that might be applied for cardiac decision making in this population. This framework incorporates cancer-related factors such as the need for uninterrupted cancer treatment; the risk of intervention-related complications in this population; and quality of life, which is magnified in importance as an outcome if longevity is limited.

◎ **参考译文**：有创性心脏介入可以降低患有急性冠状动脉综合征、严重瓣膜疾病、心力衰竭和室性心律失常的特定患者的死亡率和发病率。然而，显示出心脏结果改善的随机试验排除了晚期恶性肿瘤的患者，例如正在接受持续治疗的晚期实体器官癌症和预后谨慎的无法治愈的血液系统肿瘤。缺乏直接的临床试验证据来告知这些患者有创性心血管介入的风险和益处。

在开展各种开创性的心血管试验的同时，癌症治疗也取得了突破性进展，包括靶向生物疗法和免疫疗法。这些疗法显著改善了许多晚期癌症患者的生存率。随着靶向癌症疗法的不断发展，无事件生存率和总生存率都有所提高，这使得患者面临更高的风险，即经历与癌症治疗相关的心血管毒性以及无关的不良心血管后果等竞争风险。医疗保健提供者一直不愿意将晚期癌症的患者转诊接受有创性心脏手术，因为这些患者很可能在接受有创性心脏介入治疗之前就死于癌症。然而，许多患者的预期寿命更长，这对这一观点提出了挑战。

鉴于对晚期癌症患者进行有创性心脏介入的临床试验数据有限，对这些患者进行循证决策需要了解患者的预期癌症特异性生存期。如果预期生存期超过从有创性心脏介入中获益所需的时间，那么可以推断患者可能从心脏介入中获益。我们的目标是总结当前数据，以指导有常见转移性癌症或恶性肿瘤且预后不良、适合接受癌症特异性治疗(称为晚期癌症)且有严重心血管疾病的患者作出决策。为了实现这一目标，我们描述了支持在一般人群中进行有创性心脏介入的证据，并整合了癌症人群中这些介入措施的现有文献。晚期癌症患者的一个关键考量因素是癌症死亡的竞争风险，这可能会影响患者从有创性心脏介入中获益的可能性。因此，我们描述了几种最常见癌症的生存预期。最后，我们描述了一个可能适用于该人群心脏治疗决策的概念框架。该框架涵盖了与癌症相关的因素，例如不间断癌症治疗的必要性，该人群发生介入相关并发症的风险，以及生活质量(如果寿命有限，生活质量的重要性就会凸显)。

第六单元 心脏瓣膜

第一节 心脏瓣膜口译知识点

正常心脏有四个瓣膜(valve)，右心房(right atrium, RA)与右心室(right ventricle, RV)之间的瓣膜被称为三尖瓣(tricuspid valve)，其有三个瓣叶(valve leaflet)，瓣叶下有腱索及乳头肌(papillary muscle)作支撑。右心室与肺动脉之间的瓣膜被称为肺动脉瓣(pulmonary valve)，其有三个瓣叶，与三尖瓣不同，它没有腱索及乳头肌。左心房(left atrium, LA)与左心室(left ventricle, LV)之间的瓣膜被称为二尖瓣(mitral valve，也被称为僧帽瓣)，它有两个瓣叶，瓣叶下有腱索及乳头肌作支撑。左心室与主动脉之间的瓣膜被称为主动脉瓣(aortic valve)，其与肺动脉瓣类似，有三个瓣叶，没有腱索及乳头肌。

正常状态下，在心脏收缩期(systole)，血液由左右心室分别经过主动脉瓣及肺动脉瓣，打入主动脉及肺动脉。此时，主动脉瓣及肺动脉瓣呈打开状态，而左心的二尖瓣及右心的三尖瓣呈关闭状态，只有保持这样，才能将血液充分射出。在心脏舒张期(diastole)，二尖瓣及三尖瓣呈打开状态，这样才能使血液充分注入心室以进行下一周期，此时主动脉瓣及肺动脉瓣呈关闭状态，以确保在心脏收缩期射出的血液能灌流到全身各处包括肺部。

如果各种疾病造成瓣膜的瓣叶打开不完全，即狭窄(stenosis)；关闭不完全，即反流(regurgitation)，或者两者均存在，就会使得在其上游的心房或心室受到压力增加或血容积(volume)负担的增加，情况若无改善，逐渐会造成整个心脏的衰竭，因此所谓的瓣膜性心脏病，就是指这四个瓣膜单一或合并出现瓣膜狭窄、反流或两者合并的病变而导致的心脏疾病。

心脏瓣膜病(heart valve disease)是常见的心脏疾病，现代心脏超声可明确诊断。严重的心脏瓣膜病会显著缩短患者寿命。因为确诊时，心脏瓣膜的解剖形态(morphology)已发生改变，因而一般情况下心脏瓣膜病无法通过药物治疗得到根治，需要机械物理的治疗方式才能获得显著的疗效。

过去，心外科的开胸手术(thoracotomy, open-chest operation)是治疗心脏瓣膜病的标准方式。而近年来，随着医学技术和材料学的进步，心脏瓣膜病也可以通过介入的方式得到有效治疗，这种方式也被称为经导管、经皮、经血管治疗。

总体而言，心脏瓣膜的手术治疗可分为采用传统的胸骨正中切口手术(1.0时代)、微创外科(小切口)瓣膜手术(2.0时代)和经导管瓣膜介入治疗(3.0时代)。其中,微创外科瓣膜手术采用小切口、非胸骨全部劈开方式以减小手术创伤,通过电视胸腔镜和外科手术机器人辅助进行手术。微创外科瓣膜手术虽然造成的切口小,但术中心脏仍要停跳,仍需要体外循环辅助(extracorporeal circulation)。研究显示,其虽然能降低手术创伤,但并不能降低手术风险。

心脏瓣膜病的介入治疗,简而言之,其基本原理是采用导管介入方式,将治疗器械压缩到一根很细的导管(直径4~10mm),然后穿刺外周血管(通常是股动脉或股静脉)或者心前区,插入导管,并将器械输送到所要治疗瓣膜的位置,在超声或者X线透视指导下,对瓣膜进行修复或者更换,从而达到治疗目的。心脏瓣膜介入治疗伤口较微创外科手术进一步缩小,且是在心脏跳动情况下进行手术,无需心脏停跳及体外循环,从而避免了这两者引发的不良反应,故手术安全性明显提高。

目前心脏瓣膜介入治疗有以下几类:

第一,球囊扩张术(balloon dilatation):采用一个可膨胀的球囊,通过导管输送到狭窄的瓣膜进行扩张,撕开瓣叶在交界处的粘连而不损伤瓣叶,因此可以治疗狭窄但并不导致瓣膜反流。代表技术为经皮二尖瓣球囊扩张及经肺动脉瓣球囊扩张。经皮二尖瓣球囊扩张(percutaneous balloon mitral valvuloplasty,PBMV)是1976年日本医生井上宽治(Inoue)等设计出由两层乳胶夹一层尼龙网组成的、具有自身定位能力的二尖瓣球囊导管,称为Inoue球囊导管,将球囊导管沿股静脉、右心房并经房间隔穿刺送至狭窄的二尖瓣口,然后充盈球囊使狭窄的二尖瓣口扩张成形,并于1984年进行首次临床报道,之后该器械成为PBMV的全世界标准器械,沿用至今。大量研究结果显示,PBMV即刻可产生血流动力学改善,二尖瓣瓣口面积增加,跨瓣压、左心房压及肺动脉压下降,心排血量增加,生活质量提高。由于效果确切,微创安全,欧美及我国指南都将PBMV推荐为解剖合适的风湿性二尖瓣狭窄患者首选的治疗选择(Ⅰ类指征,A类证据)。风湿性二尖瓣狭窄在西方很少见,在我国仍常见,因此我国在这方面积累了丰富经验。

经皮肺动脉瓣球囊扩张(PBPV),1982年,Kan首先报道采用球囊扩张技术治疗先天性肺动脉瓣狭窄(PS),这种技术被称为经皮球囊肺动脉瓣成形术(PBPV),其因简便、有效、安全而得到广泛应用。随着现代工业和导管技术的发展,大量关于PBPV的临床应用研究得以进行,这些研究结果证实PBPV可为大部分PS患者的首选治疗手段,可替代外科开胸手术,成为各大指南首选推荐的治疗手段(Ⅰ类指征)。2020年ESC先心指南推荐的PS进行PBPV手术主要指征为(具有以下之一):出现相关症状,峰值跨瓣压差大于64mmHg,右心室功能下降三尖瓣反流,合并右向左分流(right-to-left shunt)。

第二,经导管主动脉瓣置换术(transcatheter aortic valve replacement,TAVR):其通过股动脉送入瓣膜介入导管,将人工瓣膜送至主动脉瓣区打开,完成人工瓣膜置入,恢复瓣膜功能,从而实现对原先病变的瓣膜的功能替代。

2002年进行了世界首例TAVR,由此,心脏瓣膜病经导管介入治疗取得突破,心脏瓣膜介入时代的序幕正式拉开。而在 TAVR 之前，经导管肺动脉瓣置换术（transcatheter pulmonary valve replacement，TPVR）在 2000 年已有报道，但患者多为法洛四联症（tetralogy of Fallot，TOF）术后患者，发病率低，影响有限。而在主动脉瓣介入治疗出现之后，经导管二尖瓣、三尖瓣介入治疗得到了迅速发展，国内外创新器械研发日新月异，使得大创伤高风险的外科手术逐渐让路于微创低风险的经导管介入操作。

TAVR 也称作经导管主动脉瓣置入术（transcatheter aortic valve implantation，TAVI），其基本原理是狭窄坚硬的主动脉瓣构成了一个狭窄管道，该解剖特点可为 SAVR 瓣膜的金属支架提供良好的支撑固定作用。起初，TAVR 只用于三叶式的主动脉瓣狭窄患者，但随着研究进展，发现对于二叶式主动脉瓣狭窄患者，TAVR 也是适用的，目前已得到指南推荐。随着器械的改进，目前部分 TAVR 器械带有锚定功能。因此，部分解剖合适的主动脉瓣反流（aortic regurgitation，AR）患者也可以使用 TAVR 治疗。TAVR 发展迅速，对于重度（severe）主动脉瓣狭窄（aortic stenosis，AS）的患者，其临床适应证（clinical indication）已放宽至外科手术高、中、低危的患者。2020 年美国心脏协会/美国心脏病学会（American Heart Association/American College of Cardiology，AHA/ACC）瓣膜疾病管理指南以及 2021 年欧洲心脏病学会/欧洲心胸外科学会（European Society of Cardiology/European Association for Cardio Thoracic Surgery，ESC/EACTS）瓣膜疾病管理指南中，对于不同危险分层的患者，TAVR 获得了代替外科主动脉瓣置换术（surgical aortic valve replacement，SAVR）的Ⅰ类推荐。在部分国家，TAVR 的量已经超过 SAVR 的量。

TAVR 生物瓣膜的使用寿命有限，因此要考虑患者年龄。目前指南的最低推荐年龄为 65 岁。首次手术选择 TAVR 的患者相较于 SAVR，可获得更大的有效瓣口面积（effective orifice areas，EOA），TAVR 瓣中瓣（在人工瓣膜中再置入一个人工瓣膜）置入时发生人工瓣膜-患者不匹配（prosthesis-patient mismatch，PPM）的风险较小。目前大多数耐久性（durability）研究中的 TAVR 瓣膜是一代瓣膜，无抗钙化处理，而新一代 TAVR 瓣膜对于不同瓣叶材料（牛心包或猪心包）采用脱细胞处理（decellularization）方式，以延缓钙化（calcification）并增加耐久性。此外纯聚合物材料心脏瓣膜也有进展，其中有代表性的生物聚合物材料是 LifePlolymer，比生物瓣膜更为耐用，并具有更好的抗血栓性能。TAVR 也可用于治疗二叶式主动脉瓣（bicuspid aortic valve，BAV）狭窄，总体上与三叶瓣有着可比的（comparable）手术成功率。

第三，经导管缘对缘修复术（transcatheter edge-to-edge repair，TEER）：主要用于治疗二尖瓣反流/二尖瓣关闭不全（mitral regurgitation，MR），MR 是最常见且发病机制较为复杂的心脏瓣膜疾病。TEER 是一项基于外科二尖瓣缘对缘修复手术的经导管介入操作，其使用二尖瓣夹合装置（MitraClip），在超声及 X 线引导下夹住 MR 区的前瓣叶和后瓣叶并使之接合，使心脏收缩期时瓣叶之间间隙减少或消失，而舒张期时瓣口变成双孔或多孔，从而达到减少或消除 MR 的效果。

TEER 要考虑以下临床因素（clinical factor）：

心功能状态：纽约心脏病协会（New York Heart Association，NYHA）心功能分级可以为心衰（heart failure）伴中重度或重度继发性二尖瓣反流（functional mitral regurgitation，FMR）患者提供预后（prognosis）依据，而无论患者的基线（baseline）心功能状态如何，相较于单纯药物治疗，TEER 治疗能够带来获益。也有研究显示，基线 N 末端 B 型利钠肽原（NT-proBNP）的水平与全因死亡率（all-cause mortality）或 1 年内因心衰住院相关。

手术风险（surgical risk）：针对患者术前的状况，之前对于外科手术有各种各样的手术风险评估系统，但对于 TEER 患者，目前尚缺乏有针对性的风险分层工具（specific risk stratification）。

肾功能（renal/kidney function）：肾功能不全会严重影响心衰合并 MR 患者的预后。但多项研究显示，与单纯药物治疗相比，无论患者是否存在肾功能不全，植入 MitraClip 均能改善临床结局（clinical outcome），并降低终末期肾病（end-stage renal disease，ESRD）和透析治疗的发生率。

虽然 TEER 技术的安全性较高，但约 4.35% 患者可能出现相关并发症，包括术后二尖瓣狭窄（mitral stenosis，MS）、残余反流、急性肾衰等，这些并发症都会影响到患者的疗效。二尖瓣学术研究联盟（MVARC）推荐对 MVA 和二尖瓣跨瓣压差（transmitral pressure gradients，TMPG）进行测量以评估植入装置的"功能失效"。此外，TEER 术后也会出现左心室逆重构、医源性房间隔缺损（iatrogenic atrial septal defect，iASD）等问题，同样值得探讨。

目前有一种说法，即心脏瓣膜手术治疗可分为：传统的胸骨正中切口手术（1.0 时代）、微创外科（小切口）瓣膜手术（2.0 时代）以及经导管瓣膜介入治疗（3.0 时代）。作为译员，我们不能将对这三种技术的表述简单地理解为如同时代更迭一样的技术更替，这仅是一种说法而已。这三种方法，虽然在适应证方面彼此有重叠，但绝非互相替代的关系，应将其视为技术的创新与互相补充，而不应形成"当代社会只有经导管瓣膜介入治疗（3.0 时代）"的想法，传统的胸骨正中切口手术，根据患者的具体情况，仍然是挽救患者生命的重要手术。

经导管三尖瓣介入治疗最近也发展迅速，虽然三尖瓣反流发病率高，但因大多继发于左心瓣膜病变、房颤以及无症状期较长而被临床忽视，在心脏瓣膜介入治疗中起步最晚。之前经导管三尖瓣介入治疗的重点主要在于将二尖瓣修复器械应用于三尖瓣，而自 2019 年，两款经导管原位置换瓣膜显示出不俗的临床结果，使得经导管三尖瓣置换术（transcatheter tricuspid valve replacement，TTVR）成为三尖瓣介入治疗的亮点。

第二节　真实世界口译情境

一、主题会议

现在涉及心脏瓣膜主题的医学会议口译主要包括：人工瓣膜公司与国家监管机构间的咨询会议、国家监管机构对瓣膜生产公司的 GMP 核查、大型心脏会议中瓣膜分论坛、国外瓣膜医生在国内的学术路演、专门以瓣膜为主题的会议、心脏瓣膜外科会议、心外科会议等。

二、行业特点

心脏瓣膜疾病主题的医学会议口译,目前相较于其他心脏介入主题会议少一些,这可能是因为这一领域的部分内容正在快速发展或刚刚起步,另一个原因则在于专攻于此领域的医生,大多有海外学习/培训的经历,整体英文水平较好。有时部分会议中的海外讲者较少,那会议便不一定会专门安排翻译,与会者直接听英文,或由英文流利的专科医生代劳。这也是近些年的部分主题医学会议口译的一个新兴现象,即专业英语不错且对口译/同传感兴趣的专科医生,有时会积极主动地参与一些涉外会议的翻译/口译工作。这些医生大多没有经过专门的同传训练,但其对专业知识技能的熟稔、对专业英语的了解以及本身自己作为会议主办方成员的优势,大多时会抵消听力和翻译能力欠佳的劣势,部分会议赞助方有时也是乐见其成。

心脏瓣膜疾病主题的临床医学会议,主题主要在于介入与手术的比较,即 TAVR 与 SAVR 的比较、技术改良的介绍与探讨、临床试验/研究的介绍等。

三、口译难点

心脏瓣膜主题医学口译会议的难点与上一章的心脏介入主题会议的难点类似,因为瓣膜介入治疗本身也属于心脏介入的一大类,但有其更独特的难点,现介绍如下:

一是更大量的英文名词及缩略语的使用(部分内容已在前文提及,此处不再赘述),大量的解剖结构以及缩略语,大量的术式在会议演讲讨论时都是以英文缩略语的形式出现,再加上大量的英语器械名称,以及不少在此领域作出卓越贡献的国外专家教授,其名字也时有提及,还有欧美和我国的监管机构以及各类学术团体,例如 FDA/EMA/NMPA、ESC/EACTS、AHA/ACC 和各种指南、分级标准、分类标准、各类评估表单等。此外,各类临床专科概念,例如 EOA、PPM 等,无论是英译中还是中译英,都需要译员有一定的此主题相关经验或者极好的会前准备,才能分辨哪些内容跟读即可,哪些内容需要进行准确的翻译。

在会议提前提供讲者课件供译员提前预习的情况下,同译难度尚可,但对于经验缺乏的译员,最难的部分在于问答和点评讨论环节,此时若没有一定的专科素养储备,口译难度极大。

此外在部分国内讲者进行发言时,有时因为个人口音原因,加之译员对发言主题不熟悉,会导致译员难以听清具体的英文发音,导致漏译或错译。同传时效果尚可,交传时则压力极大。

二是瓣膜介入医生在操作时因为难度更大,大会手术直播时会更加"屏气凝神",发言往往更加简短快速,此时译员须及时跟上且翻译准确,也要对操作本身的原理和步骤有一定了解,否则很难跟上讲者的思路与节奏。

第三节　中英对照篇章及分析

一、英译中

These were adult patients 18 years old or older with aortic valve disease, concomitant procedures, such as a coronary bypass grafting or ascending aortic replacement were allowed. The exclusion criteria were emergency surgery, endocarditis, multiple valves, and patients with prior valve surgery or what we call redo operations. Now, the demographics of the initial cohort are listed here. You'll note there were 689 patients. The mean age was 66.9, with mean follow-up 5.3 years. On the right there, note in the green circle that 82% of these patients had a full sternotomy. In the left lower quadrant of the slide, you'll see the valve distribution, and 78% of patients had of size 23 mm or larger. On the right hand side, you'll see that most patients were male and the STS, Society of Thoracic Surgeons mortality risk was two, the European Score mortality risk was 2.5. The New York Heart Association Classification was mostly class two at 50% of patients. Note that most patients were aged 66 to 79. Now, from these original, there were originally 694 enrolled patients. Though five patients did not receive the valve due to anatomic or procedural complexities. There were subsequently 689 patients that I just shared with you, these were then followed through five years. Now, the Food and Drug Administration or FDA, which is the government regulatory body in the United States, asked that the top three enrolling centers continue following their patients. （本段内容选自2023年一位美国医生的学术演讲，有删改调整。）

◎ **参考译文**：首先是成年患者，18岁或者以上，有主动脉瓣疾病，一些同步操作，例如冠脉搭桥、降主动脉置换是可以的。排除标准是急诊手术、心内膜炎、多个瓣膜以及曾经做过瓣膜手术，或者我们称之为redo手术的患者。这里是初始队列的人口统计特征，看到一共有689位患者。平均年龄是66.9岁，平均随访5.3年。在右边，注意到在绿色圈内，82%的患者都接受过开胸手术。在幻灯片左下角，可以看到瓣膜的尺寸，78%的患者用的是23毫米或更大的。右手边还可以看到大部分患者是男性患者，STS，即胸外科医生协会死亡风险是2，欧洲评分死亡风险是2.5，NYHA分级，大部分的是分为二级，50%的患者。注意到大部分的患者是66岁到79岁。从最开始，最开始有694位患者入组。尽管有五位患者，因为一些解剖性或操作复杂的情况没有接受瓣膜。后来还是有689位患者，我刚刚分享给大家，他们之后进行了5年的随访。现在，食品药品监督管理局，FDA，也是美国的政府监督管理机构，要求前三的入组中心持续随访这些患者。

◎ **分析**：
1. "demographics"译作"人口统计特征"，此处也可处理为"特征/数据"；
2. "sternotomy"此处错译为"开胸手术"，其真正意思是"胸骨切开术"，

"thoracotomy"才是"开胸手术"。胸骨切开术是特指通过切开胸骨进入胸腔的手术,与更广泛的"开胸手术"概念有所区别,这种区分在医学文献中至关重要。

3. "In the left lower quadrant of the slide"译作"在幻灯片左下角",应避免将"quadrant"译作"象限";

4. "New York Heart Association"处理为"NYHA",全称是"纽约心脏病协会";

5. "enroll"译作"入组","top three enrolling centers"指入组患者最多的三家中心。

Here is the important seven year data to share with you today. In the green, on the left hand side, in the first column are the variables. And the second column are the number of patients at risk. In the third column are the events. And now in the fourth column, we're looking at the probability events free. Note that the event free mortality in the first row there is 85% or essentially survival is 85% at seven years. Freedom from stroke was 94% at seven years. There were a few bleeding events, most of these were related to anti-coagulation for atrial fibrillation. There were 15 endocarditis events, and seven of these did require a re-operation. There were three perivalvular leaks, one resolved, and I talked about the one that had required an early re-operation. Note that structural valve deterioration was 99.3%. There were 12 re-operations, which I'll share with you here. The early paravalvular leak patient. There were seven patients with endocarditis, most of these were strep or staph organisms. There was one patient that had paravalvular leak that required a catheter-based plug. There were two patients that had structural valve deterioration. One patient that had an aneurysm that required replacement, and at that time, its valve was replaced.

◎ **参考译文**:这里是七年的数据,也是很重要的,今天和大家来分享。绿色的左手边,第一列是变量,第二列是有风险的患者数量,第三列是事件,在第四列中,我们看到的是无事件的可能性。请注意无事件死亡率在第一行,是85%,也就是说在七年的时候生存率是85%。无卒中率是94%,是第七年的结果。只有几例出血事件,大多数是因为房颤使用了抗凝剂。有15例心内膜炎事件,其中7例需要再次手术。有3例瓣周漏,1例解决了,这就是那例我说的需要早期二次手术的。注意到结构性瓣膜衰败是99.3%。还有12例再次手术,我想跟大家分享。早期瓣周漏患者,有7例患者有心内膜炎,大部分是链球菌或金葡菌;有1例瓣周漏患者,需要基于导管的plug;有2例患者出现瓣膜结构性衰败;1例患者有动脉瘤,需要置换,此时瓣膜已经置换。

◎ **分析**:

1. "probability"意思是统计学中的"概率",但很多时候不少讲者都将其与"possibility"即"可能性"混用;

2. "Note that"是欧美讲者常用的表达,可译作"请注意、可以看到";

3. "essentially"意思是"本质上、实质上",此处处理为"也就是说",这是口译中常见的处理方式;

4. "Freedom from stroke was 94% at seven years."按照顺句驱动法处理为"无卒中是

94%，是第七年的结果。";

5. "structural valve deterioration"译作"结构性瓣膜衰败"，指瓣膜永久性的内在改变，例如瓣叶撕裂、钙化、血管翳沉积、连枷样改变或瓣叶纤维化等，导致退行性改变以及功能障碍，导致瓣膜狭窄或瓣膜反流；

6. "strep or staph organisms"指的是"streptococcus and staphylococcus"，是口语中不规则的表达，可译作"链球菌或葡萄球菌"；

7. "catheter-based plug"译作"基于导管的 plug"，此处"plug"是一款封堵器械，跟读即可。这里的"跟读即可"是指，在翻译这个术语时，由于"plug"在这里是一个相对专业的医疗器械名称，直接按照字面意思翻译为"封堵器"或"塞子"等可能不够准确或不够常用，而"基于导管的 plug"已经是一个相对明确且专业的表述，因此在不了解更具体的中文术语时，可以直接按照英文原词或这种直译的方式读出，即"跟读即可"。然而，在实际翻译中，如果有可能找到更贴切的中文术语来替代"plug"，那么使用中文术语会更为准确和易于理解。但在这个特定的例子中，"plug"作为封堵器械的一种，且与"catheter-based"（基于导管的）这一特定技术结合使用时，直接翻译并保留"plug"一词可能是一种可行的选择，尤其是在缺乏更精确中文对应词的情况下。

Back to the fact, we still take into special consideration when treating patients with low-risk group. I usually do the CT scan first because I want to take into account whether those patients have very high risk or ultra high risk anatomy. That would be very rare and because nowadays new technology, new devices can overcome those obstacles, but in case of patients have extreme size of aortic annulus, for example, very very small aortic annulus. Then you may need to use a very small size with some annulus expansion. Because they're young and think about they may need one or more procedure in the future. I may consider to discuss with surgeons and to think about to have, first would be a SAVR. And patient may have other heart valve problems and we will actually take into consideration of future coronary access and um, so all the things will be taken into consideration before we talk to the patient whether they will fit for TAVI in a low-risk group. And I think it would be heart team based, patient centered decision-making process is always the key for managing patients with severe aortic stenosis. We want to minimize the risk of procedure. We bring the patient back to the normal life and also improve quality of life as soon as possible.

◎ **参考译文**：回到事实，我们还是需要特别考虑一下，在治疗低风险组患者的时候，通常我会先做 CT，因为我想考虑这些患者是否有很高风险或者极高风险的解剖。这可能非常罕见，因为现在的新的技术、新的器械可以克服这些障碍，但是万一患者有极端大小的主动脉瓣环，比如非常非常小的主动脉瓣环，那你就需要使用非常小的瓣膜，还要做些瓣环扩张。因为他们很年轻，还要考虑到他们可能需要一次或更多次的手术，未来还要做手术。我可能要考虑和外科医生讨论，考虑首先进行 SAVR。而患者可能还有其他的瓣膜问题，我们还要考虑未来的冠状动脉通路等，所以所有方面都要考虑

第六单元　心脏瓣膜

到，然后再和患者去沟通，他们是不是适合 TAVI，是不是低风险。我想这应该是基于心脏团队，以患者为中心的决策过程，这对于严重主动脉瓣狭窄患者的管理而言非常重要。我们要把操作的风险降到最低。我们要让患者恢复正常的生活，还要提高生活质量，这一切都要尽快实现。

◎ 分析：

1. "they may need one or more procedure in the future" 处理为"他们可能需要一次或更多次的手术，未来还要做手术"，其中"未来还要做手术"是听到"in the future"后补充的；

2. "SAVR" 是 "Surgical aortic valve replacement" 的缩写，即"主动脉瓣置换手术"，因为缩略语中有字母 R，涉及儿化音，不同讲者发音略有不同；

3. "before we talk to the patient" 译作"然后再和患者去沟通"，将"before"译作"然后"是非常实用的同传处理方法；

4. "minimize" 一般可以灵活处理，"maximize" 也是一样，通常不译作"最小化"和"最大化"，应带入具体语境，否则翻译腔过重。

The reason our valves don't last as long as I've shown in the accelerated durability testing is because of the biological response to the valves. Biological response results in leaflet tearing, pannus or fibrous tissue overgrowth and calcification. In fact, for a pulmonic valve, the primary failure mode, when a pericardial valve is placed in the pulmonic position, is fibrous tissue overgrowth, as you see, in these sections of leaflets on the right hand, upper corner of the slide. But for aortic and mitral valves, our pericardial valves predominantly failed as a result of calcification with occasional failures related to pannus tissue overgrowth. What are the causes of calcification? The very first generation valves that were treated in glutaraldehyde failed in a period of seven to ten years. Those failures were examined both by Edwards and by other researchers. We found that calcification was associated with phospholipid cells that were left in the tissue. Both Edwards and Medtronic, the two leading producers of tissue valve in the early 80s produce processes using alcohol and a surfactant to wash most of the phospholipid out of the tissue. This made a dramatic difference in durability and started the shift from predominant use of mechanical valves, as in the days when I was working Carbon Medics, to the predominant use of tissue valves with now over 80% of the valves in most parts of the United States and Europe being tissue valves.

◎ 参考译文：为什么我们的瓣膜没办法维持那么长时间，就像我跟大家展示的测试那样，是因为对瓣膜的生物反应。生物反应会导致瓣叶撕裂、血管翳、纤维组织增生和钙化。事实上，对于肺动脉瓣，最主要的衰败模式，如果心包瓣膜放到了肺动脉瓣的位置的时候，会有纤维组织增生，可以看到，这些瓣叶的截面，在右手边，幻灯片的右上角。但对于主动脉和二尖瓣，我们的心包瓣膜主要的衰败原因是钙化，偶尔是血管翳组织的增生。那为什么会导致钙化呢？第一代瓣膜是经过戊二醛处理的，会在七到十年的时间衰败。这些衰败由爱德华和其他研究者人员进行检查，我们发现钙化是与磷脂细胞相关，是留在组织上的磷脂细胞。爱德华和美敦力，两家都是领先的组织瓣生产商，在20世纪80年代，生产过程中使用酒精和表面活性剂去把组织上大多数的磷脂细胞清掉。这就使得耐久性出现极大的差异，也开始从主要使用机械瓣，就像我在Carbon Medics工作时那样，转变为主要使用组织瓣，现在美国和欧洲大部分地区80%以上的瓣膜都是组织瓣。

◎ 分析：

1. "accelerated durability testing"译为"加速耐久性测试"；

2. "when a pericardial valve is placed in the pulmonic position, is fibrous tissue overgrowth"译作"如果心包瓣膜放到了肺动脉瓣的位置的时候"，此处的"when"译作了"……的时候"，这是比较典型的翻译腔，可以处理为"如果把心包瓣膜放到肺动脉瓣的位置，就……"；

3. "sections"译作"截面"，指断面图或剖面图，该词也很常见；

4. "glutaraldehyde"译作"戊二醛"，但译者如果没有提前作准备，极难会译出，同传时可根据发音通过在线词典迅速查词，或者也可以考虑跟读。

We started our clinical investigation in 2011, I had the opportunity to observe this case at the London Valves meeting, where a 23 mm Sapien was deployed inside a 19 mm porcine valve. That was quite amazing to see such a large transcatheter valve put inside such a small surgical valve. At that same time, information was coming out that showed when a valve-in-valve procedure was done in a small valve, the patient survival was not very good. It was much better when the valve-in-valve procedure was done in a larger valve. One solution to this was demonstrated in Germany in 2014, and that is to use a high-pressure balloon and break the valve open. So a larger transcatheter valve can be inserted, but just last year at the TCT meeting, transcatheter valve network data was investigated, and in a propensity matched group, it was found that although the gradients were much better, the all cause mortality, cardiac death, and life threatening bleeding was significantly worse when balloon fracturing was done in valve-in-valve procedures. We took a different path. We designed a valve that will expand in a very controlled manner, uniformly around all the struts and created radiographic markings.

◎ **参考译文**：我们也开始了我们的临床调查，是在2011年，当时我有机会参加了London Valves会议，看到了这个病例，一个23毫米的Sapien瓣膜置于19毫米的猪瓣膜当中。非常令人震惊，看到这么大的一个经导管瓣膜能放进这么小的一个外科瓣膜内。同时有一些其他的信息展示出来，瓣中瓣在一个小瓣膜当中进行的时候，这个患者的生存不是很好，如果瓣中瓣能在一个更大的瓣膜当中操作的话，那效果会更好。一个解决方案是，德国在2014年的时候，用一个高压球囊来打开这个瓣膜，这样就可以放入更大的经导管瓣膜。但在去年的TCT的会议上，经导管瓣膜网络数据调查显示，在倾向性匹配的小组当中，发现尽管梯度好得多，但全因死亡率、心脏死亡还有危及生命的出血其实会更糟糕，如果球囊在瓣中瓣操作时破裂的话，以上的情况会更糟糕。我们采取了不同的路径。我们让瓣膜能够以可控的方式扩张，均匀地围绕在所有网丝上，而且还做了影像标记。

◎ 分析：

1. "clinical investigation"译作"临床调查"，此处应处理为"临床研究"，更符合行业内的语言表达习惯；

2. "deploy"译作"置于"，根据不同语境，也可以处理为"释放""放"等；

3. "amazing"译作"令人震惊"，此处并未译出其褒义层面，应处理为"非常了不起"，近年来，"amazing"一词频繁见于各类医学会议；

4. "patient survival was not very good"处理为了"患者的生存不是很好"，其中"患者的生存"可能会让听众觉得拗口，但确实可以这样表达；

5. "break the valve open"译作"来打开这个瓣膜"，这样的处理作为现场同传译文是可以接受的，但这样的处理并未将"break"一词的意思完全表达出来，"break"此处指的是用高压球囊将之前的瓣膜破坏扩大，以容纳后续更大的瓣中瓣，此处可处理为"来破开并扩大这个瓣膜"。

Today we are gonna talk about the choice between surgical aortic valve replacement versus transcatheter aortic valve replacement within the landscape of 2020, ACC/AHA valvular heart disease guidelines. Key takeaways of this talk are reviewing the indications for surgical aortic valve replacement versus transcatheter aortic valve replacement, reviewing the outcomes of transcatheter aortic valve replacement in patients with bicuspid aortic valve stenosis, and reviewing antithrombotic therapy after aortic valve replacement. With the remarkable advances in transcatheter treatment of aortic stenosis, we now have shown that TAVR is a safe and effective procedure in old adults, regardless of their estimated surgical risk. In this meta-analysis of all TAVR trials, the mortality rate for transfemoral transcatheter aortic valve replacement is lower than that of the surgical aortic valve replacement with a hazard ratio of 0.88. （本段内容选自2020年一位美国医生的演讲，有删改调整。）

◎ **参考译文**：今天，我们来讨论外科主动脉瓣置换术与经导管主动脉瓣置换术之间的选择，背景是2020年ACC/AHA瓣膜性心脏病指南。本次演讲的重点是回顾外科主动脉瓣置换术与经导管主动脉瓣置换术的适应证，回顾经导管主动脉瓣置换术对二叶式主动脉瓣狭窄患者的治疗结果以及回顾主动脉瓣置换术后的抗血栓治疗。随着经导管治疗主动脉瓣狭窄的显著进步，我们现在已经证明，TAVR是老年人安全有效的手术，无论估计的手术风险如何。在这项对所有TAVR试验的荟萃分析中，经股动脉经导管主动脉瓣置换术的死亡率低于外科主动脉瓣置换术，风险比为0.88。

◎ 分析：

1. "landscape"可处理为"背景是"；

2. "ACC/AHA"为"美国心脏协会"（American Heart Association）与"美国心脏病学会"（American College of Cardiolog），都是心脏病学领域重要的学会；

3. "takeaway"在近年的医学会议当中出现率越来越高，意思是"要点、重要信息"；

4. "bicuspid aortic valve"译作"二叶式主动脉瓣"，正常的主动脉瓣共有三个瓣膜；若主动脉瓣先天性只有两个瓣膜，则被称为"二叶式主动脉瓣"，这是最常见的先天性主动脉瓣狭窄畸形；

5. "hazard ratio"指"风险比"，也被称为"危险比"，是一个比率，指的是两个风险率的比值，风险率是单位时间内发生的事件数占受试总体的百分比。

TAVI is also associated with a lower risk of stroke, major bleeding and atrial fibrillation, as well as shorter hospital length of stay, less pain and more rapid return to normal activities. Compared to surgical aortic valve replacement, SAVR results in higher rates of vascular complications, perivalvular regurgitation and permanent pacemaker implantation, along with valve reintervention. The only caveat is that we have accumulated data for about 50 years for surgical aortic valve replacement durability, whereas the longest durability data for TAVR about go up to only five years. We need to keep in mind that the earlier trials comparing surgical aortic valve replacement and transcatheter aortic valve replacement included only older patients with a mean age of mid-80s. The more recent trial studying patients at low and intermediate risk had a mean age of mid-70s with a very few number of patients less than 65 years of age.

◎ 参考译文：TAVI也能够降低卒中、大出血和心房颤动的风险，并缩短住院时间，减轻疼痛，更快恢复正常活动。与外科主动脉瓣置换术相比，SAVR的血管并发症、瓣周反流和永久性起搏器植入以及瓣膜再介入的发生率更高。唯一需要注意的是我们已经积累了约50年的外科主动脉瓣置换术耐久性数据，而TAVR的最长耐久性数据最多只有五年。我们需要记住，早期的试验，比较外科主动脉瓣置换术和经导管主动脉瓣置换术的试验，仅包含了老年患者，平均年龄80多岁的老年患者。最近的试验研究低风险和中风险患者，平均年龄是70多岁，只有极少数患者年龄不到65岁。

◎ 分析：

1. "TAVI is also associated with a lower risk of stroke, major bleeding and atrial fibrillation"处理为"TAVI也能够降低卒中、大出血和心房颤动的风险"，其实更准确的表达应该是"TAVI与较低风险的卒中、大出血和房颤相关"，或者"TAVI相关的卒中、大出血和房颤风险较低"；

2. "hospital length of stay"译作"住院时间"，这是医学口译中的基础概念，length of stay（LOS），指"住院时长"，是衡量住院患者的一个基础指标。

With this data in mind the concern of lack of data on valve durability in younger patients, SAVR is recommended for adults younger than 65 years of age. Both TAVR and SAVR are effective approaches to AVR in adults between 65 and 80 years of age. For symptomatic patients with severe aortic stenosis who are older than 80 years of age, or for younger patients with a life expectancy less than 10 years, and no anatomical contraindications to transfemoral TAVI. Transfemoral TAVI is recommended in preference to surgical aortic valve replacement. SAVR is recommended for patients who do not have suitable anatomy for transfemoral transcatheter aortic valve replacement. For those who have an expected survival of less than 12 months, or for whom who are expected to have minimal improvement in quality of life, palliative care is recommended after shared decision making.

◎ 参考译文：记住了这些数据，考虑到缺乏关于年轻患者瓣膜耐久性数据的担忧，建议对65岁以下的成年人进行SAVR。TAVR和SAVR都是AVR有效的方法，对于65到80岁的成人AVR都是有效的。对于有症状的重度主动脉瓣狭窄患者，年龄超过80岁的，或对于较年轻的患者，预期寿命不到10年且没有经股动脉TAVI解剖禁忌证的年轻患者，建议经股TAVI而非外科主动脉瓣置换术。对于不具有合适的经股动脉经导管主动脉瓣置换术的解剖结构的患者，建议进行SAVR。对于预期生存不到12个月，或者预期生活质量改善极小的患者，建议进行姑息治疗，在共同决策后进行姑息治疗。

◎ 分析：

1. "younger patients"译作"年轻患者"，其实不妥，应处理为"较年轻患者"。结合上下文，此处的"younger patients"指的也是60岁左右的患者，并非一般意义上的"年轻"。不过医学会议的听众也都是专业人士，此处细微的表达不会影响听众理解。比较级的处理要根据具体语境，要么把"较为"译出，要么省略"比较级"，直接翻译形容词；

2. "shared decision making"指的是医患双方共同决策，患方包含患者本人、患者家属等。

The early pivotal TAVR trials excluded patients with bicuspid aortic valve. Initial studies showing early generation valves suggested a higher rate of perivalvular leak in the bicuspid population. But data from the SDS-ACC transcatheter valve registry suggests that with the use of newer generation prosthetic valves, the rate of perivalvular leak is no different among the groups. This registry also showed no significant difference in mortality rate at 30 days and one year between bicuspid patients and tricuspid valve groups. However, the stroke rate at 30 days was higher in the bicuspid group. It's also important to note that patients with bicuspid aortic valve are often much younger, and long-term outcomes beyond five years is unclear after transcatheter aortic valve replacement. Low dose aspirin is recommended after transcatheter or surgical aortic valve replacement, and if there is no bleeding risk, a vitamin K antagonist can be used for three to six months after surgical AVR, if there is no bleeding risk, dual antiplatelet therapy for three to six months post transcatheter aortic valve replacement, or a Vitamin K antagonist for three months can be considered, and this carries the class ⅡB indication in the current guideline.

◎ 参考译文：早期的关键 TAVR 试验排除了二叶式主动脉瓣患者。初步研究表明早期瓣膜提示二叶式人群的瓣周漏率更高。但 SDS-ACC 经导管瓣膜登记的数据表明，使用新一代人工瓣膜后，各组之间的瓣周漏率并无差异。这一登记还显示，二叶组和三叶组患者在 30 天和 1 年时的死亡率没有显著差异。然而，二叶组的 30 天卒中率更高。值得注意的是，二叶式主动脉瓣患者通常更年轻，经导管主动脉瓣置换术后的 5 年以上的长期结果尚不明确。经导管或外科主动脉瓣置换术后均推荐使用小剂量阿司匹林，如果没有出血风险，可使用维生素 K 拮抗剂，在外科 AVR 术后用 3 到 6 个月，如果没有出血风险，经导管主动脉瓣置换术后可以使用 3 到 6 个月的双联抗血小板治疗，或者可考虑使用维生素 K 拮抗剂用 3 个月，这是当前指南中的ⅡB类指征。

◎ 分析：

1. "bicuspid patients and tricuspid valve groups"指的是主动脉瓣二叶或三叶，此处灵活处理即可；

2. "dual antiplatelet therapy"指"双联抗血小板治疗"，一般简称为"双抗"。

Patients who did not have any other indication for anticoagulation were randomized to low dose rivaroxaban plus low dose aspirin or clopidogrel 75 milligrams plus low dose aspirin. The primary efficacy outcome was the composite of death and thromboembolic events. The primary safety outcome was major or disabling or life-threatening bleeding. The trial, interestingly, was stopped early at a median follow up of 17 months because of safety concerns. In the rivaroxaban group, there were higher rates of death or first thromboembolic event and all-cause mortality compared with the antiplatelet only group. Major bleeding was more frequent in the rivaroxaban group, but the rates of life-threatening or disabling bleeding were actually similar in these two groups.

◎ 参考译文：没有其他抗凝指征的患者被随机分配接受低剂量利伐沙班加低剂量阿司匹林，或是氯吡格雷 75 毫克加小剂量阿司匹林。主要疗效结局是死亡和血栓栓塞事件的复合。主要安全性结局是大出血、致残性或危及生命的出血。该试验，有趣的是，被提前停止，中位随访 17 个月时提前停止，是出于安全性考量。利伐沙班组内，死亡率或首次血栓栓塞事件发生率和全因死亡率更高，相较于仅抗血小板治疗组。大出血在利伐沙班组更为常见，但危及生命或致残性出血的比率两组间实际上相似。

◎ 分析：

1. "safety concern"处理为"安全性考量"，此处的"concern"可灵活处理，译作"问题"也可以；注意虽然"safety concern"在广义上可以理解为"对安全问题的关注"，但直接译作"问题"可能在某些情况下略显笼统或不够准确。因为"concern"通常带有一种"担忧"或"关注"的情感色彩，而不仅仅是描述一个客观存在的问题。然而，在某些口语化或非正式的场合，或者当上下文已经明确指出了具体的安全问题时，将"safety

concern"简译为"安全问题"或"安全上的顾虑"等，也是可以接受的。

2. "antiplatelet only group"处理为"仅抗血小板治疗组"，有些国内医生会把"抗血小板治疗"简称为"抗板治疗"，口译时译员应予以注意。

二、中译英

那么，这么多的试验有一个共同点，就是永久起搏器的植入，在这个人群当中，它是高风险的。看一看近年来起搏器的植入，这个蓝线是住院期间的起搏器植入，红线是30天起搏器的植入。30天从10.9%降到10.8%，几乎没有变化。住院期间9.9%降到8.3%，也不是一个很明显的降低，所以说起搏器植入在TAVI组还是一个不可忽视的问题。那么起搏器植入对病人的生存有没有影响呢？其实是有影响的，看一下德国的数据。外科植入组17,700多位患者，起搏器植入率是3.6%，而TAVI组20,000多例患者，它是16.6%，很明显有一个增加的趋势。而装了起搏器的，一年的生存率，是这个虚线。没有装永久起搏器的是这个实线，这个统计学是高度的差异，所以装起搏器一年生存率，都有很明显的不良影响。（本段内容选自2022年一位国内医生的演讲，有删改调整。）

◎ 参考译文：So many trials have one thing in common, which is the implantation of permanent pacemakers. In this population, it is a high risk. Let's take a look at the implantation of pacemakers in recent years. The blue line is the implantation of pacemakers during hospitalization, and the red line is the implantation of pacemakers at 30 days. In 30 days, it dropped from 10.9% to 10.8%, almost no change. It dropped from 9.9% to 8.3% during hospitalization, which is not a very obvious decrease. So pacemaker implantation is still an issue that cannot be ignored in the TAVI group. So does pacemaker implantation have an impact on patient survival? Actually, it does have an impact. Let's take a look at the data from Germany. In surgical implantation group, there are more than 17,700 patients, the pacemaker implantation rate was 3.6%. While in TAVI group, there are more than 20,000 patients, it was 16.6%, which is a very obvious increasing trend. Those with pacemakers, their one-year survival rate is the dotted line. For those without permanent pacemakers, it is the solid line. The statistical difference is highly significant, so the one-year survival rate of pacemakers has a very obvious adverse effect.

◎ 分析：

1. "住院期间"译作"during hospitalization"，也可处理为"during hospital stay"；

2. "30天从10.9%降到10.8%"，此类的无主句，同传时只能是用it来处理，此处处理为"In 30 days, it dropped from 10.9% to 10.8%"。

那么，哪些病人可以考虑转到外科，或者是介绍进行导管治疗呢？综合因素，无可争议，一定要看患者的年龄，外科手术的风险，病人的虚弱程度，瓣膜的具体情况，股动脉有没有问题,是不是有其他瓣膜的问题,是不是有冠脉的问题。综合所有的因素去考虑。比如说,这个钙化,瓣膜如果钙化的程度并不是那么严重或很严重,尤其是有可能影响到左室流出道的钙化,或者是影响到传导系统的压迫。那么在这种情况下,可能选择外科手术比选择TAVI要合适。如果是二叶瓣,这个钙化的分析,是一个比较敏感的条件,而且也要看是不是有升主动脉的扩张,如果有,选择外科手术可能要比选择TAVI更合适。股动脉的钙化的程度,很明显也会影响到你选择TAVI。

◎ **参考译文**:Well, which patients can be considered for transfer to surgery, or transferred for catheter treatment? Comprehensive factors, no doubt, must check patient age, the risk of surgery, the patient's frailty, the specific condition of the valve, whether there is something wrong with the femoral artery, whether there are issues with other valves, and whether there are coronary artery issues. Consider all factors comprehensively. For example, for this calcification, if the valve calcification is not so severe or very severe, especially if the calcification may affect the left ventricular outflow tract or the compression of the conduction system. In this case, it may be more appropriate to choose surgery than TAVI. If it is a bicuspid valve, the analysis of calcification is a more sensitive condition, and it also depends on whether there is dilatation of the ascending aorta. If there is, surgery may be more appropriate than TAVI. The degree of calcification of the femoral artery will obviously also affect your choice of TAVI.

◎ **分析**:

1. "病人可以考虑转到"中的"转"译作"transfer",也可考虑将其译作"refer",意思是"转诊";

2. "左室流出道"译作"left ventricular outflow tract",指"左心室流出道"。

我其实非常关心另外一个话题,就是我们在外科做瓣膜置换的时候,特别担心有瓣周漏,但是一旦做介入瓣膜的时候,瓣周漏大量存在。只要是轻度的,甚至轻到中度,可能就已经被接受了,只要不是中到重度的瓣周漏就能够接受,这个患者没有太大问题。所以颠覆了我们整个外科,从最早的介绍说介入瓣,可以接近百分之五十都有瓣周漏。那个时候我们就说,即使有一点瓣周漏也是可以接受的。但到底能接受到什么程度,我不知道,介入瓣这种瓣周漏和心内膜炎的关系。因为外科一旦有瓣周漏,大量的病人就会合并心内膜炎。不知道介入瓣里面这个瓣周漏和心内膜炎到底有没有一个正向的关系?因为所有的介绍里大多数都不太介绍这个并发症。那么我们从外科医生的角度,问一下外科的教授,你是怎么来思考这个瓣周漏的,我们外科的瓣周漏和介入瓣的瓣周漏,到底是怎么样来重新定位或者思考的?

◎ **参考译文**:I am actually very concerned about another topic. That is when we do valve replacement surgery, we are particularly worried about paravalvular leaks. However, once an interventional valve is performed, a large number of paravalvular leaks exist. As long as it is mild, or even mild to moderate, it may have been accepted. As long as it is not moderate to severe paravalvular leak, it can be accepted, and this patient is OK. So it has overturned our entire surgery. From the earliest introduction of interventional valves, it was said that nearly 50% of interventional valves have paravalvular leaks. At that time, we said that even a little paravalvular leak was acceptable. But to what extent it can be accepted, I don't know. The relationship between paravalvular leaks in interventional valves and endocarditis. Because once there is paravalvular leak in surgery, a large number of patients will have endocarditis. I don't know if there is a positive relationship between paravalvular leaks in interventional valves and endocarditis? Because most of the introductions don't mention this complication. So from the perspective of a surgeon, let's ask the professor of surgery, how do you think about paravalvular leaks? How do we reposition or think about paravalvular leaks in surgery and paravalvular leaks in interventional valves?

◎ 分析：

1. "我们在外科做瓣膜置换的时候"译作"we do valve replacement surgery"，其中的动词用了"do"，其实用"perform"更好一些，但同传情况下也可接受。近些年，部分美国医生也会使用"do surgery"这样的表达；

2. "瓣周漏"可以译作"paravalvular leakage"，也可以译作"perivalvular leakage"；

3. "这个患者没有太大问题"处理为"this patient is OK"，没有必要译作"This patient doesn't have any major problems."。

完全同意刚才这位外科主任讲的，低危和低龄完全是两回事儿。你看我们今年这个XX的瓣膜批准用于低危患者，平均年龄是74岁。像国内在50多岁去给病人做，这就有很大的争议。那另外一点我们从这个美国的指南里面也可以看到，我们其实是在65岁，这是我们的底线年龄。那65岁到80岁作何选择，其实还要看患者的基本状态和预期寿命。那现在中国大概，一般除了在上海人均寿命要高一点，高于全国，大概是75到78岁。那这个生命周期管理，今天谈到这个话题，我觉得非常重要。那就是说我们现在看到，我作为一个内科医生，看到很多的患者在外科第一次瓣膜，50多岁就给了生物瓣，甚至四十八九岁，我都接触过这种患者。所以说各个地区的认识和发展也不平衡。

◎ 参考译文：I totally agree with what the director of surgery just said. Low risk and low age are two completely different things. You see, this year, our XX valve was approved for low-risk patients, and the average age is 74 years old. For example, in China, patients in their 50s are treated, this is quite controversial. Another point we can see from the U.S. guidelines is that we select the age of 65, this is our bottom line age. Then what to choose between 65 and 80 years old, actually it depends on the patient's basic condition and life expectancy. Now in China, except for Shanghai, the average life expectancy is higher than the national average, it's about 75 to 78 years old. Well, this life cycle management, we talk about this topic today, I think it is very important. That is to say, we now see that as an medical physician, many patients have their first valve in surgery department, they receive a bioprosthetic valve in their 50s, and even at the age of 48 and 49. I had such patients before. So the understanding and development in different regions are also uneven.

◎ 分析：

1. "完全是两回事儿"译作"two completely different things"。此表述在前些年口译中似乎不妥，但近几年不少美国讲者也会在演讲中使用"things"之类的表达；

2. "我们其实是在65岁"处理为"we select the age of 65"，其实是补出了讲者想表达的意思。如果译作"We are actually 65 years old"，就可能导致听众无法理解；

3. "50几岁就给了生物瓣"处理为"they receive a bioprosthetic valve in their 50s"，进行了清晰简化处理，否则在同传的情况下，直译让听众不容易理解。

真实世界的数据显示，近年来TAVR患者逐渐低危化、年轻化。根据《中国结构性心脏病年度报告（2023）》的数据，截至2023年11月30日，国内已开展TAVR手术达13万例之多，外科手术高危患者占比17.38%，中危患者44.18%，低危患者达到38.43%。与此同时，中国TAVR患者总体相对年轻，不到70岁的患者约占30%，他们有更长的预期寿命。低危、年轻患者虽然合并症较少，但对手术效果的期待更高，其全生命周期管理也更有挑战性。对于这部分患者，我们既需要重视短期手术效果，也需要着眼于未来。因此，在首次治疗时即要考虑重度主动脉狭窄患者的终身管理原则，为患者未来的多次干预提前制定方案。由于首次治疗决策对于主动脉瓣狭窄患者的长期未来具有决定性作用，首枚TAVR瓣膜的选择需要对以下五大影响低危年轻患者预后的因素进行充分考量：二叶瓣治疗难度、瓣周漏及2V-TAVR预防、传导阻滞风险、未来冠脉再介入或主瓣再干预以及耐久性的需求。XX球扩瓣在多个国内外随机对照试验中展现出优异的安全性与耐久性。XXX研究的五年随访研究结果显示，接受XX球扩瓣TAVR的患者全因死亡率仅为10%，致残性卒中、中重度瓣周漏、永久起搏器植入发生率分别为1.9%、1%、10%，患者五年内再入院率仅有10%。

◎ 参考译文：Real-world data show that TAVR patients have gradually become low risk and younger in recent years. According to the data from the "China Structural Heart Disease Annual Report（2023）", as of November 30, 2023, in China 130,000 TAVR surgeries have been performed, with 17.38% of patients with high risk for surgery, 44.18% of patients with moderate risk, and 38.43% of patients with low risk. At the same time, Chinese TAVR patients are relatively young overall, with about 30% of patients under the age of 70, and they have a longer life expectancy. Low-risk and young patients although have fewer comorbidities, they have higher expectations for surgical results, and their life cycle management is more challenging. For these patients, we need to pay attention to both short term surgical results and the future. Therefore, during the first treatment, we need to consider the lifelong management principles for patients with severe aortic stenosis, and develop plans in advance for multiple interventions in the future. Since the first treatment decision plays a decisive role in the long-term future of patients with aortic stenosis, the selection of the first TAVR valve needs to fully consider the following five factors that affect the prognosis of low-risk young patients: the difficulty of bicuspid valve treatment, paravalvular leak and 2V-TAVR prevention, conduction block risk, future coronary re-intervention or aortic valve re-intervention, and durability requirements. The XX balloon-expandable valve has shown excellent safety and durability in multiple randomized controlled trials at home and abroad. The five-year follow-up results of the XXX study showed that the all-cause mortality rate of patients who received XX balloon-expandable valve TAVR was only 10%, and disabling stroke, moderate to severe paravalvular leak, and permanent pacemaker implantation incidence rate are 1.9%, 1%, and 10%, respectively. The patient's readmission rate within five years is only 10%.

◎ 分析：

1. "合并症"译作"comorbidity"，指与原发疾病同时存在的、相互独立的一种或多种疾病或临床状态；

2. "球扩瓣"指需要用球囊扩张的瓣膜，译作"balloon-expandable valve"；

3. "再入院"译作"readmission"。

中国 TAVR 患者中二叶瓣占比显著高于其他国家。二叶瓣 TAVR 与三叶瓣相比存在较多不利解剖因素，可能导致瓣周漏、瓣膜耐久性受损和更多并发症发生，且患者的长期需求更多。针对复杂二叶瓣解剖结构，XXX 球扩瓣能够针对二叶瓣解剖难点和术后全生命周期管理的需求提供治疗方案。多项循证研究表明，球扩瓣 TAVR 在二叶瓣中可达到与三叶瓣相当的临床结果。TVT 注册研究收集了八万多名经 XXX TAVR 治疗的主动脉瓣狭窄患者，倾向配对三千对中高危患者，二叶瓣和三叶瓣的一年全因死亡或卒中发生率分别为 10.9% 和 11.2%，各项临床结局并无显著差异。XXX 二叶瓣低危患者登记研究中，二叶瓣和三叶瓣的一年主要复合终点、死亡、卒中、心血管再住院率等发生率同样并无差异。Type-0 型二叶瓣研究入选了来自中国 28 家中心的 Sievers 分型 0 型 BAV 且接受 XXX 球扩瓣进行 TAVR 治疗的患者共 112 例。随访结果显示手术技术成功率达到 99%，术后 30 天死亡或致残性卒中率仅为 0.8%，无中度及以上瓣周漏，并且为患者带来了持续的血流动力学和 NYHA 改善。

◎ 参考译文：The proportion of bicuspid valves in TAVR patients in China is significantly higher than that in other countries. Compared with tricuspid valves, bicuspid valves TAVR have more unfavorable anatomical factors, which may lead to paravalvular leak, impaired valve durability and more complications, and patients have more long-term needs. In view of the complex bicuspid valve anatomical structure, the XXX balloon-expandable valve can provide a treatment plan for the anatomical difficulties of the bicuspid valve and the needs of post-op full life cycle management. Multiple evidence-based studies have shown that balloon-expandable valve TAVR can achieve clinical results comparable to tricuspid valves in bicuspid valves. The TVT registry collected more than 80,000 patients with aortic stenosis treated with XXX TAVR, and in propensity match 3,000 pairs of medium to high risk patients, the one-year all-cause mortality or stroke incidence for bicuspid valves and tricuspid valves was 10.9% and 11.2%, respectively, and there was no significant difference in various clinical outcomes. In the XXX bicuspid valve low-risk patient registration study, there was also no difference in the one-year incidence of the primary composite endpoint, death, stroke, cardiovascular rehospitalization rate between bicuspid valves and tricuspid valves. The type-0 bicuspid valve study enrolled patients with Sievers type 0 BAV from 28 centers in China who underwent TAVR with the XXX balloon-expandable valve, in total there were 112 cases. Follow-up results showed that the technical success rate of the surgery reached 99%, the death or disabling stroke rate within 30 days after surgery was only 0.8%, there was no moderate or above level paravalvular leak, and it brought sustained hemodynamic and NYHA improvements to the patients.

◎ 分析：

1. "可达到与三叶瓣相当的临床结果"中的"相当的"译作"comparable"，这一表述在今年的会议中越来越多；

2. "Type-0 型二叶瓣研究入选了来自中国 28 家中心的 Sievers 分型 0 型 BAV 且接受 XXX 球扩瓣进行 TAVR 治疗的患者共 112 例"一句处理为"The type-0 bicuspid valve study enrolled patients with Sievers type 0 BAV from 28 centers in China who underwent TAVR with the XXX balloon-expandable valve, in total there were 112 cases."，先是预测先说出"patients"，最后补充"112 cases"；

3. "无中度及以上瓣周漏"译作"no moderate or above level paravalvular leak"，其中"以上"可用"above"来译出。

第四节　补充练习

一、中译英

目前，经导管主动脉瓣置换术（transcatheter aortic valve replacement，TAVR）已经取代外科主动脉瓣置换手术（surgical aortic valve replacement，SAVR），成为高危主动脉瓣狭窄患者首选的治疗方法，且越来越多地应用于低风险患者。与 SAVR 相比，低危和中危主动脉狭窄患者在 TAVR 术后 1 年的卒中和死亡率显著降低。有研究显示，早期 TAVR 对严重主动脉狭窄的无症状患者有明显获益。然而，在接受四维多探测器计算机断层扫描（four-dimensional multidetector computed tomography，4D MDCT）检查的患者当中，越来越多地发现 TAVR 术后经导管心脏瓣膜（transcatheter heart valve，THV）血栓的形成，其通常指瓣膜小叶上的血栓形成。

第六单元 心脏瓣膜

THV 血栓形成的临床结果可以分为瓣膜阻塞的血流动力学效应、血栓栓塞并发症以及死亡。由于病例数及临床事件较少，迄今尚无研究系统地报告所有的临床后遗症。瓣膜阻塞的血流动力学效应通常在临床上表现为心力衰竭症状，如劳力性呼吸困难。超声心动图可以确定继发于 THV 血栓形成显著瓣膜阻塞的患者。血栓栓塞，尤其是短暂性脑缺血发作（transient ischemic attack，TIA）或脑血管意外（cerebrovascular accident，CVA）是最可能被报道的临床事件。某一研究使用 MDCT 检查发现，106 例 THV 血栓形成的患者，其血栓栓塞总发生率较低；THV 血栓形成和无血栓形成患者的血栓栓塞发生率存在显著差异；THV 患者非手术 TIA 发生率较高，但缺血性卒中发生率无差异。部分其他发表的研究显示，TIA 和 CVA 发生率并无差异。THV 血栓形成的诊断和处理应基于解剖学及患者临床症状等来进行评估。

◎ **参考译文**：Currently, transcatheter aortic valve replacement (TAVR) has replaced surgical aortic valve replacement (SAVR) as the preferred treatment for patients with high-risk aortic stenosis and is increasingly being used in low-risk patients. Compared with SAVR, patients with low-risk and intermediate-risk aortic stenosis have significantly lower stroke and mortality rates 1 year after TAVR. Studies have shown that early TAVR has significant benefits for asymptomatic patients with severe aortic stenosis. However, in patients undergoing four-dimensional multidetector computed tomography (4D MDCT), the formation of transcatheter heart valve (THV) thrombosis after TAVR is increasingly found, which usually refers to thrombosis on the valve leaflets.

The clinical consequences of THV thrombosis can be divided into the hemodynamic effects of valve obstruction, thromboembolic complications, and death. Due to the small number of cases and clinical events, no study has systematically reported all clinical sequelae to date. The hemodynamic effects of valve obstruction often manifest clinically as symptoms of heart failure, such as dyspnea on exertion. Echocardiography can identify patients with significant valve obstruction secondary to THV thrombosis. Thromboembolism, particularly transient ischemic attack (TIA) or cerebrovascular accident (CVA), is the most likely clinical event to be reported. In one study using MDCT, the overall incidence of thromboembolism was low in 106 patients with THV thrombosis; there was a significant difference in the incidence of thromboembolism between patients with THV thrombosis and those without thrombosis; the incidence of nonoperative TIA was higher in THV patients, but the incidence of ischemic stroke was not different. Some other published studies have shown no difference in the incidence of TIA and CVA. The diagnosis and management of THV thrombosis should be based on anatomy and the patient's clinical symptoms.

二、英译中

More than a million people in the United States have aortic stenosis, a condition in which the aortic valve doesn't open fully because of a thickening of the valve leaflets. As a result, blood isn't adequately pumped, and pressure increases in the left ventricle, the main pumping chamber of the heart. The heart compensates by thickening its walls in order to maintain adequate pumping pressure. Without proper treatment, heart function can deteriorate.

A recent study found that when it comes to treating calcified aortic stenosis in patients with end-stage renal disease (ESRD) and heart failure with reduced ejection fraction (HFrEF), transcatheter aortic valve replacement (TAVR) and surgical aortic valve replacement (SAVR) offer distinct advantages at different stages of care. According to the research, which was published in *The American Journal of Cardiology*, TAVR was linked to better short-term outcomes while SAVR led to better long-term outcomes.

TAVR has emerged as the preferred standard of care for patients dealing with calcified aortic stenosis. However, a significant gap in knowledge existed, particularly concerning patients with ESRD on hemodialysis, as they were often excluded from pivotal trials that established TAVR's safety and efficacy. Data from a national registry also demonstrated that this vulnerable population experienced notably higher in-hospital and 1-year mortality rates compared with patients not on hemodialysis. Additionally, limited information was available regarding outcomes for patients with ESRD and HFrEF who underwent surgical interventions compared to transcatheter procedures.

To bridge this critical knowledge gap, researchers used the United States Renal Data System to identify all patients with ESRD, aortic stenosis, and HFrEF who had undergone TAVR, SAVR, or initiated dialysis after 2012, and compared survival. A comprehensive analysis was conducted using Kaplan-Meier survival curves.

The results showed that patients who underwent TAVR experienced improved survival rates compared with those under medical management. Additionally, in-hospital outcomes were in favor of TAVR, with lower in-hospital mortality rates and fewer complications observed compared with SAVR.

"This is consistent with seminal trials in TAVR and is likely a result of a minimally invasive approach and avoidance of cardiopulmonary bypass," the study authors said. On the other hand, TAVR was linked to a higher rate of pacemaker implantation.

According to the authors, the reason for this change over time is unclear, though it has been found in other similar studies comparing TAVR to SAVR with other major comorbidities. "In part, the decision to proceed with TAVR in our cohort may be based on unmeasured risk factors but all co-morbidities were similar between groups after propensity matching," they said. "The improved survival with SAVR could be explained by reduced durability of TAVR valves, however, recent studies have shown lower rates of structural valve degeneration when comparing bioprosthetic SAVR to TAVR."

They also noted that this may be due to the increased risk of paravalvular leak in TAVR, though the incidence of significant paravalvular leak is very low based on current available data.

Additionally, 19 patients who underwent SAVR and fewer than 11 patients who underwent TAVR required reintervention (P = 0.09).

"Randomized controlled trials are needed to definitively determine the best method of AVR in patients with ESRD," the authors added. "These trials should include patients with HFrEF to evaluate mortality and quality of life benefits in this patient population."

◎ **参考译文**：美国有超过一百万人口患有主动脉瓣狭窄，这是一种由于瓣叶增厚导致主动脉瓣无法完全打开的疾病。因此，血液无法充分泵送，左心室（心脏的主要泵送腔）的压力就会增加。心脏通过增厚壁来进行补偿，以保持足够的泵送压力。如果没有适当的治疗，心脏功能可能会恶化。

最近的一项研究发现，在治疗终末期肾病（ESRD）和射血分数降低的心力衰竭（HFrEF）患者的钙化主动脉瓣狭窄时，经导管主动脉瓣置换术（TAVR）和外科主动脉瓣置换术（SAVR）在不同的治疗阶段具有明显的优势。根据发表在《美国心脏病学杂志》上的研究，TAVR与更好的短期结果相关，而SAVR可带来更好的长期结果。

TAVR已成为治疗钙化性主动脉瓣狭窄患者的首选标准治疗方法。然而，知识方面存在着巨大的差距，特别是对于接受血液透析的ESRD患者，因为他们经常被排除在确定TAVR安全性和有效性的关键试验之外。来自国家登记处的数据还表明，与未接受血液透析的患者相比，这一脆弱人群的住院和1年死亡率明显更高。此外，与经导管手术相比，接受外科手术的ESRD和HFrEF患者的预后信息有限。

为了弥补这一关键的知识差距，研究人员使用美国肾脏数据系统识别了所有接受TAVR、SAVR或2012年后开始透析的ESRD、主动脉瓣狭窄和HFrEF患者，并比较了生存率。使用Kaplan-Meier生存曲线进行了全面分析。

研究结果显示，接受TAVR治疗的患者与接受医疗管理的患者相比，存活率有所提高。此外，TAVR的住院结果更佳，与SAVR相比，住院死亡率更低，并发症更少。"这与TAVR的开创性试验一致，可能是微创方法和避免体外循环的结果。"研究作者说。另一方面，TAVR与更高的起搏器植入率有关。据作者称，这种变化的原因尚不清楚，尽管在其他类似的研究中也发现了这种变化，这些研究将TAVR与SAVR与其他主要合并症进行了比较。"在某种程度上，我们决定继续进行TAVR可能是基于未测量的风险因素，但在倾向匹配后，各组之间的所有合并症都相似，"他们说，"SAVR的存活率提高可能是由于TAVR瓣膜耐久性降低所致，然而，最近的研究表明，与TAVR相比，生物瓣膜SAVR的结构性瓣膜退化率较低。"

他们还指出，这可能是由于TAVR瓣周漏风险增加，尽管根据目前可用的数据，严重瓣周漏的发生率非常低。

此外，19 名接受 SAVR 的患者和不到 11 名接受 TAVR 的患者需要再次干预（P = 0.09）。

"需要进行随机对照试验，以最终确定 ESRD 患者的最佳 AVR 方法。"作者补充道，"这些试验应包括 HFrEF 患者，以评估该患者群体的死亡率和生活质量效益。"

第七单元 神经介入

第一节 神经介入口译知识点

神经介入(neurointervention)技术,又称"神经血管介入技术",是指在医学影像设备,即数字减影血管造影(digital subtraction angiography,DSA)系统的支持下,经血管或经皮穿刺途径对中枢神经系统(大脑和脊髓)各种血管病变进行诊断及治疗的技术。神经介入技术主要用于治疗脑血管和脊髓血管病,在脑肿瘤、脊柱肿瘤等疾病的治疗上也有一定的涉及。作为目前脑血管疾病的前沿技术,该技术能针对神经系统血管疾病进行诊断和治疗,发展至今在安全性和有效性上较之前已有质的飞跃。

脑血管病(cerebrovascular disease,CVD),指各种原因导致的一个或多个脑血管病变引起的短暂性或永久性神经功能障碍,在中国已成为危害中老年人身体健康和生命的主要疾病,其死亡率和致残率位居前列,并给众多家庭带来沉重的经济负担。脑血管病的发生与发展过程受多种危险因素影响,临床上以急性发病居多。

最为普通人所熟知的脑血管病便是"中风",即"脑卒中"(stroke),特指急性脑血管病,为脑血循环障碍病因导致的突发局限性或弥散性神经功能缺损的脑部疾病的总称。随着我国居民生活方式、饮食结构的改变以及人口老龄化进程的加快等,脑卒中危险因素暴露增加,导致脑卒中发病率不断攀升。

脑血管病按病因可分为出血性(hemorrhagic)和缺血性(ischemic)两大类,按病情程度及发病特征又分为急性(acute)及慢性(chronic)两大类。

出血性脑血管病包括急性与慢性两类,急性出血性脑血管病又包括蛛网膜下腔出血(subarachnoid hemorrhage,简称"蛛血")与脑出血(intracerebral hemorrhage,ICH)。慢性脑血管病包括颅内动脉瘤(aneurysm)、脑动静脉畸形(arteriovenous malformation,AVM)和颅内异常血管网症。

缺血性脑血管病也包括急性与慢性两类,急性缺血性脑血管病包括短暂性脑缺血(transient cerebral ischemia)和急性缺血性卒中。慢性缺血性脑血管病包括动脉粥样硬化、脑动脉炎等引发的动脉狭窄和堵塞。

缺血性脑卒中相关的病灶或常见病源于颅内动脉狭窄。短暂性脑缺血发作(transient ischemic attack,TIA)指脑血管循环障碍导致的突发短暂(数分钟至数十分钟多见)的脑、脊髓或视网膜神经功能障碍。

急性缺血性卒中(acute ischemic stroke,AIS)也称"脑梗死",指因脑血循环障碍导致的脑血管病堵塞或严重狭窄，致使脑血流减少或脑供氧不足，造成脑血管供血区脑组织死亡。

颅内动脉粥样硬化性狭窄（intracranial atherosclerotic stenosis，ICAS）相关卒中的机制包括斑块破裂后引起动脉栓塞或闭塞、重度狭窄引起的血流动力学障碍、内膜增厚引起的分支闭塞性疾病，以及这些机制的组合。

ICAS 是导致我国缺血性卒中的重要原因之一，比例高达 46.6%，而在西方国家，该比例仅为 10%~15%。此外，伴有 ICAS 的患者症状更严重、住院时间更长，卒中复发率更高，且随狭窄程度的增加复发率升高，且可增加痴呆、阿尔茨海默病风险。

急性缺血性卒中是最常见的卒中类型，致死率及致残率极高，其治疗的关键是急性期，静脉溶栓（intravenous thrombolysis）可以改善患者预后，但是对大血管闭塞效果欠佳。随着血管内治疗技术及材料的发展，已有研究证实血管内治疗能显著改善颅内大血管闭塞患者预后，降低致残率和死亡率。此外，由于急性缺血性卒中治疗时间窗狭窄，高效评估病情和及时干预治疗至关重要。

出血性脑卒中相关的病灶或常见病因为颅内动脉瘤和脑动静脉畸形。蛛网膜下腔出血指在覆盖大脑（脑膜）的组织内层（软脑膜）和中间层（蛛网膜）之间的空间（蛛网膜下腔）出血。脑出血指非外伤性脑实质内的出血，是目前中老年人主要致死性疾病之一。

颅内动脉瘤（intracranial aneurysm，IA）指颅内动脉壁的囊性膨出，而并非传统意义上真正的实体肿瘤，大多是由动脉壁局部薄弱和血流冲击形成，极易破裂出血。颅内动脉瘤是出血性脑血管病中最常见且引起后果最严重的疾病之一。

脑动静脉畸形（cerebral arteriovenous malformation，cAVM）指因脑血管发育障碍导致的连接动脉和静脉的一团扩张血管，且绕过了毛细血管，并且对正常脑血流产生影响。脑出血是脑动静脉畸形最常见的临床表现。

颅内动脉瘤的治疗主要有两种方式：开颅手术及介入栓塞治疗。

开颅手术（craniotomy），即开颅后经由脑组织间的自然间隙分离脑组织，从血管外暴露动脉瘤，用动脉瘤夹从瘤颈处夹闭（clip）动脉瘤瘤颈（neck），阻断血流进入动脉瘤体内，从而去除了动脉瘤破裂与生长的风险以达治疗目的，这就是最为经典的动脉瘤瘤颈夹闭术，开颅手术也包括动脉瘤孤立术及血管搭桥术等。

介入手术则是通过血管内途径，通过股动脉或桡动脉将弹簧圈（coil）或支架送至动脉瘤内或载瘤动脉（parent artery）处释放（deploy），弹簧圈团可以直接闭塞（occlusion）动脉瘤；支架可起辅助作用或血流导向作用（flow diversion），从而降低弹簧圈团从瘤体中"掉出"的可能；也可使用血流导向装置（flow diverter，FD，或称"密网支架"），将其置于动脉瘤内或载瘤动脉处，可以减少进入瘤体的血流量，达到血流导向、血管重塑的作用；也可使用囊内扰流装置，将其直接置于动脉瘤内，起到治疗效果。动脉瘤治疗从使用技术和使用器械上可分为：单纯弹簧圈栓塞（coil embolization）、支架辅助弹簧圈栓塞（stent-assisted coiling）、密网支架植入术、载瘤动脉栓塞术等。

动脉瘤根据形态分类，可分为囊性动脉瘤（saccular）、梭形动脉瘤（fusiform）、夹层动脉瘤(dissecting)、不规则型动脉瘤(irregular shape);根据发生部位可分为前循环动脉瘤(anterior circulation),包括颈内动脉动脉瘤(ICA)、后交通动脉动脉瘤(posterior communicating artery,P-com)、脉络膜前动脉动脉瘤(anterior choroidal artery)、大脑前动脉动脉瘤(anterior cerebral artery,ACA)、前交通动脉动脉瘤(anterior communicating artery,A-com)、大脑中动脉动脉瘤(middle cerebral artery,MCA);以及后循环动脉瘤(posterior circulation),包括椎动脉动脉瘤(vertebral artery,VA)、基底动脉动脉瘤(basilar artery)、大脑后动脉动脉瘤(posterior cerebral artery,PCA);按照是否破裂分为破裂动脉瘤(ruptured)与未破裂动脉瘤(unruptured)。此外,动脉瘤还可按照病因、大小、结构等进行分类。

动脉瘤是神经介入治疗中最为常见的疾病,未破裂动脉瘤90%的患者无症状,仅仅通过常规检查可发现。动脉瘤的治疗,受到多方面因素的影响,包括动脉瘤大小、位置、破裂与否、患者意愿、就诊医院医生的技术能力等。动脉瘤的治疗极为复杂,尤其考验治疗医生的经验与技巧,动脉瘤介入治疗的出现并非完全替代了开颅手术,而是提供了一种创伤更小的方法,大多数的动脉瘤都靠介入治疗,而对于某些特定动脉瘤,还是需要开颅治疗。

脑动静脉畸形(cAVM)会造成多种严重后果,最危险的就是由于持续的高血流负荷,最终导致畸形团出血。对于检查出脑动静脉畸形的患者,应该进行积极的干预及治疗。脑动静脉畸形结构复杂,是最为复杂的脑血管疾病,治疗相对困难。针对脑动静脉畸形的治疗方法主要包括微创血管内介入栓塞、显微外科手术切除和立体定向放射治疗(stereotactic radiotherapy,SRT)三大方法。

开颅手术切除畸形团是最彻底的治疗手段,切除彻底,同时可清除血肿,但这种方法创伤大、风险高。立体定向放射治疗是利用射线照射畸形团,使其发生慢性闭塞,从而达到治疗的目的,伽玛刀(gamma knife)就是最常用的立体定向放射治疗系统,但对于体积较大的畸形团,治疗效果较差,且SRT起效慢。

血管内介入治疗则是治疗脑动静脉畸形最常用的方法,主要是将栓塞剂(embolic agent)打入供血动脉(feeding artery)和引流静脉(drainage vein),阻塞血管,以达到治疗目的。

缺血性脑卒中是因为脑血管被血栓或血块堵塞,造成血流无法通过,进而导致脑组织缺血缺氧,最终导致脑细胞死亡,造成无法恢复的伤害。过去的治疗方式大多是注射溶栓药物,即溶栓治疗(thrombolysis)。现在随着技术的进步,除了溶栓,还可进行动脉取栓(thrombectomy),即可以通过介入使用机械方式将血管内血栓取出,使用的器械一般为取栓支架,或称支架取栓器(stent retriever)。在明确诊断后,将导丝(guidewire)穿过血栓部位,然后释放支架取栓器,待取栓器与血栓充分连接或嵌入(engage)后,将支架取栓器连带血栓一同拉出,以达到取栓并恢复血管通畅的治疗效果。在这一过程中,经常需要与其他器械与技术联用,例如有时需要使用球囊,有时取栓需要与抽吸(aspiration)技术共同使用等。

第二节　真实世界口译情境

一、主题会议

随着最近四十年医学技术的发展，神经介入"从无到有"，对于颅内血管瘤、动静脉畸形、卒中、狭窄性病变等疾病的治疗，神经介入有其独到的优势，近年来神经介入领域蓬勃发展，相关器械和操作技术的更新换代速度很快，以下主题的医学会议可能涉及神经介入：

介入器械公司与国家监管机构间的咨询会议、国外神经介入大型会议的实时转播、国内各类神经介入大会、国内神经介入主题会议的操作展示、国外神经介入医生在国内进行学术路演以及神经介入器械临床应用的国内外医生交流会议等。

二、行业特点

神经介入主题会议中，最基础、最常见的是动脉瘤的治疗，但随着这一行业技术的飞速发展，医学会议中的主题早已不是动脉瘤一家独大，还包括囊内扰流装置、血流导向装置、动静脉瘘、动静脉畸形、支架取栓、颅内支架植入、人工智能的应用、新器械、新理念，神经介入医学会议中主题极为丰富。

而且这一领域会议口译主题演变的速度也令人咋舌，以动脉瘤介入治疗为例，几年之前，大量的会议还在讨论应用各类"支架辅助弹簧圈"技术来治疗动脉瘤，当时的讨论侧重于各种手法及技巧，医生的经验与技巧得到极大的重视；而近两年的同类会议中，支架辅助弹簧圈以及介入医生的经验和技巧仍然重要，但更多的演讲讨论主题则关注于血流导向装置、动脉瘤囊内扰流装置、术前规划软件的应用、介入机器人的使用等，而这些主题几年前则罕有讨论，正是因为这一行业年复一年技术的快速推陈出新，使得会议口译主题快速地更新换代。

全球多个国家的神经介入领域都发展迅速，有些特定国家的讲者，例如来自阿根廷、智利、埃及、白俄罗斯等国的医生讲者，在其他医学主题会议中难得一见，但神经介入主题会议中时有出现。随之而来的就是不同的口音、不同的理念、以及风格迥异的演讲。

三、口译难点

神经介入主题的医学会议口译难点颇多。

第一，此主题虽然名为"神经介入"，但真正的治疗操作发生于神经系统，即大脑、脊髓内部或表面的血管当中，动静脉皆有。而神经系统的血管解剖相对于其他系统的解剖，理解方式并不相同，其更加立体，对于无医学背景的译员而言难度相对较大，需要有非常好的空间想象能力。

神经介入主题会议口译中经常涉及的血管解剖名称约为四十个，偶尔会提到的还有约三十个，还有不少使用频率较低的，而其中不少血管解剖名称除完整名称之外，还有相应的缩略语。这些大量的名词与缩略语对于初涉此主题的译员无疑是一场噩梦，在会前准备不充分或没有熟悉此领域译员搭档帮助的情况下，甚至会出现难以开口的情况。

第二，因为影像技术与通信技术的发展，现在的神经介入主题会议中，"干巴巴"讲课的比例越来越少，越来越多的讲者都会在演讲时展示神经介入操作中各类血管造影、血管/器械操作的影像或图片，乃至视频；而且现在很多神经介入会议都会有手术直播的环节，即大会会场直接连线医院，将医院导管室内神经介入操作过程的关键步骤进行直播（此过程不涉及患者隐私）。直播视频中的血管解剖与影像，相较于解剖图谱上所绘制的标准血管解剖图形差异颇大，译员如果希望能够看懂甚至熟悉此类影像内容的话，只能在针对性培训后靠着一定量的会议实践积累才能有望实现。

而在进行介入操作直播时，大会会安排讨论或点评嘉宾进行实时讨论与点评，此类发言内容一般并无幻灯片或发言稿可供参考，直播画面一般为实时血管造影，译员如果看不懂，只能纯粹进行听译，这对译员的听力和口译能力提出了相对较高的要求。

第三，神经介入操作的治疗理念有别于其他治疗方式，不同于外科手术以切除、吻合或放置内植物的治疗方式。主要是使用各种器械进行栓塞（弹簧圈栓塞动脉瘤、用胶栓塞畸形团）、支撑（各类支架支撑血管壁从而影响血液流动）、调整（使用球囊进行成形或辅助其他设备）、去除（用取栓支架取出血管中的血栓），而这些操作都是在透视下进行的，并非直视，所以译员要对这些操作提前有所了解，否则纯靠听力的话，会难以理解，同传难度较大。

而且随着技术和理念的不断发展，治疗的范围越来越广，现在不仅是针对动脉系统疾病进行诊断治疗，针对静脉系统的静脉狭窄、静脉内血栓等情况，也都有相应的治疗，而这些主题在近些年的会议中也时有提及，而动脉和静脉虽然都是血管，但其结构、功能、解剖差异巨大，译员应进行额外的学习和准备。

第四，与其他介入会议非常类似，在神经介入主题的会议中，讲者会使用大量的不规则用语及英文缩略语。在中文发言时，为了表达简单快速或出于各种原因，讲者在发言时也会混杂不少英文单词及缩略语、不规则中英文表达，涉及血管解剖名称、具体操作方法、耗材/器械名称、药名等，再加上各自的口音，这需要译员有一定的相应经验或者较好的会前准备，才能快速应对。例如国内医生经常习惯讲"冒个烟"，指的是微导管进入相应血管后，想推注少量造影剂以观察血管形态、血流状态及导管位置等信息，在显示屏上动态观察之下可以看到，造影剂显示的血流由近向远，墨色渐淡，及至丝缕，宛如烟雾，俗称"冒烟"，而英语中对应的表达则是"do/give/show me an angio"。

第五，神经介入的治疗原理有其独到之处，有时理解起来有一定困难，例如治疗动静脉畸形时所用的"高压锅技术"，以及众多支架的设计原理，扰流装置型号选择时的考量等，译员均需要一定的会议经验，并结合不断的自我学习，才能有一定的理解。

第三节 中英对照篇章及分析

一、英译中

We also always recommend to do an ultrasound guide puncture. Why ultrasound? For sure you may do the puncture without ultrasound. But at the end, you don't know what is the arterial diameter, and you don't know the potential sort of complication source. For us, we always perform this with ultrasound. And we have a minimum diameter for placing, for example, 8F catheter, and the minimum will be 2.5 mm. If we have a radial artery, which is less than 2.5 mm, we normally, we don't place an 8F catheter in that location. Another point is that you need to use a dilator cocktail. The dilator cocktail contains heparin, verapamil, nitroglycerin, which is diluted in blood. And then you flush the radial artery, with this type of maneuver, you may dilate the artery 0.5 mm after 5 minutes after the cocktail, which is a lot if you consider the external diameter of the catheter. This is the typical position of the patient. We normally use this type of tools that keep the arm very close to the body of the patient. We have this position of the hand to expose the radial artery to the operator. You see how we have connected the table in order to have the catheters located in a good position. If you wanna do the radial, I recommend you to use these type of tools. Otherwise, you may have problems because you see the catheter, which is over the patient, will be with no stability. (本段内容选自2023年一位美国医生的演讲，有删改调整。)

◎ **参考译文**：我们一般都建议做超声引导穿刺，为什么要做超声呢？当然你可以做穿刺，不用超声引导，但是你不知道桡动脉的直径，就不知道潜在的并发症来源。对于我们，我们做的时候一直用超声。我们置管有最小直径，比如8F的导管，最小要2.5毫米。如果桡动脉是小于2.5毫米，通常我们就不会在这一位置用8F的导管。另外一点是你需要用扩张鸡尾酒，扩张鸡尾酒包括肝素、维拉帕米、硝酸甘油，它会在血液当中稀释。然后冲桡动脉，通过这个操作，你可以把桡动脉扩0.5毫米，大概是在使用鸡尾酒后5分钟，这个扩大的程度就很大了，如果你考虑到导管的外径。这是一个比较经典的患者体位，我们常规应用这些工具保证患者胳膊非常贴近身体，手的位置摆成这样，从而把桡动脉暴露给术者。你们也看到我们是如何把操作台连接在一起的，这样就可以确保导管的位置良好。如果你想做桡动脉的话，我建议大家用这些工具。否则的话就可能会出问题，因为你们看到导管就会在患者的身上，就不是很稳固了。

◎ **分析**：

1. 近年来，"do the puncture"这样的表达在非英语母语讲者的讲话中屡见不鲜，非常符合中文的习惯，可将其处理成"做穿刺"；

2. "arterial diameter"译作"桡动脉的直径"，增加了重要的信息，但因为上下文语义明确，并不会让听众造成误解；

3. "placing"译作"置管",如果译作"放置"或"插管",感觉稍显不足或过度;

4. 以"8F"为例,其中的"F"的意思为French,是单位,有时也写作"Fr"。国外讲者有时将其读作"eight F",有时读作"eight French",口译时译员直接将其读作"八F"即可,切勿读作"八French"甚至"八法国"等;

5. "which is a lot"译作"这个扩大的程度就很大了"。其中,"扩大"最好改为"扩张",更符合这一主题的语言表达习惯。同传中,其实译得越多,出错的概率就越大,此处译作"这就很多了",要比多译更好,同时也能节省一半的时间;

6. "typical position"译作"比较经典的患者体位";

7. "no stability"译作"不是很稳固了",其实就是"就不稳定了"。这就是同传时的随口语义弱化,将讲者明确的意义习惯性地弱化或加上怀疑,抑或加上一些副词,例如"就可能不稳了""可能就不很稳了"等。

And this is an example of the CTA but it's only to show that even the radial has different anatomical variations. So we need to understand which artery you are facing in order to decrease the potential complications. This is an example of the elongation of the artery. The way to do this is only to push the wire and then do a straight at the artery. And this is the most frequent type of navigation that we have in their radial approach. This is the typical setup that we use for radial navigation. We don't do exchange maneuver. We normally use a long, 130 cm, Simmons 1 or Simmons 2 for co-axially navigated a very big catheter, like in 088 Ballast or similar. This is an example of my fellow that was performing her first approach of 8F system. She already performed before, as mentioned, 100 diagnostic angio. So this is the regular technique. Again, even a very young fellow may do this, so the complexity is not significant. But at the end, you see that we are very precise with the puncture with a guide ultrasound. We previously place there. And you see how precise is during the ultrasound. You don't require multiple maneuvers for doing that. And at the end, that means that you are decreasing the rate of vasospasm, which may limits the technique.

◎ **参考译文**:这是一个CTA的例子,但是只是给大家展示一下,桡动脉也有不同的解剖变异。所以我们必须了解,我们所处理的动脉到底是什么样的,这样才能够减少并发症的发生。这是一个动脉延长的例子,做法就是,你只需要推进导丝,然后拉直就行。这是最常见的一种操作,桡动脉入路的方式。这个是我们桡动脉操作常用的一种设置。我们不做交换操作,通常就是用一个比较长的、130厘米的Simmons 1或Simmons 2,同轴输送进一个大导管,像088的Ballast或者类似的。这里举个例子,是我的fellow,正在做她第一次的8F系统的入路。她之前已经做过,就像之前说过的,做过了100多例诊断造影。所以这就是一个常规的技术,甚至一个非常年轻的从业人员也可以完成,所以也不是很复杂。最后,你们可以看到,我们的穿刺在超声的引导下是非常准确的。我们之前放在那里,你可以看到它是多么地精准,用超声引导。这么做不需要很多复杂的操作。最后,这意味着你能够减低血管痉挛率,血管痉挛可能会限制这一技术。

◎ **分析**：

1. "facing"译作"所处理的"，表面上并不影响理解，但稍作分析就知不妥，桡动脉只是血管通路，真正要"处理"的病灶是颅内的血管病变，只是在选择桡动脉入路时，桡动脉会有解剖变异，而术者在面对不确定的血管解剖结构时，需要提前有所了解。所以译作"处理"并不妥，但同传时这样的处理也可接受，并不影响沟通；

2. "navigation"译作"操作"。"navigation"的本义是"导航"，但在此处译作导航不符合此主题的表达习惯，故处理为"操作"；

3. "fellow"直接跟读即可，因为此处指代意义不明，可能是指代进修医生，也可能是接受培训的住院医生，也可能是学生，也可能是讲者医疗组内的低年资医生。近年来，国内医生对于fellow的概念接受程度也越来越高，直接跟读不会造成听众的理解障碍；

4. "may do this"译作"也可以完成"，这其实又是译员口译时的随口近义词替换。"可以做"并不意味着"能够完成"，区别还是有的。

We normally use for a stroke, long sheath for the left side. Sorry, for the right side. And for the left side, we use ballon-guide catheter. And I will see some images of that. So this is the typical image of bovine anatomic variation with the radial approach is used in the first line. But compared with the right femoral approach, you see how tractable is the catheter. And you may achieve a very distal navigation with no problems. So, it's very important also to do a good compression after finish. So what after finish? We use this type of bandages, I think it's highly recommended to do this, because a good compression may be significant, because you may have a radial artery enough for doing a second procedure. If you don't do a good compression, what is gonna happen is you're gonna have a thrombosis of the artery after all, which maybe needs a potential secondary treatment. It's very important to achieve a very distal position, be proximal is not enough, because you may have failures of recanalization of a stroke. That's why we try to recommend to achieve a distal position even over the tortuosity. This is a good example to see how this long sheath of the Ballast navigated through the tortuosity in this super kind of occlusion through the radial approach, you may achieve this type of distal navigation of the catheter.

◎ **参考译文**：我们处理卒中一般都会用比较长的鞘，用于左侧，啊抱歉是右侧。而左侧是用球囊引导导管。我给大家展示几张影像，这个是一个典型的牛型动脉变异，桡动脉入路一线应用。但相比于右侧股入路，你可以看到导管更容易操作，而且上到远端完全没有问题。非常重要的就是结束后好好加压包扎。所以结束之后该怎么做呢？我们用这种绷带。我强烈推荐这么做，因为好的加压非常重要，因为你可能还有一根桡动脉足够做第二次的操作。如果你加压不好，就可能在动脉中出现血栓，那可能就会需要二次治疗。还有一点很重要，就是我们要做到非常远端的到位，近端到位是不够的，因

第七单元 神经介入

为你可能无法卒中再通。这就是为什么我们建议远端到位，即使要经过迂曲解剖。这是一个很好的例子，可以看到 Ballast 的长鞘管是如何通过这种超级闭塞的迂曲解剖，用的是经桡入路，你可以实现这种类型的导管的远端到位。

◎ 分析：

1. "long sheath"译作"长鞘管"，"比较长的鞘"也能理解，但并非专业表达；

2. "ballon-guide catheter"译作"球囊导引导管"，但一般不说"球囊引导导管"，常用 BGC 作为其简称；

3. "compression"指"加压包扎"，用得比较少，一般用"pressure bandaging/dressing"表示"加压包扎"。"加压包扎"指软组织损伤处理后，用弹力绷带包扎伤口，可以控制水肿，较少炎症反应充血等；

4. "tortuosity"意思是"迂曲"，此处处理为"迂曲解剖"，多出解剖二字，是为了符合中文表达习惯。

So if you wanna place the vein, I will show you what is the technique, but it's a little bit different. It's recommended to use this. If you want to avoid this type of complication. This is a case, a patient that we embolize intracranial dural fistula. And we do a jugular approach and we had this tremendous hematoma after the embolization. That's why we tried to adapt their arm approach into the venous side. This is the venous variation, as you see, our selection was the cephalic vein, or the basilic vein. This is the two different anatomical variations. We don't recommend to puncture below the elbow, because there veins are very small. So we recommend to puncture over the elbow. Again, basilic or cephalic. So this will be the typical setup, for example, embolizing an intracranial AVM or intracranial dural fistula, will be one radial and two veins, for example. This is a typical approach only through the arm. You may do whatever you want. Basilic vein is bigger, but it's less comfortable because it's in the inner part of the arm. The cephalic vein is a little bit smaller, but is much comfortable for us to be punctured. The good news is that the veins are super big, normally are more than 3 mm. So it's very easy, much easier than arterial site.

◎ 参考译文：如果你想放静脉的话，我来给大家展示一下这个技术，但有点不一样。建议用这个，如果你想避免这种并发症的话。这个病例，我们给患者栓塞颅内硬膜瘘。我们做颈静脉入路，有一个巨大的血肿，是在栓塞后出现的。这就是为什么我们要去调整到手臂入路进入静脉。这个是静脉变异，可以看到我们的方案是头静脉或者是贵要静脉。这是两个不一样的解剖变异，我们不建议在肘下穿刺，因为那里的静脉非常细。我们建议是在肘上穿刺，再强调一次，是头静脉或者是贵要静脉。这是一个典型的处理方法，比如栓塞颅内的 AVM 或者是硬膜瘘，会用一条桡动脉入路，两条静脉入路。比如这是典型的入路，只过手臂，你想做什么都可以。贵要静脉更粗，但是不舒服，因为它是在手臂的内侧。头静脉细一点，但是对我们来说穿刺舒服得多。好消息是静脉很粗，一般都超过三毫米，所以是很容易的，要比动脉穿刺容易得多。

◎ 分析：

1. "if you wanna place the vein"，指的是穿刺静脉进行颈静脉介入治疗，此处处理为"如果你想放静脉的话"；

2. "typical setup"处理为"典型的处理方法"，此处的"setup"指的是一系列的操作、器械和方法的组合；

3. "The cephalic vein is a little bit smaller"和"Basilic vein is bigger"译作"头静脉细一点"和"贵要静脉更粗"，更符合此语境。

This is, for example, a large P-com aneurysm. It looks an easy case for flow diverter. For example, that's why we placed the flow diverter. But in the last picture with a yellow arrow there, that right after the deployment of the device and after retrieving the micro catheter, we do the run and all the proximal of the stent migrated into the aneurysm. This is a trivial complication and very difficult to solve. So we were spending three or four hours trying to renavigate it again through the micro, so through the stent, we use different types of wires, micro catheters, everything maneuvers. It was a real nightmare for me, and I remember this case as a nightmare. So I spent, I think, five hours and at the end, we found out one possible solution was to inflate a balloon between the stent and the lumen, there are two lumen of the aneurysm, inflated very gently, at the same time, we pulled back very gently the balloon. And with the second microwire, we navigate it inside of the stent and we pull everything back in order to leave the stent just at the level of the neck. And after that, we placed, I think, was two flow diverters in order to do a fully reconstruction. This is an example of a very complex maneuver. At the end, the results were good, but they were really complex to fill this.

◎ **参考译文**：这个是一个大的 P-com 动脉瘤。看起来很简单，用血流导向装置就行，所以我们就放置了血流导向装置。但是在最后一张图，黄色的箭头那里。就在器械释放之后，我们收回微导管之后，我们做了造影，看到支架的全部近端都移位到了动脉瘤内。这是一个很小的并发症，但是很难解决，我们花了三四个小时努力重新调整，通过微导管调整，穿支架，我们用了不同的导丝、微导管，所有的操作。对我来说真的是个噩梦，我一直记得这个病例，就是一场噩梦。我花了大概五个小时，最后呢，我们找到了一个可行的解决方案，就是打一个球囊，放在支架和管腔之间，这个动脉瘤有两个管腔，非常小心地把球囊打起来，与此同时，我们把球囊轻轻地拉出来。然后用第二根微导丝，把它上到支架内，然后把所有东西都向后拉，从而把支架留在瘤颈的位置。在这之后，我们又放了两根血流导向装置，目的是完全重建。这个例子的操作非常复杂，最后结果是很好的，但是确实非常复杂，很难填上。

◎ 分析：

1. "a large P-com aneurysm"译作"一个大的 P-com 动脉瘤"，在同传的语境下是可

以接受的，但也可直接译作"大的后交通动脉瘤"，"P-com"是"posterior communicating artery"的简称，即"后交通动脉"，这是神经介入主题中的基础词汇；

2. "flow diverter"译作"血流导向装置"，没有问题，但现在不少国内医生也将其称为"密网支架"，两者是一个概念；

3. "renavigate it again through the micro, so through the stent"处理为"重新调整，通过微导管调整，穿支架"，此处的两个"through"意义不同，第一个指"通过"，同"by/via"；第二个指的是"穿过"，同"go through/across"。这里的"micro"指的是微导管，也是简称，译员须结合上下文补出，否则听众无法理解。此处的翻译有一定难度，译员需要理解讲者的逻辑，能够基本理解讲者展示的图片。

The S stent device is a stent made of woven nitinol stents with low porosity folded in a plastic sheath, characterized by its flexibility and self-expanding properties. Its porosity is 45%~60%, and it has a 9mm distal radiopaque tip. It is deployed by careful pressure on the retraction of the delivery line and microcatheter; an advantage of the device is that it can be re-sheathed, even if it has been deployed up to 90%. Also, the conveying system has an improved pusher profile to achieve the best compromise between flexibility and pushability. Since the introduction of auxiliary stent implantation for the treatment of fusiform aneurysms in the 1990s, in the past decade, S stents have been used to maintain blood flow in arteries, excluding aneurysms sacs. These instruments were known as the flow diverter devices, FD, and they have become critical instruments; several kinds have been used to treat intracranial aneurysms (IAs) over recent years. （本段内容选自2024年一篇论文，有删改调整。）

◎ **参考译文**：S支架是一款镍钛诺的编织支架，孔隙率低，支架折叠在塑料鞘管中，它的特点是它的灵活性和自膨特性。它的孔隙率是45%~60%，并且有9毫米的远端不透射线尖端。通过仔细地对输送器材和微导管的回退和加压来释放这款导管；它的一个优势是可回收，哪怕支架已经释放了90%也可回收。此外，输送系统的推进器大小也有改进，来获得最佳的灵活性和推送性间的平衡。自从引入辅助支架植入用于治疗梭形动脉瘤以来，这始于20世纪90年代，在过去的10年中，S支架已被用于维持动脉血流，封堵动脉瘤囊。这些器械被称为血流导向装置，FD，它们已经成为了重要的器械；已有数种被用于治疗颅内动脉瘤(IAs)，这是近几年的情况。

◎ **分析**：

1. "nitinol"译作"镍钛诺"，镍钛诺是镍和钛的非磁性合金，有记忆形状、超弹性等特性，在医疗领域应用广泛；

2. "porosity"译作"孔隙率"，是所有支架的一个客观指标，指支架的孔洞空隙所占据的比例，用百分比表示；

3. "radiopaque"译作"不透射线"，意思是此部分器械的材料不透射线，即通过透视可以显影，因此在造影时可以看到，也可直接译作"显影"；

4. "re-sheath"意思是"重新入鞘"，这里可直接译作"回收"；

5. "compromise"意思是"折中、妥协",此处译作"平衡"较好;

6. "exclude"此处指"将……排除在外",此处译作"封堵"。此处同传难度较大,可能被译员随口译作"不包括"或"排除",导致听众理解困难。

The first FD to obtain European Commission approval was the S flow diverter in 2008. Eventually, short-and mid-term findings have been reported. FDs redirect blood flow from the aneurysm, prevent thrombosis development, promote neo-intimal growth along with the mesh, and reconstruct the parent artery. The safety and efficacy of FD treatment for many complex IAs have been recorded in numerous studies. In the Briganti and collaborators systematic review, more than half of small IAs were treated with FDs. Despite the vast number of studies on the effectiveness of FDs in treating aneurysms, numerous unexpected adverse effects have also been reported. In addition, there is a lack of research on the problems associated with this approach. Few studies have examined clinical and technological incidents in the use of FDs to treat IAs systematically.

◎ 参考译文:首个获得欧盟委员会批准的 FD 是 2008 年的 S 血流导向装置。最终,短期和中期结果有所报道。FD 可以改变动脉瘤的血流方向,防止血栓形成,促进新生内膜沿网孔生长,并重建载瘤动脉。FD 治疗众多复杂颅内动脉瘤的安全性和有效性在大量研究中都有记录。在 Briganti 及其合作者的系统综述中,超过一半的小型颅内动脉瘤都使用 FD 治疗。尽管有大量的研究聚焦于 FD 治疗动脉瘤的有效性,但也有大量的意想不到的不良反应有所报告。此外,也缺乏对这种方法相关问题的研究。很少有研究分析过使用 FD 治疗动脉瘤的临床和技术事故,进行系统性的分析。

◎ 分析:

1. "mesh"指代支架/血流导向装置表面的网格/网孔样结构;

2. "parent artery"译作"载瘤动脉",这是神经介入主题的基础词汇,是其唯一的译法;

3. "systematic review"译作"系统综述",系统综述是一种方法,指系统地汇总、评估并综合研究文献,从而回答特定的问题或评估特定治疗方法的效果;

4. "IA"指"intracranial aneurysm",即"颅内动脉瘤";

5. "approach"在医学口译中有多重含义,最主要的是"(手术)入路",此处可处理为"方法"。

The S Flow Diverter is a self-expandable stent braided from 48 nitinol wires. The DIVERSION registry is a prospective multicenter study covering all consecutive FD patients in French participating centers between October 2012 and February 2014. IAs care remains a significant obstacle for modern medicine. In massive subarachnoid dissections and in using multiple clips for artery reconstruction in cases of dysplastic and giant aneurysms, surgical developments have been introduced. However, the S FD has shown mounting evidence in the management of this disease; therefore, the primary goal of this study was to determine the effect of the S flow diverter device on neurological prognosis and mortality in intracranial aneurysms.

◎ **参考译文**：S血流导向装置是一种自膨式支架，由48根镍钛诺合金丝编织而成。DIVERSION登记是一项前瞻性多中心研究，涵盖了法国的参与中心的所有连续FD患者，时间是从2012年10月到2014年2月。颅内动脉瘤的诊疗仍然是现代医学的一大障碍。对于巨大的蛛网膜下腔夹层，以及使用多个动脉瘤夹进行发育不良及巨大动脉瘤的动脉重建，外科手术的进展也已经介绍过了。但是，S血流导向装置在这种疾病的管理中显示出越来越多的证据；因此，本研究的主要目标是确定S血流导向装置对颅内动脉瘤的神经系统预后和死亡率的影响。

◎ **分析**：

1. "self-expandable stent"译作"自膨式支架"或"自膨胀式支架"，自膨式支架是超弹性支架，通过输送导管到达病变处，释放后支架自动膨胀扩张；

2. "clip"在此处译作"动脉瘤夹"，补充了"动脉瘤"，要比译作"夹子"更符合这一语境。

The S diverter device has a good safety and efficacy profile for treating intracranial aneurysms with high complete occlusion rates. With appropriate mortality and morbidity rates in complicated aneurysms, it is a safe care option that is unlikely to be handled with other techniques. There is, however, a chance of neurologic morbidity and ischemic incidents due to the procedure. It is essential to study the mechanism of delayed rupture after flow diversion to determine the required perioperative medication and optimal implantation method. Further studies are needed to provide reliable data on the technique's safety and delayed rupture after the procedure.

◎ **参考译文**：S血流导向装置治疗颅内动脉瘤具有良好的安全性和疗效，完全闭塞率高。在复杂动脉瘤中死亡率和发病率较合适，是一种安全的治疗选择，不大可能用其他技术处理。然而，由于存在神经系统发病率和缺血事件的可能性，这一操作有这些可能性，至关重要的就是研究血流导向后延迟破裂的机制以确定所需的围手术期用药和最佳的植入方法。需要进一步研究，以提供这一技术的安全性和术后延迟破裂的可靠数据。

◎ **分析**：

1. "safety and efficacy profile"中的"profile"一般不用译出，译作"安全性和疗效"即可。

二、中译英

它的穿刺效率相对来说也更加提高了。可以说，借用××医院的一个同事的话就是，因为我们的这个翻台率非常快，每天能够完成的任务就非常多。所以说，我们私下里来谈，就是说前一个病人下去以后，后面一个病人上来，然后我们踩下去第一脚，我们叫这个给"图像"。图像第一脚踩下去，这个时间5分钟。就是说下一个病人上去以后，消好毒，穿好刺，第一脚看你导丝送进去了，比较理想的时间是5分钟，把消毒算在内了。所以，这个目前来说，我们对于桡动脉穿刺的要求，逐渐地从手术成功，变成一个高效的手术成功。这个目前来说，这是我们在桡动脉穿刺方面的进展。对于心内科，我们对于时间上的要求相对来说更加严格。（本段内容选自2023年一位国内医生的演讲，有删改调整。）

◎ **参考译文**：Its puncture efficiency has been relatively improved. To quote a sentence from a colleague from XX Hospital, he said that because our room turnover is very fast, we complete a lot of tasks every day. We privately say that the previous patient leaves, the next patient comes, and then we step down for the first time, we say to have the angio, the first step for the angio, and this time is 5 minutes. That is to say, after the next patient comes, after disinfection, after puncture, the first step, the guidewire is sent in within the specified time, the ideal time is 5 minutes, including disinfection. At present, our requirements for radial artery puncture have gradually changed from being successful to efficient. At present, radial artery puncture, compared with cardiology, our requirements for time are more strict.

◎ **分析**：

1. 本段文本除了隐去敏感信息外，保留了讲者大量的口头禅，这位讲者代表了一类讲者的风格，在演讲时会掺杂大量的口头禅以及重复无用的信息，此时译员最好能做到"过滤式翻译"，对于"一个""这个"之类的表达，无须"忠实于讲者"，否则会导致译语凌乱不堪，下面总结出了本段"过滤无用信息后"所提取的有用信息："它的穿刺效率相对来说提高了。借用××医院的一个同事的话，他说因为我们的翻台非常快，每天完成的任务非常多。我们私下里说，前一个病人下去，后一个病人上来，然后我们踩下去第一脚，我们说给图像，图像第一脚踩下去，这个时间是5分钟。就是说下一个病人上去以后，消好毒，穿好刺，第一脚，导丝送进去，规定时间，比较理想的时间是5分钟，算消毒在内。目前我们对桡动脉穿刺的要求，逐渐从成功变成高效，目前桡动脉穿刺，相对于心内科，我们对于时间的要求更加严格。"

2. "翻台率"译作了"room turnover"，room指operation room，即手术室，翻台意思是在手术室完成一台手术后，将前一位患者送出，完成手术室的清洁和下一台手术的准备，再将下一台手术的患者送入手术室的过程，现代大型医院都致力于提升手术室的利用率，美国医院尤甚。

冠脉介入当中确实有很多有挑战性的病变。目前来说，非常公认的最有挑战的一个病变，冠脉介入，这个CTO病变，就是指我们血管100%堵塞了。那么，它的一个远端血管或者远端心肌的供血，实际上是通过侧支循环来供应的，这种病变我们目前来说还是非常有挑战性，也被誉为冠脉介入领域的"最后的堡垒"。针对这个病变，目前来说，全球的手术成功率的普遍情况是这样的，差不多在比较大的顶级医院，基本上它的手术成功率，差不多在 80% 到 85% 之间。所以说，这个水平已经是全球顶级的医院能够达到的一个 level，对于一些普通的一些相对来说等级差一点的医院，它的手术成功率甚至只有百分之四五十的样子。所以，对于这种病变，如果说出现了影响我们手术成功率的情况，那我们这个桡动脉还是不能考虑。因为会把我们手术成功率的最初情况给改变了，那是不行的。

◎ **参考译文**：So in coronary intervention, there are many challenging lesions. And this is a generally acknowledged most challenging lesion. Coronary intervention, CTO lesion means that the vessel is 100% occluded. And the distal vessel and distal myocardium blood supply, actually is supplied by the collateral circulation. This lesion, for us, currently is very challenging and it is regarded as "the last fortress" in coronary intervention. And for this lesion, currently, the global procedure success rate is, for top-level big hospitals, the surgical success rate, is around 80% to 85%, around this level. And this level is the top-level hospitals around the world, and for some lower-level hospitals, the surgical success rate is only 40% to 50%. So for this lesion, if it disturbs the success rate, we still cannot consider radial artery. Because this, the success rate is actually the priority, so if it's against it, it's not acceptable.

◎ **分析**：
1. "病变"译作"lesion"，这是医学口译中的词汇；
2. "心肌"译作"myocardium"，也可译作"cardiac muscle"。

另外就是出血方面的问题。出血颈动脉颅内动脉瘤治疗。因为我本身是做缺血的医生，所以这一块还不是了解得特别深入。但是可以看到似乎是出血性疾病，更适合经桡去做。因为我们知道经桡在缺血里头有好多病人年龄大，他有很多这个严重血管迂曲，或者是有严重的血管动脉粥样硬化，这个在通路中还是有些问题的。但是出血性疾病可能更年轻，可能血管弹性更好，那更适合去做，现在看起来这个是更适合的，也有大量文献，不管是做栓塞还是做导流装置这些，这个都是有很好的结果的。最后就是经桡在取栓中的应用，这一块可能是最后的挑战。如果说把急诊的这个取栓能够去克服的话，那么经桡在神经介入领域的地位就没什么阻碍了，实际上我们可以知道确实有一些取栓病号儿是非常适合经桡的。

◎ **参考译文**：Another issue is bleeding, the treatment of intracranial aneurysms. Since I am a doctor who specializes in ischemia, I am not particularly in-depth in this area. However, it seems that hemorrhagic diseases are more suitable for transradial approach. Because we know that many patients with ischemia are older, have severe vascular tortuosity, or have severe vascular atherosclerosis, which still has some problems in the access. Patients with hemorrhagic diseases may be younger, and their blood vessels may be more elastic, so they are more suitable for this. Now it seems that this is more suitable. There are a lot of literatures, whether it is embolization or flow diverters, there are very good results. Finally, the use of transradial approach in thrombectomy may be the last challenge. If emergency thrombectomy can be overcome, then there will be no obstacles to transradial approach in the field of neuro intervention. In fact, we know that there are indeed some thrombectomy patients that are very suitable for transradial thrombectomy.

◎ 分析：
1."经桡"指"经桡动脉入路"，译作"transradial approach"；
2."出血性疾病"译作"hemorrhagic diseases"。

再提一下路径的并发症。一个是罕见的上肢筋膜间隙综合征。第二个呢，桡动脉的痉挛。那么痉挛跟刚刚鸡尾酒这个地方，已经阐述过了。这个是强烈推荐使用硝酸甘油，维拉帕米的组合，包括肝素以及组合的这样的一个鸡尾酒的使用。这样的话呢，可以非常显著地降低桡动脉痉挛的风险。但这个地方呢，也要注意，就这些经验是来自冠脉，冠脉的手术都是局麻，而我们现在是大量全麻的手术，我们全麻手术过程中使用这个鸡尾酒会导致血压偏低，所以我们在做出血性的疾病一般不太会有问题。但当你是做一个颅内的狭窄全麻手术，如果你已经麻好了一支鸡尾酒进去，血压掉到六七十，可能会诱发术中的缺血事件，所以这个是需要你跟麻醉医生之间要形成个非常好的沟通，甚至在局麻下完成鸡尾酒的给药，再进行全麻，这也是个选择。

◎ 参考译文：I would like to mention the complications of the pathway. One is the compartment syndrome of the upper limb, which is rare. The second is radial artery spasm. We have already explained. For this one, it is highly recommended to use the combination of nitroglycerin and verapamil, including heparin and the cocktail. This can significantly reduce the risk of radial artery spasm. However, we should also remind you that these experiences come from coronary artery. Coronary artery surgery is all done under local anesthesia, while we are now doing a lot of general anesthesia. The use of cocktails during general anesthesia surgery can cause lower blood pressure, so we generally do not have problems with hemorrhagic diseases. However, if you are doing general anesthesia surgery for intracranial stenosis, after anesthesia, if you give a cocktail injection, the blood pressure will drop to 60 or 70, which may induce intra-op ischemic events. So, this requires very good communication between you and anesthesia physicians. Even to complete the cocktail administration under local anesthesia and then perform general anesthesia, is also an option.

◎ 分析：
1."桡动脉的痉挛"译作"radial artery spasm"，"动脉痉挛"译作"artery spasm"，是指因导丝、导管等腔内器械反复刺激血管，或管腔内停留时间过长，导致动脉中层平滑肌的持续收缩，从而导致管腔缩小或闭塞的现象；
2."鸡尾酒"译作"cocktail"，医学口译中的鸡尾酒指的是"鸡尾酒疗法"，就是将不同药物混合后使用，比如传染病领域有 HIV 的鸡尾酒治疗，骨科领域有鸡尾酒镇痛。此处指的是将部分药物混合后，用于预防或解除动脉痉挛。

第七单元 神经介入

神经介入的范畴是整个的脑血管，关联三大类疾病——动脉性疾病，包括动脉瘤和动脉管腔的狭窄、静脉疾病和动静脉畸形。脑血管领域高质量的研究很多，但是依然远远少于心血管。2002年美国发表了相关指南，并于2009年做了简单的更新。2012年，得益于材料、技术的发展，该指南再一次更新。在美国，80%的医生首选介入治疗动脉瘤，从2007年开始颅内动脉瘤的介入栓塞已经超过了开颅。在中国，受经济发展、医保政策的关联，在东部一些发达的地区，神经介入栓塞动脉瘤成为了首选的治疗方式，但是在一些西部欠发达的地区，这一选择可能会少一些。在我们医院，介入动脉瘤栓塞的比例在90%以上。颅内狭窄是我们中国人特有的发病率非常高的一类疾病。2005年之后，我们认识到，颅内狭窄似乎应该更积极地做介入干预，因为再发卒中的风险高达23%。（本段内容选自2018年一位国内医生的演讲，有删改调整。）

◎ **参考译文**：The scope of neuro intervention is the entire cerebrovascular system, which is related to three major types of diseases: arterial disease, including aneurysms and stenosis of the arterial lumen, venous disease, and arteriovenous malformations. There are many high-quality studies in the field of cerebrovascular diseases, but they are still far less than cardiovascular diseases. In 2002, in the United States relevant guidelines were published and a simple update was made in 2009. In 2012, thanks to the development of materials and technology, the guidelines were updated again. In the United States, 80% of doctors prefer interventional treatment for aneurysms. Since 2007, interventional embolization of intracranial aneurysms has exceeded craniotomy. In China, due to economic development and medical insurance policies, neurointerventional embolization of aneurysms has become the preferred treatment method in some developed areas in the east, but in some underdeveloped areas in the west, this selection may be less. In our hospital, the percentage of interventional aneurysm embolization is over 90%. Intracranial stenosis is a type of disease with a very high incidence rate that is unique to us Chinese. After 2005, we realized that intracranial stenosis should be treated with more active interventions because the risk of recurrent stroke is as high as 23%.

◎ **分析**：
1. "开颅"译作"craniotomy"，指"开颅手术"，是医学神经领域的一个基础词汇；
2. "积极"译作"active"，有时也可译作aggressive。

在美国的指南中，大家也可以看到，对于中度的狭窄，即70%以下的狭窄，无论怎么发生卒中，都不建议采用介入干预。在颅内狭窄的研究中，给我们一些提示：对于神经内科的医生，80%的医生会选择保守治疗，而神经介入的医生，选择介入的医生会显著地下降，这个数量会有非常明显的变化。在西方，当你碰到了一个病人药物治疗无效的时候，你会考虑对这个病人做什么呢？18%的人会仍然考虑维持原来的药物治疗，82%的人会采用新的单纯球囊扩张来治疗。所以颅内狭窄是不是变成了一滩死水？很显然不是，我们根据不同的病人要探索不同的策略，采用合适的介入策略。

◎ **参考译文**：In the U. S. guidelines, you can also see that for moderate stenosis, that is stenosis less than 70%, no matter how the stroke occurs, interventional treatment is not recommended. In the study of intracranial stenosis, some suggestions were provided: for neurologists, 80% of them will choose conservative treatment, while for neurointerventional physicians, the number of physicians who choose intervention will drop significantly, and this number will change significantly. In the West, when you encounter a patient who doesn't respond to drug treatment, you will consider what to do with the patient. 18% of people will still consider maintaining the original drug treatment, and 82% will use the new simple balloon dilatation for treatment. So has intracranial stenosis become a stagnant pool? Obviously not, we need to develop different strategies according to different patients and adopt appropriate interventional strategies.

◎ **分析**：

1. "保守治疗"译作"conservative treatment"，就是不用介入或手术治疗，主要靠药物治疗；

2. "探索不同的策略"在此处译作"develop different strategies"，更符合语境，优于"explore"。

在各国的指南中，对于症状性的颅内狭窄，大家相对的争议比较少，而无症状的颅内狭窄争议非常大。对于无症状性的颅内狭窄，很多人的建议是只有在并发症的发生率小于3%的情况下，才可以考虑做介入的干预。我们发现强化的药物治疗对于颅内狭窄的治疗非常好。那么，强化的药物治疗对颈动脉狭窄的疗效是否积极呢？美国数据显示，整个颈动脉狭窄的治疗量是下降的，我们现在的最佳药物治疗的疗效有了显著的改进。

◎ **参考译文**：In the guidelines of various countries, there is relatively less controversy about symptomatic intracranial stenosis, but there is a lot of controversy about asymptomatic intracranial stenosis. For asymptomatic intracranial stenosis, many people suggest when the incidence of complications is less than 3%, the interventional treatment can be considered. We found that intensive drug therapy is very good for the treatment of intracranial stenosis. So, is the effect of intensive drug therapy positive for carotid stenosis? Data from the United States show that the overall treatment volume for carotid stenosis is decreasing, and the efficacy of our current best drug therapy has improved significantly.

◎ **分析**：

1. "强化的药物治疗"译作"intensive drug therapy"，"强化"一词在不同的语境下可以译作"intensive""enhanced"或"augmented"；

2. "无症状性的"译作"asymptomatic"，后者读音的重音虽然在第二个字母 a 上，但为了与"symptomatic"区分,大多数讲者都会重度第一个字母 a,读作"A symptomatic",口译时译员应予以注意;

3. "颈动脉狭窄"译作"carotid stenosis",但某些非英语母语讲者会使用"narrowing"。

现在最热门的是颅内大血管的闭塞,在中国能下沉到县级医院,未来的十年到二十年,颅内大血管闭塞的技术会快速发展。我们都知道从最早的 1999 年发表的动脉溶栓到现在已经探索了十几年,这里面有几个标志性的事件,第一个事件是 2012 年定义了最有效的支架型取栓器,2013 年"新英格兰"连发了三篇研究,采用的是第一代的取栓器械,对我们临床的指导价值并不大,我们都在期待 2012 年以后采用的支架型取栓器。2015 年的五个 RCT 研究,同时在"新英格兰"发表,采用的都是第二代的支架内取栓器开通大血管,都得到了一致的临床结果。在神经外科领域,我们认为这是一项了不起的技术,给我们广大的脑卒中病人带来了非常大的福音。

◎ **参考译文**:The most popular one nowadays is the intracranial large vessel occlusion. In China, this can be carried out in county-level hospitals. In the next ten to twenty years, the technology for intracranial large vessel occlusion will develop rapidly. We all know that since the earliest arterial thrombolysis was published in 1999, till now, exploration has been around for more than ten years. There have been several landmark events. The first event was the definition of the most effective stent retriever in 2012. In 2013, *NEJM* consecutively published three studies using the first generation of thrombectomy devices, which were not of much value in guiding our clinical practice. We were all looking forward to the stent retriever adopted after 2012. Five RCT studies in 2015 were published at the same time in *NEJM*. They all used the second-generation stent retriever to open the large vessels, and all obtained consistent clinical results. In the field of neurosurgery, we believe that this is an outstanding technology, which has brought great benefits to our vast number of stroke patients.

◎ **分析**:

1. "县级医院"译作"county-level hospitals",国内医生发言时常提到这个表达;

2. "大血管闭塞"只能译作"large vessel occlusion",在神经介入领域中,LVO 是一个特殊的类别;

3. "标志性的事件"译作"landmark events"。近几年,"landmark"一词在会议中的使用频率越来越高;

4. "支架型取栓器"译作"stent retriever",医生一般将其称为"支架取栓器";

5. "新英格兰"译作"*NEJM*",即 *New England Journal of Medicine*,全称为《新英格兰医学杂志》,是"国际四大医学期刊"之一,另外三个期刊分别是《柳叶刀》《美国医学会杂志》以及《英国医学杂志》。

第四节 补充练习

一、中译英

1953 年，Seldinger 发明了经皮穿刺动脉置管技术，使得医生能够将微创治疗器械安全地进入和撤出血管。得益于经皮穿刺动脉置管技术，神经介入、外周介入、心脏介入等血管介入技术才得以出现。可以说，经皮穿刺动脉置管技术是所有血管介入技术的源头。基于经皮穿刺动脉置管技术，Lussenhop 在 1960 年将直径在 2.5 毫米至 4.2 毫米之间的球形甲基丙烯酸甲酯栓塞引入手术暴露的左颈动脉分叉部，成功栓塞了脑动静脉畸形；Gerard Debrun 在 1975 年应用充气可脱球囊治疗外伤性颈动脉海绵窦瘘及颅内动脉瘤。这些探索性的操作，哪怕用今天的眼光看，也是十分危险的操作，但是这些介入神经放射学先驱通过开创性的研究，为脑血管疾病的治疗开辟了新的路径。

而在神经介入技术的发展历程中，弹簧圈的发明是其中一个重要里程碑。在弹簧圈发明之前，临床常用球囊治疗颅内动脉瘤，但是球囊属于规则形状，而颅内动脉瘤则是不规则形状，两者匹配较为困难。同时，颅内动脉瘤十分脆弱，在球囊释放的过程中，有可能撑破动脉瘤，造成严重并发症。针对这一难题，Guglielmi 教授受到游离弹簧圈及电解促进血凝等试验的启发，提出了电解脱弹簧圈。1991 年，Guglielmi 教授团队入组了首例临床试验，用时约半小时才得以解脱弹簧圈。但在当时，这一结果已让他们振奋不已。在此之后，弹簧圈的解脱时间越来越短，如今已可实现即时解脱。而自电解脱弹簧圈发明之后，便开启了以弹簧圈主导的全血管内动脉瘤介入治疗时代。

受人类视野的限制，神经介入技术的发展同样离不开影像技术的支持。最初，神经介入操作是在 X 线机及显影剂的指引下进行，但是这种不连续的透视影像十分考验临床医生的技巧。而随着计算机等技术发展，1979 出现了数字减影血管造影技术（DSA），这为神经介入的发展奠定了坚实基础。DSA 是指血管造影的影像通过数字化处理，把不需要的组织影像去除掉，只保留血管影像。其特点是图像清晰、分辨率高，对观察血管病变、血管狭窄的定位测量、诊断及介入治疗提供了真实的立体图像，为各种介入治疗提供了必备条件。到了 20 世纪 90 年代，计算机技术的发展日益成熟，依托计算机技术的 3D 血管造影开始出现。此前，临床医生需要根据 DSA 影像在脑海内构建血管立体影像，确保病变部位的定位准确。而 3D 血管造影技术则是帮助医生完成了这一步骤，极大地降低了医生操作神经介入手术的难度。

在此之后，各种各样的图像处理技术陆续出现，进一步辅助神经介入手术简化。而临床医生后续提出了更高的要求，希望看到脑组织及血管之间的关系、脑组织的供血情况等。这就需要更多的技术创新，如融合 CT 技术、磁共振技术等。如今，冠脉介入领域出现了 OCT、FFR 等技术，可以使医生看到血管病变情况及供血情况。不过，脑血管比心脏血管更加脆弱，血管腔内影像技术还须继续发展，以保证其在脑血管应用中的安全性。

◎ **参考译文**: In 1953, Seldinger invented the percutaneous arterial catheterization technique, which enabled doctors to safely insert and withdraw minimally invasive treatment devices from blood vessels. Thanks to the percutaneous arterial catheterization technique, vascular intervention techniques such as neuro intervention, peripheral intervention, and cardiac intervention have emerged. It can be said that percutaneous arterial catheterization is the source of all vascular intervention techniques. Based on the percutaneous arterial catheterization technique, Lussenhop introduced a spherical methyl methacrylate embolization with a diameter of 2.5mm to 4.2mm into the bifurcation of the left carotid artery exposed by surgery in 1960, and successfully embolized the cerebral arteriovenous malformation; Gerard Debrun used an inflatable detachable balloon to treat traumatic carotid cavernous fistula and intracranial aneurysm in 1975. These exploratory operations are very dangerous even from today's perspective, but these pioneers of interventional neuroradiology have opened up new paths for the treatment of cerebrovascular diseases through pioneering research.

In the development of neurointerventional technology, the invention of the coil is one of the important milestones. Before the invention of the coil, balloons were commonly used in clinical practice to treat intracranial aneurysms, but balloons are of regular shape, while intracranial aneurysms are of irregular shape, and it is difficult to match the two. At the same time, intracranial aneurysms are very fragile, and during the release of the balloon, the aneurysm may be ruptured, causing serious complications. In response to this problem, Professor Guglielmi was inspired by experiments such as free coils and electrolysis to promote blood coagulation, and proposed the electrolytic release coil. In 1991, Professor Guglielmi's team enrolled in the first clinical trial, and it took about half an hour to release the coil. But at that time, this result had already made them excited. Since then, the release time of the coil has become shorter and shorter, and now it can be released instantly. Since the invention of the electrolytic release coil, the era of all-vascular aneurysm interventional treatment dominated by coils has begun.

Limited by the limitation of human vision, the development of neurointerventional technology is also inseparable from the support of imaging technology. Initially, neurointerventional operations were performed under the guidance of X-ray machines and developer, but this discontinuous perspective image was very challenging for clinicians. With the development of computer and other technologies, digital subtraction angiography (DSA) appeared in 1979, which laid a solid foundation for the development of neuro intervention. DSA refers to the removal of unnecessary tissue images through digital processing of angiography images, leaving only vascular images. Its characteristics are clear images and high resolution, which provide real three-dimensional images for the observation of vascular lesions, positioning measurement, diagnosis and interventional treatment of vascular stenosis, and provide necessary conditions for various interventional treatments. In the 1990s, the development of computer technology became increasingly mature, and 3D angiography based on computer technology began to appear. Previously, clinicians needed to construct a three-dimensional image of blood vessels in their minds based on DSA images to ensure accurate positioning of the lesion site. 3D angiography technology helps doctors complete this step, greatly reducing the difficulty of doctors performing neurointerventional surgery.

After that, various image processing technologies emerged one after another, further assisting in simplifying neurointerventional surgery. Clinicians subsequently put forward higher requirements, hoping to see the relationship between brain tissue and blood vessels, the blood supply of brain tissue, etc. This requires more technological innovations, such as the fusion of CT technology and magnetic resonance technology. Today, technologies such as OCT and FFR have appeared in the field of coronary intervention, which can enable doctors to see vascular lesions and blood supply. However, cerebral blood vessels are more fragile than heart blood vessels, and intravascular imaging technology needs to continue to develop to ensure its safety in cerebrovascular applications.

二、英译中

The development and implementation of robotic-assisted techniques offer significant potential for improving patient care, minimizing radiation exposure, and improving ergonomics in neuro intervention. These innovations have shown promise in treating patients with severe symptomatic carotid stenosis and aneurysms of the basilar artery. In a recent Canadian study, a patient with a basilar trunk aneurysm underwent a stent-assisted coiling procedure with nearly all steps robotically performed, except for the manual placement of the guide-sheath and coaxial catheter. The robot's ease of use and smooth, precise movements facilitated navigation, stent placement, and coiling, demonstrating the potential for even greater robotic involvement in the future.

Using robotic-assisted techniques can reduce radiation exposure and ergonomic challenges faced by neurointerventional radiologists, leading to a more diverse and inclusive field that attracts a broader range of talented physicians. Furthermore, advancements in technology, such as sophisticated simulators and artificial intelligence (AI), will likely continue to enhance patient outcomes and reduce training differences among interventional practitioners. AI algorithms may help radiologists detect life-threatening neurological conditions more rapidly, such as ruptured aneurysms, aneurysm growth, and ischemic strokes. Faster detection may lead to quicker neurovascular team notifications and improved patient outcomes.

As clinical trials continue to investigate the efficacy of robotic-assisted endovascular procedures, the adoption of this modality among practitioners has the potential to increase care coverage across the nation. Remote care delivery through robotic systems can provide access to specialty care in underserved areas. However, healthcare facilities must address potential challenges, such as converting a robotic case to a manual case in case of complications or connectivity issues, before investing in this technology.

The implementation of robotic devices will require updates to the medical-legal framework and consideration of federal logistics and regulations regarding licenses, hours of coverage, and liability. As remote care becomes more widespread, it is essential to ensure that specialists are available to take over patient care in case of complications.

In summary, embracing robotic-assisted techniques and technology in neuro intervention holds promise for improving patient care, attracting a more diverse pool of trainees, and expanding care coverage to underserved areas. By overcoming the challenges associated with implementing these advancements, the field of neuro intervention can continue to grow and innovate.

◎ **参考译文**：机器人辅助技术的开发和实施为改善患者护理、最大限度地减少辐射暴露和改善神经介入的人体工程学提供了巨大的潜力。这些创新在治疗患有严重症状性颈动脉狭窄和基底动脉瘤的患者方面显示出了良好的前景。在最近的一项加拿大研究中，一名基底动脉瘤患者接受了支架辅助栓塞手术，除了手动放置导鞘和同轴导管外，几乎所有步骤都是由机器人完成的。机器人易于使用，动作流畅、精确，便于导航、放置支架和栓塞，这表明未来机器人参与的可能性更大。

使用机器人辅助技术可以减少神经介入放射科医生面临的辐射暴露和人体工程学挑战，从而使该领域更加多元化和包容，吸引更多优秀医生。此外，技术进步，例如复杂的模拟器和人工智能（AI），可能会继续改善患者的治疗效果并减少介入从业人员之间的培训差异。人工智能算法可以帮助放射科医生更快地检测危及生命的神经系统疾病，例如动脉瘤破裂、动脉瘤生长和缺血性中风。更快地检测可以更快地通知神经血管团队并改善患者的治疗效果。

随着临床试验继续研究机器人辅助血管内手术的疗效，从业者采用这种方式有可能增加全国的医疗覆盖率。通过机器人系统进行远程护理可以为医疗服务不足的地区提供专科护理。然而，医疗机构在投资这项技术之前必须解决潜在的挑战，例如在出现并发症或连接问题时将机器人病例转换为手动病例。

机器人设备的实施将需要更新医疗法律框架，并考虑有关许可证、覆盖时间和责任的联邦物流和法规。随着远程护理变得越来越普遍，确保在出现并发症时有专家接手患者护理至关重要。

总之，在神经干预中采用机器人辅助技术有望改善患者护理，吸引更多不同的受训人员，并将医疗覆盖范围扩大到医疗服务不足的地区。通过克服与实施这些进步相关的挑战，神经干预领域可以继续发展和创新。

第八单元 神经内科

第一节 神经内科口译知识点

神经内科(neurology)是关于神经方面的二级学科,并非属于传统内科的概念,主要收治脑血管疾病(脑梗死、脑出血)、偏头痛(migraine)、脑部炎症性疾病(脑炎、脑膜炎)、脊髓炎、癫痫(epilepsy)、阿尔茨海默病(Alzheimer disease, AD)、帕金森病(Parkinson's disease, PD)、代谢病和遗传倾向疾病(例如庞贝氏病, Pompe's disease)、三叉神经痛、坐骨神经痛、周围神经病(peripheral neuropathy)、神经肌肉疾病(neuromuscular disease,例如重症肌无力, myasthenia gravis, MG)、脱髓鞘疾病(demyelinating diseases)以及部分罕见病(rare diseases)等。

主要检查手段包括头颈部MRI、CT、ECT、PETCT、脑电图、TCD(经颅多普勒超声)、肌电图、诱发电位及血流变学检查、基因诊断等,同时与心理科交叉进行神经衰弱、失眠(insomnia)等功能性疾患的诊治。

一、癫痫

癫痫是大脑神经元突发性异常放电(abnormal discharge),导致短暂的大脑功能障碍,是影响所有年龄人群的一种脑部慢性非传染性疾病(chronic non-communicable diseases, NCD)。癫痫发作(epileptic seizure)是指脑神经元异常和过度超同步化放电所造成的临床现象。其特征是突然和一过性的症状,异常放电的神经元在大脑中的部位不同,临床表现也不同。发作从极短暂的意识丧失或肌肉反射,到严重持续性抽搐(convulsion)不等,发作的频率也存在差异,从每年发作少于一次,到每天发作几次不等。全世界大约有5000万癫痫患者,近80%的癫痫患者生活在低收入和中等收入国家。相较于普通人群(general population),癫痫患者的过早死亡风险要高出3倍。

当脑部受到刺激,如外伤、药物、睡眠不足、感染、发热,或脑部缺氧或能量异常,例如心律异常、血氧水平过低或血糖水平过低(低血糖症),无论既往有无癫痫病史均可诱发单次癫痫发作。此类刺激所引起的惊厥称作"诱发性惊厥"(非癫痫性惊厥)。

癫痫分类复杂,可分为局灶性、全面性、全面性合并局灶性、不明类型四类。国内,病因明确的,称为继发性癫痫(secondary epilepsy);病因不明确的,称为特发性癫痫(idiopathic epilepsy);部分对于药物、手术、迷走神经刺激(vagus nerve stimulation)等治疗方法应答不佳(poor response)的患者,称为难治性癫痫(intractable epilepsy, IE)。

常用的抗癫痫药物包括传统抗癫痫药物，有卡马西平（carbamazepine，CBZ）、丙戊酸（valproic acid，VPA）、苯妥英钠（phenytoin sodium，PHT）、苯巴比妥（phenobarbital，PHB）、氯硝西泮（clonazepam，CZP）等；以及新抗癫痫药物，有左乙拉西坦（levetiracetam，LEV）、拉莫三嗪（lamotrigine，LTG）、托吡酯（topiramate，TPM）、奥卡西平（oxcarbazepine，OXC）、加巴喷丁（gabapentin，GBP）等。

二、帕金森病

帕金森病是一种神经系统退行性疾病（degenerative disease），会导致行动不便以及心理健康问题、睡眠障碍、疼痛和其他健康问题。随着时间的推移，症状会逐步恶化。没有治愈方法，但可以通过一些疗法和药物减轻症状。常见症状有特异性运动症状（motor symptoms），包括静止性震颤（static/resting tremor）、动作迟缓（bradykinesia）、僵硬（rigidity）、步态姿势不稳（postural instability）等，以及非运动症状（non-motor symptoms），包括认知功能障碍（cognition impairment）、睡眠障碍（sleep disorders）、感觉障碍（sensory disorder/disturbance）和言语困难（speech difficulty）等。帕金森病导致高残疾率和医护需求。许多帕金森病患者还会发展为痴呆（dementia）。此病通常发生在老年人身上，但年轻人也可能受到影响。男性比女性更易受到影响。帕金森病的病因尚不清楚，但有该疾病家族史的人患病风险较高。暴露于空气污染、杀虫剂和化学溶剂可能会增加风险。研究显示，帕金森病可能与黑质多巴胺能神经元变形死亡相关，但根本原因并不明确。

帕金森病的治疗措施包括：营养支持、一般支持治疗、心理支持治疗。药物治疗包括：复方左旋多巴（compound levodopa）、多巴胺受体激动剂（dopamine receptor agonists，DA）、单胺氧化酶B型抑制剂（monoamine oxidase type B inhibitor，MAO-B）、金刚烷胺（amantadine）等。手术治疗包括神经核毁损术以及脑深部电刺激术（Deep brain stimulation，DBS）。

三、阿尔茨海默病

阿尔茨海默病是一种中枢神经系统的退行性病变，主要发生在老年或老年前期。疾病的主要特征包括进行性的认知功能障碍和行为损害。阿尔茨海默氏病是痴呆症最常见的形式，可能占病例数的60%~70%。阿尔茨海默病是老年期最常见的一种痴呆类型，并且随着年龄的增长，患病的风险也在增加。

阿尔茨海默病的症状包括记忆障碍、失语、失用、失认以及视空间能力损害等。此外，患者的抽象思维和计算力也会损害，常伴随人格和行为的改变。这种疾病不是传染的，而是由基因、生活方式和环境因素共同作用的结果。

该疾病通常需要长期治疗，目前医学界主要通过药物和心理治疗等方法控制病情发展，延缓症状恶化。尽管阿尔茨海默病目前尚无彻底根治的方法，但患者通过良好的生活习惯，包括规律的体育锻炼、科学的饮食、适当的社交活动可以预防疾病的发生和发展。

阿尔茨海默病的命名来源于首次描述这种疾病的德国医生阿尔茨海默。近年来，阿尔茨海默病的研究取得了重大进展，基因技术、脑成像技术等在阿尔茨海默病的早期诊断方面发挥了重要作用，同时也为理解疾病的发生机制提供了新的视角。然而，阿尔茨海默病的确切发病机制仍不清楚，如何有效预防和治疗阿尔茨海默病仍然是科学家们需要努力探索的问题。

阿尔茨海默病患者人群庞大，根据不同的流行病学研究，全球可能有5000万患者人群，而其起病先于症状出现，随着人均寿命的延长、人口老龄化的加剧，预计未来会有更多的患者，阿尔茨海默病又给患者家庭和社会带来了沉重的负担，因此全球多家制药公司在此领域都投入了大量的资源进行药物研发。

四、神经肌肉病

神经肌肉病是可分为周围神经疾病（peripheral nerve diseases）、神经肌肉接头疾病（neuromuscular junction disorders）以及肌肉疾病（muscular disease, myopathy）。会议口译中可能遇到的有肌萎缩侧索硬化症（amyotrophic lateral sclerosis, ALS）、包涵体肌炎（inclusion body myositis）、运动神经元病（motor neuron disease）、肌营养不良（myodystrophy）、重症肌无力（myasthenia gravis, MG）、周围神经病等。

重症肌无力为获得性自身免疫疾病（acquired autoimmune disease），主要症状为神经肌肉传递障碍引起的骨骼肌收缩无力，即附着于人体骨骼上做出动作的肌肉逐渐失去力量。患者会感到疲劳，活动后劳累感更加明显，休息后能得到缓解，其临床表现（clinical manifestation）包括眼睑下垂（blepharoptosis）、吞咽困难，乃至呼吸困难。

在作出诊断后，药物治疗包括胆碱酯酶抑制剂（cholinesterase inhibitors）；免疫抑制剂（immunosuppressor），包含糖皮质激素（glucocorticoid）、硫唑嘌呤（azathioprine, AZA）、环磷酰胺（cyclophosphamide, CTX/CYC）、他克莫司（tacrolimus）、吗替麦考酚酯（mycophenolate mofetil, MMF）；静脉注射用丙种球蛋白（intravenous immune globulin, IVIG）。除了药物治疗，还可以进行血浆置换（plasma exchange）。

五、脱髓鞘疾病

脱髓鞘疾病的广义概念是神经纤维髓鞘的破坏、崩解和脱失导致的一系列疾病。狭义的脱髓鞘疾病一般指中枢神经系统特发性炎性脱髓鞘疾病（idiopathic inflammatory demyelinating diseases, IIDDs），包括多发性硬化（multiple sclerosis, MS）、视神经脊髓炎谱系疾病（neuromyelitis optica spectrum disorder, NMOSD）、抗髓鞘少突胶质细胞糖蛋白免疫球蛋白G抗体相关疾病（myelin oligodendrocyte glycoprotein antibody-associated disease, MOGAD）等。

多发性硬化（MS）患者可能会出现肢体无力、感觉异常、眼部症状、共济失调（ataxia）、发作性症状（持续时间短暂的感觉或运动异常）等症状；视神经脊髓炎谱系疾病（NMOSD）患者可能出现视神经炎（optic neuritis）、脊髓炎（myelitis）、人脑综合征等症状。

脱髓鞘疾病在诊断时往往需要较多检查，包括磁共振成像（magnetic resonance imaging，MRI）、脑脊液（cerebrospinal fluid，CSF）检查、肌电图（electromyography，EMG）检查、组织活检（tissue biopsy）等，耗时耗力，而往往诊断困难。治疗手段主要包括糖皮质激素、血浆置换以及免疫球蛋白。

六、罕见病

罕见病，或称孤儿病（orphan disease），全球范围内并无统一定义，世界卫生组织（World Health Organization，WHO）对罕见病的定义是患病人数小于总人口0.65‰至1‰的疾病，美国及欧盟的定义略有差异，标准更加严格一些。

罕见病种类繁多，欧美国家目前发现有7000多种。我国多部委也发布了《罕见病目录》，截至2023年，共有207种罕见病纳入目录，我国人口基数大，罕见病患者在我国约有2000万人，即所谓"罕见病并不罕见"。

其中医学会议口译中能遇到的包括戈谢氏病（Gaucher disease）、庞贝氏病（Pompe disease）、威尔森氏症（Wilson's disease）、脊髓性肌萎缩症（spinal muscular atrophy，SMA）等。在众多罕见病中，只有不到1%的疾病有有效治疗方案，如戈谢氏病、庞贝氏病。

罕见病因其总体患者群体相对较小，除特殊临床症状外，其他都属于一般意义的疑难杂症，因此诊断往往相对困难，而且针对性的药物研发进展较慢，因此罕见病的科研、治疗及用药有别于常见病。而近年来，随着社会的发展进步，罕见病患者中的名人效应，以及其他原因，罕见病领域得到了越来越多的关注，也有了相应的医学会议口译需求。

第二节　真实世界口译情境

一、主题会议

神经内科主题会议范围很广，而现代医学专科及亚专科越分越细，需要口译的神经内科会议的主题往往非常明确。近年来，随着人口的老龄化，阿尔茨海默病患者越来越多，相应的研究和会议也相应增多，医学研究领域针对AD发病机制、重要相关分子研究、药物研发、临床研究、临床治疗的会议层出不穷。

神经内科中也有很多疾病为罕见病，近些年来，综合性的罕见病会议以及具体的某一罕见病会议也偶有举办，例如庞贝氏病或脊髓性肌萎缩病会议等。

二、行业特点

神经内科主题相关会议中，主题演讲中基础研究内容比较多，这就导致中文表达中掺杂了较多的英文名称及英文缩略语，主要涉及分子名称、通路名称、基因名称等，比如Tau protein（发音为"陶"蛋白）、STING、cGAS、P301S、Trem2、Mef2c、IFN （interferon，干扰素）等。这些信息无须翻译，直接听辨后跟读即可。

很多神经内科主题会议中，虽然很多会议现场安排同声传译，但仍有不少国内或华人讲者会选择用英文发言。整体而言，相较于其他专科，讲者往往语速较快。

此外，神经内科医学会议中的病例汇报环节，在介绍病历时，讲者往往介绍得非常细致，详细程度远超外科系统，其中涉及病史、用药史、具体体检结果、鉴别诊断等，而且进行病例汇报的医生一般相对年轻，其所制作的课件往往信息量大，介绍时一般语速较快，译员如果不作充分准备，交传和同传难度均较大。

很多神经内科的会议口译，相对其他专科会议而言，显得"小而精"，对口译准确度和专业表达的要求反而更高，并未因会议小而降低要求。

在脱髓鞘疾病领域，还存在"谱系疾病"和"相关疾病"的命名，说明该领域部分疾病鉴别分类和命名仍未完全明确及统一，所以会议口译经常会对翻译疾病名称的准确性有着很高的要求，有时会特别关注疾病名称与鉴别，而这些疾病名称，无论中英文，都冗长拗口。

三、口译难点

本章介绍的医学英语中存在一个现象，同一诊断和症状很多时候有两套词语，一套为更加专业的医学专业名词，另外一套相对容易理解。典型的例子如高血压，有 hypertension 和 high blood pressure 两种表达；还有高血糖，有 hyperglycemia 和 high blood glucose/sugar 三种表达方式，sugar（糖）比 glucose（葡萄糖）更容易被听众理解。这类情况在医学会议口译中不胜枚举，近年来，越来越多的海外讲者和讨论嘉宾倾向于使用后者，尤其是美国讲者，因为对于非英语母语者，后者显然更加容易记忆和交流。

例如，笔者在一次会议口译中，甚至听到哈佛的教授使用"more good"这样的表述来替代"better"，可能的主要目的也是为了强调以及保证非英语母语者更好地理解。

但在特定国家讲者和特定专科会议中，不少讲者仍然会选择使用更专业的医学词汇，尤其在涉及神经主题时，例如"运动迟缓"一词，专业词汇是"bradykinesia"，而更通俗易懂的表达则有多种，包括"slow movement""slowed movement""slow muscle movement""slowness of movement"；再如"言语困难"对应的英文专业词汇是"dysphasia"，而简单的表达则为"speech difficulty"；"感觉异常"的英文是"paresthesia"，而简单的表达则为"abnormal sensation"。

这一现象在神经内科的会议口译中尤其明显，加之神经内科部分疾病属于普通人理解的"疑难杂症"，其症状相较于大众常见的呼吸道、消化道症状更为少见，因此在口译的时候，面对更专业的表达，译员如果积累或准备不足，会面临一定的困难，算得上是一个难点。这里不谈词根词源，只谈会议口译前准备的实际情况，这一现象确实给译员带来一定挑战。

这一现象在汉语中也有，汉语中部分对于症状的描述颇有古风遗蕴，例如"纳差"表示食欲不佳，"盗汗"表示入睡后异常出汗，"里急后重"表示下腹部不适的一种症状等。但相较于英语成套的"专业"与"非专业"的诊断及症状的表述，现代医学汉语中这一语言现象给译员带来的挑战相对有限。

此外，很多以神经内科为主题的会议，会讲到基础研究及药物研发，在此语境下，很多英文名称是可不译的，直接跟读即可，所以译员需要对相关内容有一定的积累，在同传过程中才能迅速判断哪些翻译，哪些跟读。

神经内科治疗会使用各种药物，无论是英文还是中文，药名都拗口且不容易记忆，而且英文药名如前所示，经常也有缩略语形式。有些专科，例如传染病领域和肿瘤领域，甚至会出现一种药物既有标准化学名，又有商品名，或有三个英文字母的缩略语名称，还有单字母名称，这些对于专科医师而言已习以为常，早已烂熟于胸，但对于译员而言，又是另外一重挑战。神经内科部分主题会议，例如罕见病会议、神经肌肉病及脱髓鞘疾病，其病因有遗传性或特发性，病理机制理解相对其他常见疾病稍微困难一些，对此译员也须做较好的会前准备。

第三节　中英对照篇章及分析

一、英译中

Alzheimer's disease is named after Dr. Alois Alzheimer. In 1906, Dr. Alzheimer noticed changes in the brain tissue of a woman who had died of an unusual mental illness. Her symptoms included memory loss, language problems, and unpredictable behavior. After she died, he examined her brain and found many abnormal clumps, now it's called amyloid plaques, and tangled bundles of fibers, now it's called neurofibrillary, or tau tangles. These plaques and tangles in the brain are still considered some of the main features of Alzheimer's. Another feature is the loss of connections between neurons in the brain. Neurons transmit messages between different parts of the brain, and from the brain to muscles and organs in the body. Alzheimer's disease is a brain disorder that slowly destroys memory and thinking skills, and eventually, the ability to carry out the simplest tasks. In most people with Alzheimer's, symptoms first appear later in life. Estimates vary, but experts suggest that more than 6 million Americans, most of them age 65 or older, may have Alzheimer's. （本段内容来自网络，有删改调整。）

◎ **参考译文**：阿尔茨海默病是以阿洛斯·阿尔茨海默博士的名字命名。在1906年，阿尔茨海默医生注意到脑部组织的改变，是一位女性，其死于并不常见的精神疾病。她的症状包括记忆力减退、语言问题以及不可预测的行为。她死后，他检查了她的大脑，发现了许多异常团块，现在被称为"淀粉样斑块"，以及缠结的纤维束，现在被称为"神经原纤维"或"tau缠结"。大脑内的这些斑块和缠结仍然被认为是阿尔茨海默病的一些主要特征。另一个特征是大脑内神经元间的连接丧失。神经元在大脑的不同部位之间传递信息，并从大脑传递到体内的肌肉和器官。阿尔茨海默病是一种大脑的疾病，会慢慢破坏记忆力和思维能力，而最终，破坏执行最简单任务的能力。在大多数阿尔茨海默病患者中，症状在晚年才首次出现。尽管预计有差异，但专家认为超过 600 万的美国人，其中大多数年龄是 65 岁或以上，可能患有阿尔茨海默病。

◎ 分析：

1. "Dr. Alois Alzheimer"译作"阿洛斯·阿尔茨海默博士"，此处的"Dr."其实应该译作"医生"；

2. "noticed changes in the brain tissue of a woman who had died of an unusual mental illness."按照顺句驱动的方法处理为"注意到脑部组织的改变，是一位女性，其死于并不常见的精神疾病。"可与"注意到一位死于罕见精神疾病的妇女的脑组织发生了变化。"进行对比，除了语序之外，几处也有口语化的调整；

3. "After she died"直接译作"她死后"，医学会议演讲与讨论时讲者对于"die/death""死/死亡"并不避讳。这是学术交流，非文学翻译，直译即可，无须调整为"pass away/on""不在/逝去"等；

4. "tau"无须翻译，直接跟读即可，读音同"陶"，指"tau 蛋白"，这是现代 AD 会议中的基础词汇；

5. "and eventually, the ability to carry out the simplest tasks"此处译为"而最终，破坏执行最简单任务的能力。"重复补充了"破坏"二字，听起来更加流畅；

6. "but experts suggest that"译作"但专家认为"，"suggest"一词，在医学口译中其"建议"的含义较少用到，更多的时候则表示"显示、提示"，常见的用法例如"the results of the study suggested"，不同语境下可灵活处理。

Memory problems are typically one of the first signs of cognitive impairment related to Alzheimer's. Some people with memory problems have a condition called mild cognitive impairment, MCI. With MCI, people have more memory problems than normal for their age, but their symptoms do not interfere with their everyday lives. Movement difficulties and problems with the sense of smell have also been linked to MCI. Older people with MCI are at greater risk for developing Alzheimer's, but not all of them do so. Some may even revert to normal cognition. The first symptoms of Alzheimer's vary from person to person. For many, decline in nonmemory aspects of cognition, such as word finding, vision/spatial issues, and impaired reasoning or judgment may signal the very early stages of the disease. Researchers are studying biomarkers, which are biological signs of disease found in brain images, cerebrospinal fluid, and blood, to detect early changes in the brains of people with MCI and in cognitively normal people who may be at greater risk for Alzheimer's. More research is needed before these techniques can be used broadly and routinely to diagnose Alzheimer's in a health care provider's office.

◎ **参考译文**：记忆问题通常是阿尔茨海默病相关认知障碍的早期征象之一。一些有记忆问题的人会有轻度认知障碍，即 MCI 的问题。患有 MCI 的人记忆问题更严重，相较正常的同龄人，但他们的症状不会影响日常生活。而运动困难和嗅觉问题也是与

MCI 相关。老年人，患有 MCI，他们患阿尔茨海默病的风险更大，但并非所有人都如此。有些人甚至可能恢复正常认知。阿尔茨海默病的初始症状因人而异。对于许多人来说，认知的非记忆方面下降，例如找词、视觉/空间问题以及推理或判断能力受损可能预示着疾病的极早期阶段。研究人员正在研究生物标志物，即疾病生物学征象，可在脑部影像、脑脊液和血液中找到，以发现患 MCI 人的大脑中的早期改变，以及在认知功能正常人中，那些可能患阿尔茨海默病风险更大的人。还需要进行更多的研究，然后这些技术才能够广泛地常规用于医疗行业中阿尔茨海默病的诊断。

◎ 分析：

1. "cognitive impairment"译作"认知障碍"，这是神经内科会议中的基础词汇；

2. "at greater risk for developing Alzheimer's"处理为"患阿尔茨海默病的风险更大"，"develop"表示"得/患（病），（疾病）进展"，是医学口译中的基础词；

3. "biomarkers"大多数时候可译作"生物标志物"，也可译作"生物标记物"，但后者使用较少。

As Alzheimer's worsens, people experience greater memory loss and other cognitive difficulties. Problems can include wandering and getting lost, trouble handling money and paying bills, repeating questions, taking longer to complete normal daily tasks, and personality and behavior changes. People are often diagnosed in this stage. In this stage, damage occurs in areas of the brain that control language, reasoning, conscious thought, and sensory processing, such as the ability to correctly detect sounds and smells. Memory loss and confusion grow worse, and people begin to have problems recognizing family and friends. They may be unable to learn new things, carry out multistep tasks such as getting dressed, or cope with new situations. In addition, people at this stage may have hallucinations, delusions, and paranoia and may behave impulsively. Ultimately, plaques and tangles spread throughout the brain, and brain tissue shrinks significantly. People with severe Alzheimer's cannot communicate and are completely dependent on others for their care.

◎ 参考译文：随着阿尔茨海默病的恶化，人们会经历更严重的记忆丧失和其他认知困难。问题可能包括徘徊和迷路、难以处理金钱和支付账单、重复提问、需要更长时间才能完成正常的日常任务以及性格和行为的变化。人们通常在这个阶段被诊断出来。在这个阶段，损伤会出现在大脑控制语言、推理、有意识思维以及感官处理的区域，例如正确检测声音和气味的能力。记忆丧失和思维混乱会恶化，人们开始无法识别家人和朋友。他们可能无法学习新事物、进行多步骤任务，例如穿衣，或者应对新的情况。此外，处于这个阶段的人可能会出现幻觉、妄想和偏执，还可能表现出冲动行为。最终，斑块和缠结扩散到整个脑部，并且脑组织会显著缩小。患有严重阿尔茨海默病的人无法交流，完全依赖他人的照料。

◎ 分析：

（1）"wandering"译作"徘徊"，此处指"徘徊症状"；

（2）"hallucinations, delusions, and paranoia"译作"幻觉、妄想和偏执"，是心理精神方面的基础词汇，其中"paranoia"可表示"多疑、妄想、偏执"，需要结合上下文判断，或借由其他内容解释。

Tau is a small protein with a short name and a big reputation. Predominantly found in the brain, this protein serves multiple functions in healthy brain cells. Like most proteins, tau is vulnerable to changes in its environment and genetic mistakes. These factors can make tau no longer fit to carry out its usual job, a problem associated with many brain diseases. A buildup of the abnormal tau leads to "tangles" that cause cell damage and inflammation, contributing to Alzheimer's disease symptoms. In Alzheimer's disease, an abnormal form of tau accumulates and begins sticking together in thread-like structures called neurofibrillary tangles. These tangles are not effectively disposed of through the cell's usual ways of removing "trash". The build-up damages the microtubule, disrupting how neurons function. Tau tangles start in the brainstem, which connects the brain to the spinal cord. From the brainstem, they spread upward towards two brain regions that are key to memory.

◎ **参考译文**：Tau 是一种小蛋白，名字简短但名声显赫。主要是在大脑内，这种蛋白在健康的脑细胞中发挥多种功能。像大多数蛋白一样，tau 对于环境变化和基因错误非常脆弱。这些因素会使得 tau 蛋白不再适合发挥其正常功能，这与很多脑部疾病有关联。异常 tau 蛋白的累积会导致"缠结"，从而导致细胞损伤和炎症，并加剧阿尔茨海默病的症状。在阿尔茨海默病中，一种异常形式的 tau 会累积并会粘在一起，线状结构，称为神经原纤维缠结。这些缠结无法有效处理掉，通过细胞常规清除"垃圾"的方法无法有效处理。累积的物质会破坏微管，扰乱神经元的功能。Tau 的缠结始于脑干，其连接大脑和脊髓。从脑干开始，它们向上扩散到两个脑区，其对记忆至关重要。

◎ 分析：

1. "with a short name and a big reputation"处理为"名字简短但名声显赫"，将 and 处理为了转折语气，更符合当下语境；

2. "Predominantly found in the brain"中的"found"并未译出，一定要译出的话，可以处理为"主要见于脑内"，如果处理为"主要在大脑内发现"则稍显突兀；

3. "disrupting how neurons function"处理为"扰乱神经元的功能"，词性调整后更符合该语境下的表达需求。

Normally, tau proteins are found on the inside of neurons' axons to maintain their correct structure. This is crucial, because if the axon is compromised, the messages it carries cannot reach the next cell in the chain. In some forms of dementia, including Alzheimer's disease and frontotemporal dementia, tau proteins become damaged and detach from their axons. Now moving freely inside the neuron, the abnormal tau proteins clump together to form neurofibrillary tangles. This dysfunctional tau is toxic to neurons and causes them to die. When neurons in a chain die, that chain is broken, and messages can't be delivered as effectively through the brain. This disruption of messaging is what causes the thinking difficulties that underpin dementia. Research is now focused on why tau is damaged in these conditions and how exactly it causes the death of neurons.

◎ **参考译文**：通常情况下，tau 蛋白可见于神经元轴突的内部，以维持其正确的结构。这一点至关重要，因为如果轴突受损，它所携带的信息就无法到达链条中的下一个细胞。在某些类型的痴呆中，包括阿尔茨海默病和额颞叶痴呆，tau 蛋白会受损并从轴突分离。现在，在神经元内自由移动，异常的 tau 蛋白聚在一起形成神经原纤维缠结。这种功能失调的 tau 蛋白对神经元有毒性，会导致其死亡。如果一个链条中的神经元死亡，该链条就会断裂，信息无法有效地通过大脑传递。这种信息传递的中断是导致痴呆症的思维困难的原因。现在的研究关注是为什么 tau 蛋白在这些情况下会受损，以及它究竟是如何导致神经元死亡的。

◎ **分析**：

1. "if the axon is compromised" 译作"如果轴突受损"，"compromise" 一词在医学口译中比较常见，比如"immunocompromised" 可译作"免疫受损"；

2. "When neurons in a chain die, that chain is broken" 可处理为"如果一个链条中的神经元死亡，该链条就会断裂"，不一定非要译作"当……的时候"。

Amyloid begins life as amyloid precursor protein, APP, which is a common, normal protein in the central nervous system. It can be processed in two different ways: one that produces a healthy soluble protein, and one that produces toxic amyloid-beta. Both of these processes happen normally, and in healthy brains the amyloid-beta is cleared from the brain before it can do any damage. Scientists think that people with Alzheimer's disease overproduce amyloid-beta and/or are less able to effectively clear it from their brains. Amyloid-beta is dangerous because it clumps together, first forming small clusters called oligomers and eventually accumulating into bulky amyloid plaques. These clumps cause a variety of chemical reactions around neurons that damage and destroy them. One way is by activating the immune system to trigger inflammation, and another is by causing the production of abnormal tau.

◎ **参考译文**：淀粉样蛋白最初是淀粉样前体蛋白，简称 APP，这是一种常见的正常蛋白质，位于中枢神经系统中。它可以通过两种不同的方式进行处理：一种能产生健康的可溶性蛋白质，另一种产生毒性的淀粉样蛋白-β。这两个过程都是正常发生，在健康的大脑中，淀粉样蛋白-β 会从大脑中清除掉，在其造成任何损害之前就会被清除掉。

科学家认为，阿尔茨海默病患者过度产生淀粉样蛋白-β 以及/或许无法有效地将其从大脑中清除。淀粉样蛋白-β 很危险，因为它会聚在一起，首先形成小簇，称为低聚物，最终积聚成大块的淀粉样斑块。这些团块会导致各种化学反应，这些化学反应围绕着神经元，损害并摧毁神经元。一种方式是通过激活免疫系统触发炎症，另一种方式是导致产生异常的 tau 蛋白。

◎ 分析：

1. "the amyloid-beta is cleared from the brain before it can do any damage"按照顺句驱动的方法处理为"淀粉样蛋白-β 会从大脑中清除掉，在其造成任何损害之前就会被清除掉。"后面补充了"就会被清除掉"，符合口语的表达习惯；

2. "overproduce"译作"过度产生"，在医学口译中有一些以"over"为前缀的动词，一般都译作"过度"，例如"overtreat"译作"过度治疗"，"overdiagnose"译作"过度诊断"，"overexpress"译作"过度表达"或"过表达"等；

3. "and/or"在书面翻译时可能译作"和/或"，但在同传时可考虑译作双字词"以及/或许"，中间稍停顿，从而适当降低信息密度，使表达更加清晰，方便听众理解。

Parkinson disease is a neurodegenerative disorder that mostly presents in later life with generalized slowing of movements, bradykinesia, and at least one other symptom of resting tremor or rigidity. Other associated features are a loss of smell, sleep dysfunction, mood disorders, excess salivation, constipation, and excessive periodic limb movements in sleep, REM behavior disorder. It is estimated that Parkinson disease affects at least 1% of the population over the age of 60. The disorder is associated with the loss of dopaminergic neurons in the substantia nigra and the presence of Lewy bodies. Most cases are idiopathic. Only about 10% of cases have a genetic cause, and these cases are seen in young people. The disorder has a slow onset but is progressive. Tremor is often the first symptom and later can be associated with bradykinesia and rigidity. Postural instability is usually seen late in the disease and can seriously impact the quality of life. Also important is the presence of autonomic symptoms that may precede the motor symptoms in some patients. The diagnosis in most patients is based on history and clinical presentation. SPECT scans can be performed in doubtful cases or to rule out other neurological disorders.

◎ **参考译文**：帕金森病是一种神经退行性疾病，主要在晚年出现，表现为全身性动作缓慢，即运动迟缓，以及至少一种其他静止性震颤或僵硬症状。其他相关特征为嗅觉丧失、睡眠障碍、情绪障碍、唾液分泌过多、便秘以及睡眠中过度周期性肢体运动、REM 行为障碍。据估计，帕金森病影响了至少 1%的 60 岁以上人群。该疾病与多巴胺能神经元的损失相关，这些神经元位于黑质中，还有就是路易体的存在。大多数病例是特发性的。只有大约 10%的病例有遗传原因，这些病例见于年轻人。这一疾病发病缓慢但却是进行的。震颤通常为首发症状，后来可能与运动迟缓和僵硬相关。姿势不稳定通常见于疾病晚期，会严重影响生活质量。同样重要的是，自主神经症状的出现，这可能先于运动症状，部分患者有此表现。大多数患者的诊断是基于病史和临床表现。可进行 SPECT 扫描，用于可疑病例或排除其他神经系统疾病。

◎ **分析**：

1. "neurodegenerative disorder"译作"神经退行性疾病"，医学英语中，"disorder" "disease" "condition"在特定语境下都可以译作"疾病"；

2. "resting tremor"译作"静止性震颤"，英语中也可表达为"static tremor"；

3. "population over the age of 60"，此处的"population"译作"人群"，与"人口"相比，更偏向临床医学的语境；

4. "genetic cause"译作"遗传原因"，此处不宜译作"基因"；

5. "Also important is the presence of autonomic symptoms that may precede the motor symptoms in some patients."按照顺句驱动的方法处理为"同样重要的是，自主神经症状的出现，这可能先于运动症状，部分患者有此表现。"部分字词的添加使得语句通顺。

Over the past century, our understanding of the etiology of PD has evolved immensely. In 1919, it was first recognized that loss of pigmentation in the substantia nigra of the midbrain is a feature of the post-mortem brain examination of patients with PD. In the 1950s, it was further understood that the pigmented neurons that are lost in the substantia nigra are dopaminergic, and it is the loss of dopamine in subcortical motor circuitry that is implicated in the mechanism of the movement disorder in PD. PD is a disorder of the basal ganglia, which is composed of many other nuclei. The striatum receives excitatory and inhibitory input from several parts of the cortex. The key pathology is the loss of dopaminergic neurons that lead to the symptoms. The cause of PD is linked to the use of pesticides, herbicides and proximity to industrial plants. Some individuals have been found to develop Parkinsonian-like features after injection of 1-methyl-4-phenyl-1, 2, 3, 6-tetrahydropyridine, MPTP. This chemical accumulates in the mitochondria. There is also research suggesting that oxidation and generation of free radicals may be the cause of damage to the thalamic nuclei. Genes are important as the risk of PD in siblings is increased if one member of the family has the disorder. These cases also tend to occur much earlier in life. Abnormal levels of aggregated alpha-synuclein are a major component of Lewy bodies and are found at autopsy. It is felt that the altered function of alpha-synuclein may play a role in the etiology of PD. Current research is focused on preventing the propagation and aggregation of alpha-synuclein.

◎ **参考译文**：在过去的一个世纪中，我们对 PD 病因的理解进步巨大。1919 年，人们第一次认识到中脑黑质色素沉着的丧失是 PD 患者尸检脑部检查的一个特征。20 世纪 50 年代，人们进一步理解，黑质中丧失的色素神经元是多巴胺能神经元，而正是皮层下运动回路中多巴胺的丧失与 PD 运动障碍的机制有关。PD 是一种基底神经节疾病，基底神经节包含许多其他核团。纹状体接收兴奋性和抑制性输入，其来自皮层的几个部位。关键病理是导致症状的多巴胺能神经元的丧失。PD 的病因与杀虫剂、除草剂的使用以及邻近工厂相关。一些个体会出现类似帕金森病的特征，发生在注射MPTP后。这一化学物质会积聚在线粒体内。还有研究表明，氧化和自由基的产生可能是导致丘脑核团受损的原因。基因很重要，因为如果家族中有一个成员有此疾病，兄弟姐妹患PD的风险就会增加。这些病例往往倾向于在生命很早期就出现。异常水平的聚集的α-突触核蛋白是路易体的主要成分，在尸检中可以发现。感觉α-突触核蛋白功能的改变可能在帕金森病的病因中起作用。当前的研究聚焦在防止α-突触核蛋白的增殖和聚集。

◎ **分析**：

1. "which is composed of many other nuclei"译作"基底神经节包含许多其他核团"，此处的"nuclei"译作"核团"，而非"核"；

2. "1-methyl-4-phenyl-1, 2, 3, 6-tetrahydropyridine"一词，考虑到讲者口音和语速，如果演讲时幻灯片上有显示，译员依靠强大的医学化学素养的积累或可译出"1-甲基-4-苯基-1, 2, 3, 6-四氢吡啶"，但难度极大。译员如果素养稍差或幻灯片上不显示，则基本无法译出，但无论全程能否译出，起码要能跟读出"MPTP"。

An earlier feature of PD is tremor, typically unilateral and present at rest, which is usually the reason for seeking help at a neurology clinic. After using the hands, such as to pick up a book, the tremor may vanish for some minutes, only to return when the patient is distracted and resting once again. This is the so-called reemerging tremor that is typical of PD. Although tremor is a prominent and early symptom of PD, it is not always present and is not a necessary feature for diagnosis. Slowness, or bradykinesia, on the other hand, is a core feature of PD. Patients will notice it takes them longer to do simple tasks, their walking is slower, and their ability to respond to threats is compromised. In the clinic, patients demonstrate an inability to tap their index finger and thumb rapidly, tap their foot rhythmically on the floor, or walk steadily.

◎ **参考译文**：PD的一个早期特征就是震颤，一般是单侧，在静息时出现，这通常就是看神经内科的原因。在双手活动后，例如拿起一本书，震颤可能会消失几分钟，而在患者注意力分析且再次静息时，震颤会再次出现。这就是所谓的PD典型的复发性震颤。震颤虽然是PD的显著早期症状，但并非一直出现，也并非诊断的必要特征。动作缓慢，或运动迟缓，在另一方面，则是PD的核心特征。患者会注意到他们需要更长的时间来完成简单的任务，他们的行走速度更慢，他们对威胁的应对能力也受到损害。在门诊，患者表现为无法快速敲击食指和拇指，无法用脚有节奏地敲击地板，也无法稳定行走。

◎ **分析**：

1. "which is usually the reason for seeking help at a neurology clinic"译作"这通常就是看神经内科的原因"，"for seeking help"在此中文语境下译作"看"已经足够，译员无须字对字翻译，可与"这通常是在神经科诊所寻求帮助的原因"相比较；

2. "After using the hands"此处处理为"在双手活动后"，似乎比"在使用双手后"稍好一些；

3. "In the clinic"译作"在门诊"，符合国内的临床实际情况；

4. "patients demonstrate an inability to tap their index finger and thumb rapidly, tap their foot rhythmically on the floor, or walk steadily."译作"患者表现为无法快速敲击食指和拇指，无法用脚有节奏地敲击地板，也无法稳定行走。"此处因为讲者的语速和口语原因，补充了两个"无法"，以便于听众更好地理解。

Pharmacologically, this is typically levodopa, when combined with carbidopa, it decreases side effects and improves CNS bioavailability. A dopamine agonist, such as pramipexole, may be started in younger patients; it may not be as effective as levodopa but will have fewer side effects. Anticholinergics or amantadine may be used if the predominant symptom to be controlled is a tremor. Selegiline is often used to treat early disease and can provide mild symptom relief. Most antiparkinsonian medications provide good symptom control for 3 to 6 years. After this period, the disease progresses and is often unresponsive to medications. In general, younger patients should be treated more aggressively than older people. A multidisciplinary approach to the management of PD is essential. Patients do much better when a structured physical therapy program geared to PD is employed; they can be taught to improve their balance and gait, improve their stability, and maintain an active life. Some unique features of this movement disorder have been exploited to advantage; patients do well with music therapy in physical fitness programs, cycling, and boxing. Patients who cannot walk may find themselves able to dance. Depression, carer fatigue, constipation, REM sleep disorder, paranoia, and psychosis are often seen. They can be side effects of the medication or part of the primary disease, and all need to be addressed.

◎ **参考译文：** 从药理学角度来看，这一般是左旋多巴，与卡比多巴联用时，它能减少副作用并提高中枢神经系统的生物利用度。多巴胺激动剂，例如普拉克索，可用于较年轻的患者；它可能不像左旋多巴那样有效，但其副作用较少。可以使用抗胆碱能药物或金刚烷胺，如果要控制的主要症状是震颤的话，则可以使用这两种药物。司来吉兰通常用于治疗早期疾病，可以缓解轻度症状。大多数抗帕金森病药物能提供3到6年良好的症状控制。这一阶段之后，疾病会发展，并且通常对药物没有应答。一般而言，年轻患者，相较于老年人，应该接受更积极的治疗。多学科的方法对PD的管理至关重要。如果采用针对PD的结构化物理治疗计划，患者的情况会好得多；可以教他们改善平衡和步态，提高他们的稳定性，保持积极的生活。这种运动障碍的一些独有的特征，已经有了充分利用；有了音乐疗法，患者表现良好，体现在健身计划、骑自行车和拳击。无法行走的患者可能会发现自己能够跳舞。抑郁症、照料者疲劳、便秘、**REM**睡眠障碍、偏执和精神病很常见。它们可能是药物的副作用或是原发病的一部分，所有这些都要解决。

◎ **分析**：

1. "Patients do much better"此处灵活处理为"患者的情况会好得多"，符合国内此行业的表达习惯；

2. "carer fatigue"译作"照料者疲劳"。此处应注意听译，不要错译为"护理疲劳"。"carer"具体指日常照料PD患者的人，多为家属或护工；

3. "REM"全称是"rapid eye movement"，意思是"快动眼"，不过此处讲者并未展开，同传时跟读即可。

二、中译英

近几年AD领域发展迅速，比如AD新型靶向治疗药物的批准上市，血浆生物标志物的出色应用，以及某些个体中影像和体液生物标志物并不一致的现象等，因此亟须更新指南以满足研究和临床管理的需求。2022年初，阿尔茨海默病协会组织了一个指导委员会，领导NIA-AA框架的修订工作。来自美国梅奥诊所的CJ教授作为该委员会主席，在大会上提交了《NIA-AA阿尔茨海默病临床诊断指南修订版》的草案，以征求科学界的意见和审查。修订版指南依然强调了从生物学角度定义AD，而非基于临床表现，这将推动未来大规模地从生物学角度诊断AD。随着大数据和人工智能技术的发展，AD全球数据资源正经历着前所未有的开放与共享浪潮。这一过程促进了跨地域、跨研究机构、跨患者群体的多维度数据融合，极大地丰富了研究样本的多样性和数量，为科研人员提供了前所未有的、全面且前沿的研究资源。（本段内容来自网络，有删改调整。）

◎ **参考译文**：In recent years, the AD industry has been developing rapidly, such as the approval of new targeted therapeutic drugs for AD, the excellent application of plasma biomarkers, and the phenomenon that imaging and body fluid biomarkers are inconsistent in some individuals. Therefore, it is urgent to update the guidelines to meet the needs of research and clinical management. In early 2022, the Alzheimer's association convened a steering committee to lead the revision of the NIA-AA framework. Professor CJ from the Mayo Clinic in the United States, as the chairman of the committee, submitted a draft of the "Revised NIA-AA Clinical Diagnosis Guidelines for Alzheimer's Disease" at the conference to solicit opinions and reviews from the scientific community. This revised guideline still emphasizes the definition of AD from a biological perspective rather than based on clinical manifestations, which will promote the large-scale diagnosis of AD from a biological perspective in the future. With the development of big data and artificial intelligence technologies, AD global data resources are experiencing an unprecedented wave of openness and sharing. This process promotes multi-dimensional data fusion across regions, research institutions, and patient groups, greatly enriches the diversity and quantity of research samples, and provides researchers with unprecedented comprehensive and cutting-edge research resources.

◎ 分析：

1. "更新指南"译作"update the guidelines"，更符合此语境下英语的表达习惯；

2. "指导委员会"译作"steering committee"，是近年来讲到临床科研时的常用词汇；

3. "梅奥诊所"译作"Mayo Clinic"。梅奥诊所是美国一家医疗集团，医疗水平与行业内影响力当前位于全球前列，医学译员应有所了解。近年来，"Mayo Clinic"也被译作"妙佑医疗"，但大多数的国内医生还是习惯使用"梅奥诊所"这一称谓；

4. "前沿"译作"cutting-edge"，前几年，对于"前沿""最新前沿"类似的表达，国外讲者还较多地使用"cutting-edge""cutting the edge"等表达，但近两年，讲者更多使用的则是"latest"或"most recent"之类更加简单、更容易为非英语母语者所理解的表达。

对于AD而言"早诊早治"的重要性不言而喻，但是仅关注"筛"和"诊"还远远不够。既往实践经验提示我们，即使社会各界付出诸多努力，开展筛查，也并非所有筛查发现的可疑认知障碍者后续都会到专业机构进行诊断，更谈不上及时得到全面细致的指导和支持。因此，本次会议上，与会专家呼吁：重视"筛"与"诊"的同时，还需要更积极地关注诊断后支持，为筛查后支持及诊断后服务投入更多研究和资源。来自加拿大麦吉尔大学的FL女士，就"通过创新教育和培训改善诊断后支持和生活质量"进行了演讲，以"创新教育和培训"为切入点，以麦吉尔大学老龄研究中心的工作为例，以亲身经历为引，步步深入讲述了普及获得诊断后支持资源途径的重要性。

◎ 参考译文：The importance of "early diagnosis and early treatment" for AD is self-evident, but it is far from enough to focus only on "screening" and "diagnosis". Previous practical experience tells us that even if all sectors of society make great efforts to carry out screening, not all suspected cognitive impairments found in the screening will be diagnosed in professional institutions, let alone receive comprehensive and detailed guidance and support in a timely manner. Therefore, at this conference, experts called for: while paying attention to "screening" and "diagnosis", more attention should be paid to post-diagnosis support and invest more with research and resources in post-screening support and post-diagnosis services. Ms. FL from McGill University in Canada gave a speech on "Improving post-diagnosis support and quality of life through innovative education and training". Taking "innovative education and training" as the starting point, the work of the McGill University Center for Aging Research as an example, and her personal experience as a guide, she talked about the importance of popularizing access to post-diagnosis support resources step by step.

◎ 分析：

1. 医学会议的中文表达中经常会用到单字词，例如"筛（查）""诊（断）""治（疗）""（预）防""（临床）医（疗实践）""（临床）教（学）""（临床）研（究）"，对应的英文则是screening, diagnosis, treatment, prevention, clinical practice, clinical education, clinical

research。对于此类基础词汇，译员最好能做到"肌肉记忆"，听到后能下意识译出，才不会影响同传节奏；

2. "重视'筛'与'诊'的同时，还需要更积极地关注诊断后支持"，国内讲者发言时，很多时候会大量用此类无主句，同传时译员可用被动语态应对，此处处理为"while paying attention to 'screening' and 'diagnosis', more attention should be paid to post-diagnosis support"，而没有补充主语"we"然后用主动语态；

3. 对于发言条理清晰的中文讲者，可适当拉长 EVS，不一定要使用顺句驱动的技巧，例如本段最后一句；而对于发言较破碎、逻辑条理欠清晰、口头语较多的讲者，就算拉长 EVS 有时也无济于事，此时应使用顺句驱动的方法尽快处理每一个短句。

作为一名照料者，FL 女士发现虽然政府和很多机构在开展提高公共意识的活动，但是这些信息和海报很多时候并没有传递到需要的人手里，许多患者在被诊断时也未能获得充足的指导，所以支持教育和培训刻不容缓。FL 女士利用社区发放知识传单、宣传痴呆陪伴指南、建立关怀广播、医学院开展课程、发表演讲等多种途径在努力为 AD 患者诊断后支持事业奋斗，并且在得到社会支持后将资源以多种语言发布，为更多患者带来获益，切实提高公众意识。"这不是在孤岛上工作，完成患者支持需要包括学校、社会工作、护理、康复、法律等等多个学科共同行动。"这是 FL 女士参与的 2023 年发表的一项荟萃分析，她也反复强调多学科多元素在 AD 患者支持中的重要性，以及"数字化痴呆教育和干预可以改善护理体验，远程教育与面对面教育具有相似效果"，这项研究也是对本次会议主题的有力支持。

◎ **参考译文**：As a caregiver, Ms. FL found that although the government and many organizations are carrying out activities to raise public awareness, this information and posters are often not delivered to those in need, and many patients do not receive adequate guidance when they are diagnosed, so support education and training are urgent. Ms. FL, by distributing knowledge leaflets in the community, promoting dementia companionship guidelines, establishing care broadcasts, conducting courses in medical schools, and giving speeches, and many other channels, strives for the cause of supporting AD patients after diagnosis. After receiving social support, she publishes resources in multiple languages to benefit more patients and effectively raise public awareness. "This is not working on an isolated island. Patient support requires joint action from multiple disciplines including schools, social work, nursing, rehabilitation, law, and many other disciplines." This is a meta-analysis published in 2023 with the participation of Ms. FL, she also repeatedly emphasizes the importance of multidisciplinary and multi-element support for AD patients and "digital dementia education and intervention can improve the nursing experience, and remote education has similar effects to face-to-face education", this research is also a strong support for the theme of this conference.

◎ 分析：

1. "并没有传递到需要的人手里"处理为"not delivered to those in need"，在医学口译中，中译英的时候，"those"是一个非常有用的表达，对于"基线时有糖尿病的""有过CV事件的""那些电话随访的""那些未能入组的"之类的常用表达，译员都可以用those轻松应对；

2. 从这段话的一些表述中，例如"并没有传递到需要的人手里""许多患者在被诊断时""将资源以多种语言发布"等，我们基本可以判断这段话的原文是英文，在被简单翻译成中文后未经过润色直接讲了出来。对于此类的文本，同传时译员如果能迅速作出判断，则大可放心使用顺句驱动的方法，难度不会很大。

新西兰的KB教授提供的记忆门诊诊断后支持经验也聚焦于此。在"提升新西兰记忆门诊的诊断后支持：现状、提供理想支持的阻碍和促进因素"的汇报内容中提到，记忆门诊通常会为出现认知损害或其他可能代表痴呆诊断的人群提供专业评估服务，但是在诊断后支持的工作中，新西兰记忆门诊目前提供的信息还比较少，有巨大的潜力空间。KB教授对15位痴呆患者以及20位照料者进行了访谈，从而分析当前诊断后支持工作的现状。研究结论表明，痴呆患者和照料者目前主要的依靠是家庭支持，记忆门诊目前并未能提供理想的资源，需要新西兰政府以及多方共同的支持从而改变这一情况。

◎ 参考译文：Professor KB of New Zealand also focused on the post-diagnosis support experience of memory clinics. The report "Improving post-diagnosis support in New Zealand memory clinics: current status, barriers and facilitators to providing ideal support" mentioned that, memory clinics usually provide professional assessment services for people with cognitive impairment or other conditions that may represent a dementia diagnosis, but in terms of post-diagnosis support, New Zealand memory clinics currently provide relatively little information and have great potential. Professor KB interviewed 15 dementia patients and 20 caregivers to analyze the current status of post-diagnosis support. The study suggested that dementia patients and caregivers currently mainly rely on family support, and memory clinics are currently unable to provide ideal resources. The New Zealand government and multiple parties need to work together to change this situation.

◎ 分析：

1. "研究结论表明"处理为"The study suggested"，不一定要处理为"The study conclusion showed"，因为前者更符合英语的表达习惯；

2. 此段句子较长，信息密集，更像是讲者读稿。同传时，译员如果提前拿到稿件，可进行翻译后跟读，也可跟随视译；但如果未提前拿到稿件，同传有一定难度，可重点把握关键词的短时记忆，如"诊断后支持"，短时间内将两个词合并为一个词，可减低同传时的记忆难度。

WHO也提供了一系列线上资源，协助各国开展诊断后支持的工作，如iSupport等。

来自世界卫生组织的 HC 博士团队"全球估算 2019 年 WHO 194 个成员国痴呆患者非正式照护数据"的内容分享从经济学数据层面再次证实了痴呆后护理照料的重要性。报告提示目前大多数痴呆患者是由家庭成员或者其他无偿照料者进行照料的，如果将这部分负担转化为工作时长相当于接近 6700 万小时，并且约 70% 的照料由女性承担。所以 iSupport 等线上资源就更需要得到合理运用。

◎ **参考译文**：WHO also provides a series of online resources to assist countries in carrying out post-diagnosis support, such as iSupport. Dr. HC's team, from WHO, with "Global Estimates of 2019 194 WHO Member State Informal Dementia Patient Care Data", the content sharing, from the perspective of economic data, once again confirms the importance of post-dementia care. The report suggests that most dementia patients are currently cared for by family members or other unpaid caregivers. If this burden is converted into working hours, it is equivalent to nearly 67 million hours of working time, and about 70% of the care is undertaken by women. Therefore, online resources such as iSupport need to be used reasonably.

◎ **分析**：

1. "来自世界卫生组织的 HC 博士团队提供的'全球估算 2019 年 WHO 194 个成员国痴呆患者非正式照护数据'的内容分享从经济学数据层面再次证实了痴呆后护理照料的重要性。"译作"Dr. HC's team, from WHO, with 'Global Estimates of 2019 194 WHO Member State Informal Dementia Patient Care Data', the content sharing, from the perspective of economic data, once again confirms the importance of post-dementia care."译员将句子拆成了若干个结构，否则在同传情况下，极难译出。

仑卡奈单抗是一种用于治疗阿尔茨海默病的人源化单克隆抗体，可以选择性中和并清除导致阿尔茨海默病神经病变的可溶且有毒性的 β-淀粉样蛋白聚集体。因此，仑卡奈单抗可能对 AD 病理过程产生积极影响并减缓疾病发展进程。目前，仑卡奈单抗是唯一一款可用于治疗早期 AD 且无需剂量滴定的抗 Aβ 抗体。仑卡奈单抗与之前的药物 A 一样，是一种静脉注射抗体，旨在去除淀粉样蛋白沉积物。与 A 不同，仑卡奈单抗靶向尚未聚集在一起的淀粉样蛋白形式。仑卡奈单抗靶向的是 Aβ 的聚集形式，包括寡聚体、protofibril、fibril 和淀粉样聚集体等。

◎ **参考译文**：Lecanemab is a humanized monoclonal antibody for the treatment of Alzheimer's disease, it selectively neutralizes and clears soluble and toxic amyloid-beta aggregates that cause Alzheimer's disease neuropathy. Therefore, lecanemab may have a positive impact on AD pathology and slow the disease progression. Currently, lecanemab is the only anti-Aβ antibody that can be used to treat early AD without dose titration. Lecanemab, like the previous drug A, is an intravenous antibody, designed to remove amyloid deposits. Unlike A, lecanemab targets forms of amyloid that have not yet aggregated together. Lecanemab targets aggregated forms of Aβ, including oligomers, protofibril,

fibril, and amyloid aggregates.

◎ 分析：

1. "剂量滴定"译作"dose titration"，这个表述近年来使用得越来越多；

2. "包括寡聚体、protofibril、fibril 和淀粉样聚集体等"这种表述也是医学口译中的一大特色。在进行神经内科、肿瘤学、免疫治疗、靶向治疗等主题中译英时，译员经常会遇到中文发言中夹杂不少英文，多为药物名称、产品名称、试验名称、分子或基因名称等，口译时译员要能及时识别，哪些需要口译，哪些跟读即可。

Clarity AD 是一项为期 18 个月、多中心、双盲、安慰剂对照的平行组试验，涉及早期阿尔茨海默病患者。符合条件的参与者以 1∶1 的比例随机分配接受静脉注射 lecanemab，每 2 周 10 mg/kg，或安慰剂。随机分组根据临床亚组，包括阿尔茨海默病引起的轻度认知障碍或根据下述标准的轻度阿尔茨海默病相关痴呆；基线时是否存在经批准用于治疗阿尔茨海默病症状的伴随药物，包括乙酰胆碱酯酶抑制剂、美金刚胺或两者；载脂蛋白 E ε4 携带者或非携带者；以及地理区域。在试验期间，参与者接受了血浆生物标志物的连续血液检测，并可以参加三个可选的子研究，这些子研究评估了通过 PET 测量的脑淀粉样蛋白负荷的纵向变化、通过 PET 测量的脑 tau 病理特征和脑脊液阿尔茨海默病的生物标志物。

◎ 参考译文：Clarity AD is an 18-month, multicenter, double-blind, placebo-controlled, parallel-group trial, involving patients with early Alzheimer's disease. Eligible participants are randomized 1∶1 to receive intravenous lecanemab, 10 mg/kg every 2 weeks, or placebo. Randomization is based on clinical subgroups, including MCI due to Alzheimer's disease, or mild Alzheimer's disease-related dementia according to the criteria described below; the presence of concomitant medications approved to treat symptoms of Alzheimer's disease at baseline, including acetylcholinesterase inhibitors, memantine, or both; apolipoprotein E ε4 carriers or noncarriers; and geographic regions. During the trial, participants undergo serial blood testing for plasma biomarkers and could participate in three optional sub-studies, which evaluate longitudinal changes in brain amyloid burden measured by PET, brain tau pathology features measured by PET, and Alzheimer's disease CSF biomarkers.

◎ 分析：

1. "安慰剂"译作"placebo"，指没有治疗作用的与实际药物外观一致的制剂，其作用主要是通过心理暗示和期望效应从而产生可能的疗效。在临床试验中，用安慰剂充当对照组的参照物，从而评估新的药物或治疗方式的真实疗效。"安慰剂"是医学口译中的最基础的词汇与概念；

2. "轻度认知障碍"此处译作"MCI"，而没有译作"mild cognitive impairment"，这样的处理需要译员对于内容有较好的理解，能够判读出普通听众对于缩略语的接受程度，比如"MCI"在阿尔茨海默病诊疗领域，几乎尽人皆知，所以译员可以如此操作，以节省时间，但译员如果没有把握，最好不要如此行事；

3. "脑脊液"译作"CSF"，而非"cerebrospinal fluid"，道理同上。

第四节 补 充 练 习

一、中译英

在大型的、基于人群的加拿大健康与衰老研究（Canadian Study of Health and Aging）中，将老年人划分为以下三种状态：无认知下降、非痴呆的认知损害（CIND）和痴呆。该研究定义 CIND 为表现任一认知域的客观认知损害，评分降低范围处于正常和痴呆 2 个界值之间。总体来讲，约 16.8% 的老年人可划入此类。此类人群中显示最终进展至痴呆（在 5 年随访期间约 5% 的患者进展至痴呆）和死亡风险增加。

CIND 这一名称，对医师来说有一个好处就是只需认定存在认知损害，无须考虑认知下降程度，是否存在功能损害以及可能的基础性原因。当然采用这一术语也有几项固有局限。一个缺陷是，患者可能因基础病症（如终身的静止性脑损伤、精神发育迟滞或精神分裂症）导致认知下降而被考虑为 CIND，但这些病症在全科或专科医师实践中是很明显的。这种情况下，医师并不涉及 CIND 的预后及诊断方法，重视的只是患者新出现的记忆下降的主诉。目前在加拿大记忆门诊就诊的患者中采用如下命名方法，即显示具有异质性的病因，包括有遗忘性、血管性、精神病性、神经病性、代谢性和混合性。

MCI 这一术语体现了正常状态与痴呆之间这一灰色地带特征，并在目前广泛应用。这一术语适用于老年人群中存在短期或长期记忆损害，但无显著的日常认知功能损害者。最初 MCI 诊断标准需具备较此前认知水平下降的主观报告，且缓慢起病，症状持续 6 个月以上。目前主观报告又补充了记忆下降的客观证据，可通过简易或广泛认知测验获知，同时其他认知域一般无缺损。不过虽然强调了客观的表现，但尚无界定记忆下降的确切表述。后来的工作是又扩大了定义，除记忆之外其他认知域也可显示损害。针对所有情况，该术语排除了因明显抑郁、谵妄、精神迟滞及其他精神障碍引发相关认知损害的患者。如果患者记忆严重下降，伴明显功能损害和其他认知损害，则患者符合痴呆临床标准，而非 MCI。

一个不确定因素为是否要考虑将轻度抑郁患者排除于 MCI 之外。有研究显示，由 MCI 继续发展至 AD 的患者中有 60% 存在抑郁，而抑郁实际上是 MCI 患者中有效的预后指证。另一挑战是评估"功能活动的明显损害"，作为一条痴呆标准，其在 MCI 与痴呆鉴别中有重要作用。不幸的是，功能活动的评估标准几乎没有达成共识，而何谓"显著的"功能损害当然也无共识。约 31% 的 MCI 患者可能存在轻微功能改变，有人甚至认为有必要列入功能改变的条目。MCI 诊断要鉴别的关键点是这一改变是否影响到较高级功能，而这并不代表"显著的损害"。不过这仍是一个很粗略的界定，发现功能损害最敏感的问题是询问患者能否保持原有爱好，能否处理复杂财务事项，是否会使用新设备和工具，或者发现他们重复同样错误或忘记年月日。在客观评价记忆下降方面的争议在于，是选择简易认知测验还是全套神经心理学评定。

◎ **参考译文**：In the large, population-based Canadian Study of Health and Aging, older adults were divided into three states: no cognitive decline, cognitive impairment without dementia (CIND), and dementia. The study defined CIND as objective cognitive impairment in any cognitive domain, with scores falling between the normal and dementia boundaries. Overall, approximately 16.8% of older adults fell into this category. This population showed an increased risk of eventual progression to dementia (approximately 5% of patients progressed to dementia during a 5-year follow-up period) and death.

The term CIND has the advantage that physicians only need to identify the presence of cognitive impairment, regardless of the degree of cognitive decline, the presence of functional impairment, or possible underlying causes. However, there are several inherent limitations to this term. One drawback is that patients may be considered CIND because of underlying conditions (such as lifelong static brain damage, mental retardation, or schizophrenia) that are obvious in general or specialist practice. In this case, the physician does not address the prognosis and diagnostic approach of CIND, but only focuses on the patient's complaint of new memory loss. The current nomenclature used for patients attending Canadian memory clinics is to reflect the heterogeneous etiologies, including amnestic, vascular, psychiatric, neuropathic, metabolic, and mixed.

The term MCI captures the gray area between normal and dementia and is now widely used. The term applies to older adults who have short-term or long-term memory impairment but no significant impairment in daily cognitive function. Initially, the diagnostic criteria for MCI required a subjective report of a decline in cognitive function from the previous level, with a slow onset and symptoms lasting for more than 6 months. Subjective reports are now supplemented with objective evidence of memory loss, which can be obtained through simple or extensive cognitive tests, and other cognitive domains are generally intact. However, despite the emphasis on objective manifestations, there is no precise statement to define memory loss. Later work has expanded the definition to include impairment in cognitive domains other than memory. For all cases, the term excludes patients with cognitive impairment related to significant depression, delirium, mental retardation, and other psychiatric disorders. If a patient has severe memory loss with significant functional impairment and other cognitive impairment, the patient meets the clinical criteria for dementia but not MCI.

One uncertainty is whether to consider excluding patients with mild depression from MCI. Studies have shown that 60% of patients who go on to develop AD from MCI have depression, and depression is actually a valid prognostic indicator in MCI patients. Another challenge is to assess "marked impairment of functional activities", which is a dementia criterion and plays an important role in differentiating MCI from dementia. Unfortunately, there is little consensus on the criteria for assessing functional activities, and certainly no consensus on what constitutes "significant" functional impairment. About 31% of MCI patients may have slight functional changes, and some even think it is necessary to include a functional change item. The key point to distinguish in the diagnosis of MCI is whether the change affects higher-level functions, which does not represent "significant impairment". However, this is still a very rough definition, and the most sensitive questions to detect functional impairment are to ask patients whether they can maintain their original hobbies, handle complex financial matters, use new equipment and tools, or find that they repeat the same mistakes or forget the year. Controversy in the objective assessment of memory loss lies in whether to choose a brief cognitive test or a full neuropsychological assessment.

二、英译中

Spinal muscular atrophy (SMA) is a genetic disease affecting the central nervous system, peripheral nervous system, and voluntary muscle movement (skeletal muscle). Most of the nerve cells that control muscles are located in the spinal cord, which accounts for the word spinal in the name of the disease. SMA is muscular because its primary effect is on muscles, which don't receive signals from these nerve cells. Atrophy is the medical term for getting smaller, which is what generally happens to muscles when they're not stimulated by nerve cells. SMA involves the loss of nerve cells called motor neurons in the spinal cord and is classified as a motor neuron disease.

The age at which SMA symptoms begin roughly correlates with the degree to which motor function is affected: The earlier the age of onset, the greater the impact on motor function. Children who display symptoms at birth or in infancy typically have the lowest level of functioning (type 1). Later-onset SMA with a less severe course (types 2 and 3, and in teens or adults, type 4) generally correlates with increasingly higher levels of motor function.

SMA symptoms cover a broad spectrum, ranging from mild to severe. The muscles closer to the center of the body (proximal muscles) are usually more affected in SMA than the muscles farther from the center (distal muscles). The muscles closer to the center of the body (proximal muscles) are usually more affected in SMA than are the muscles farther from the center (distal muscles). The primary symptom of chromosome 5-related (SMN-related) SMA is weakness of the voluntary muscles. The muscles most affected are those closest to the center of the body, such as those of the shoulders, hips, thighs, and upper back. The lower limbs seem to be affected more than the upper limbs, and deep tendon reflexes are decreased. Special complications occur if the muscles used for breathing and swallowing are affected, resulting in abnormalities in these functions. If the muscles of the back weaken, spinal curvatures can develop.

There's a great deal of variation in the age of onset and level of motor function achieved in chromosome 5-related SMA. These are roughly correlated with how much functional SMN protein is present in the motor neurons, which in turn correlates with how many copies of SMN2 genes a person has. Sensory, mental, and emotional functioning are entirely normal in chromosome-5 SMA. Some forms of SMA are not linked to chromosome 5 or SMN deficiency. These forms vary greatly in severity and in the muscles most affected. While most forms, like the chromosome 5-related form, affect mostly the proximal muscles, other forms exist that affect mostly the distal muscles (those farther away from the body's center) — at least in the beginning.

Several treatments have been developed for SMA that preserve motor neurons, improve muscle function, and extend lives, but these are not cures. Treatment early in life tends to provide more benefit than treatment later in life, as older people who have been living with SMA and have experienced greater loss of motor neurons.

FDA-approved treatments for SMA include: Nusinersen increases production of the SMN protein and is approved to treat children and adults with SMA. This medication is administered via lumbar puncture. Onasemnogene abeparovec-xioi is a gene therapy for children less than two years old who have infantile-onset SMA (Type I). This therapy replaces the SMN1 gene function by delivering a new working SMN gene to the person's motor neurons. This treatment has been shown to improve muscle movement, function, and survival. Risdiplam is an orally administered drug to treat people age two months and older. Risdiplam works by increasing the concentration of SMN protein in the body.

People with SMA can benefit from physical therapy, occupational therapy, and rehabilitation to help improve posture, prevent joint immobility, and slow muscle weakness and atrophy. Stretching and strengthening exercises may help reduce joint contractures, increase range of motion, and improve circulation. Some individuals may require additional therapy for speech and swallowing difficulties. Assistive devices such as supports or braces, orthotics, speech synthesizers, and wheelchairs may be helpful to improve functional independence.

It is important that the people with SMA get proper nutrition to help them maintain weight and promote muscle function. People who cannot chew or swallow may require a feeding tube. Non-invasive ventilation can improve breathing during sleep, and some individuals also may require assisted ventilation during the day due to muscle weakness of the respiratory muscles (along the chest).

◎ **参考译文**：脊髓性肌萎缩症（SMA）是一种影响中枢神经系统、周围神经系统和随意肌运动（骨骼肌）的遗传性疾病。控制肌肉的大多数神经细胞位于脊髓中，因此该病的名称中带有"脊髓"一词。SMA之所以被称为肌肉性肌萎缩症，是因为它主要影响肌肉，而肌肉不会接收来自这些神经细胞的信号。萎缩是医学术语，表示肌肉变小，当肌肉不受神经细胞刺激时，通常会发生这种情况。SMA 涉及脊髓中称为运动神经元的神经细胞的损失，被归类为运动神经元疾病。

SMA 症状开始出现的年龄与运动功能受影响的程度大致相关：发病年龄越早，对运动功能的影响越大。出生时或婴儿期出现症状的儿童通常功能水平最低（1 型）。晚发型 SMA 的病程较轻（2 型和 3 型，以及青少年或成年人中的 4 型）通常与运动功能水平不断提高相关。

SMA 症状范围很广，从轻微到严重不等。SMA 患者中，靠近身体中心的肌肉（近端肌肉）通常比远离中心的肌肉（远端肌肉）受到的影响更大。5 号染色体相关（SMN-related）SMA 的主要症状是随意肌无力。受影响最严重的是靠近身体中心的肌肉，例如肩部、臀部、大腿和上背部的肌肉。下肢似乎比上肢受到的影响更大，并且深部腱反射减弱。如果用于呼吸和吞咽的肌肉受到影响，导致这些功能异常，则会出现特殊并发症。如果背部肌肉无力，则会出现脊柱弯曲。

5 号染色体相关 SMA 的发病年龄和运动功能水平存在很大差异。这些与运动神经元中存在的功能性 SMN 蛋白数量大致相关，而后者又与一个人拥有的 SMN2 基因拷贝数相关。5 号染色体 SMA 的感觉、心理和情绪功能完全正常。某些形式的 SMA 与 5 号染色体或 SMN 缺乏无关。这些形式的严重程度和受影响最严重的肌肉差异很大。虽然大多数形式（如 5 号染色体相关形式）主要影响近端肌肉，但也存在其他形式主要影响远端肌肉（远离身体中心的肌肉）——至少在开始时是这样。

已经开发出几种针对 SMA 的治疗方法，可以保护运动神经元、改善肌肉功能并延长寿命，但这些都不是治愈方法。早期治疗往往比晚期治疗更有益，因为患有 SMA 的老年人会经历更严重的运动神经元损失。

FDA 批准的 SMA 治疗方法包括：Nusinersen 可增加 SMN 蛋白的产生，并被批准用于治疗患有 SMA 的儿童和成人。这种药物通过腰椎穿刺给药。Onasemnogene abeparovec-xioi 是一种针对患有婴儿期 SMA（Ⅰ型）的两岁以下儿童的基因疗法。这种疗法通过将新的有效 SMN 基因传递给患者运动神经元来取代 SMN1 基因功能。这种治疗已被证明可以改善肌肉运动、功能和生存率。Risdiplam 是一种口服药物，用于治疗两个月及以上的人群。Risdiplam 通过增加体内 SMN 蛋白的浓度发挥作用。

SMA 患者可以从物理治疗、职业治疗和康复中受益，以帮助改善姿势、防止关节僵硬、减缓肌肉无力和萎缩。伸展和强化锻炼可能有助于减少关节挛缩、增加活动范围和改善血液循环。有些人可能需要额外的治疗来治疗言语和吞咽困难。辅助设备，如支架或支具、矫形器、语音合成器和轮椅可能有助于提高功能独立性。

SMA 患者获得适当的营养以帮助他们保持体重和促进肌肉功能非常重要。无法咀嚼或吞咽的人可能需要喂食管。无创通气可以改善睡眠期间的呼吸，有些人由于呼吸肌（沿着胸部）的肌肉无力，也可能需要白天辅助通气。

第九单元 血液肿瘤

第一节 血液肿瘤口译知识点

血液肿瘤是一种特殊的肿瘤疾病，与常规意义的实体肿瘤或癌症不同，其并非一块明确的实体占位病变，而主要是起源于造血系统的恶性肿瘤，临床常见的为白血病(leukemia)、多发性骨髓瘤(multiple myeloma)以及恶性淋巴瘤(malignant lymphoma)。

白血病按照细胞分化成熟度及自然病程(natural course)可分为急性白血病(acute leukemia, AL)和慢性白血病(chronic leukemia, CL)。其中，AL的细胞分化停滞在早期阶段，多为原始细胞和早期幼稚细胞，病情进展快，自然病程可能仅为几个月。CL的细胞分化停滞在较晚的阶段，多为较成熟细胞和成熟细胞，病情相对缓慢，自然病程或为数年。

按照主要受累的细胞类型，白血病可分为淋巴细胞白血病和非淋巴细胞(髓细胞)白血病。可将AL分为急性淋巴细胞白血病(acute lymphoblastic leukemia, ALL)和急性髓系/髓细胞性白血病(acute myeloid leukemia, AML)；慢性白血病可分为慢性淋巴细胞白血病(chronic lymphocytic leukemia, CLL)、慢性髓系/髓细胞性白血病(chronic myeloid leukemia, CML)及少见类型的白血病。

急性淋巴细胞白血病(ALL)是一种血液和骨髓癌症。骨髓是骨骼内生成血细胞的海绵状组织。急性淋巴细胞白血病，也称"急淋"，"急性"指病情(condition)进展迅速(rapid progression)。急性淋巴细胞白血病中的"淋巴细胞"一词是指被称为"淋巴细胞"的白细胞，也就是被ALL影响的细胞。

急性淋巴细胞白血病的临床体征和症状表现包括：骨髓受白血病细胞浸润引起的骨髓正常造血衰竭，出现贫血(anemia)、感染(infection)、出血(bleeding)等症状，以及白血病细胞的髓外浸润(extramedullary infiltration)引起淋巴结、肝脾肿大等。贫血是白血病最常见的症状，随病情进展而加重，可出现苍白、无力、头晕、心悸、浮肿等症状。出血的部位分布广泛，以皮肤、黏膜最为常见，表现为皮肤瘀点、瘀斑、齿龈及鼻出血等。患者发病时，因为淋巴细胞功能下降，以及中性粒细胞减少(neutropenia)，极易发生感染。白血病细胞增殖浸润会导致肝脾淋巴结肿大以及骨关节疼痛。

急性淋巴细胞白血病的治疗，需考虑防止感染、输血支持治疗、营养维持以及放射/化学治疗。化疗有化疗方案(chemotherapy regimen)，治疗可分为诱导期(induction period)治疗、强化治疗(intensification therapy)和巩固治疗(consolidation therapy)，所涉及的化疗药物包括：环磷酰胺（CTX）、长春新碱（VCR）、长春地辛（VDS）、柔红霉素（DNR）、左旋门冬酰胺酶（L-asp）或培门冬酶（PEG-ASP）、泼尼松（PDN）、地塞米松（DXM）、大剂量甲氨蝶呤（HD-MTX）、依托泊苷（VP-16）、阿糖胞苷（Ara-C）、6-巯基嘌呤（6-MP）等。

多发性骨髓瘤（multiple myeloma，MM）是间细胞恶性增殖性疾病，特点是骨髓中的浆细胞无限制增生，大部分病例还伴有单克隆免疫球蛋白（monoclonal immunoglobulin）分泌，导致器官或组织损伤。

多发性骨髓瘤有经典的四联征，即血钙升高（Ca^{2+} increase）、肾功能不全（renal insufficiency）、贫血（anemia）以及骨痛（bone pain），不少医生也会用四个症状的首字母缩写来描述，即"Crab"症状，很多时候医生在讲课时会在幻灯片上放一张螃蟹的照片。其他症状包括肝脾增大、淋巴结肿大、发热、感觉异常等。

骨痛与病理性骨折，骨髓瘤细胞分泌破骨细胞活性因子而激活破骨细胞，导致骨溶解与破坏，最常见的症状就是骨骼疼痛，多为腰骶处、胸骨及肋骨疼痛。由于肿瘤细胞对骨质的破坏，可出现病理性骨折，可能为多处骨折同时存在。

贫血与出血，贫血常为首发症状，早期贫血症状较轻，后期贫血情况严重，且可能出现血小板减少，引起出血症状。皮肤黏膜出血较多见，严重者可见内脏及颅内出血。

肝、脾、淋巴结及肾脏病变，肝、脾肿大，颈部淋巴结肿大，骨髓瘤肾脏病变。

神经系统症状，神经系统骨髓外浆细胞瘤的患者可出现肢体瘫痪、嗜睡、昏迷、复视、视力减退等症状。

感染，MM多见细菌感染，最常见为细菌性肺炎、泌尿系统感染及败血症。治疗后免疫受损的患者，也容易出现带状疱疹，也可见到其他真菌病毒感染。

肾功能损伤，很多MM患者会出现慢性肾功能衰竭，有高磷酸血症、高钙血症及高尿酸血症。

多发性骨髓瘤的治疗方法包括自体造血干细胞移植（autologous hematopoietic stem cell transplantation，ASCT）、免疫治疗（immunotherapy），如双特异性抗体治疗（bispecific antibodies，BsAbs）以及化疗。常见的治疗药物有蛋白酶体抑制剂（proteasome inhibitor，PI），包括伊沙佐米（ixazomib）、硼替佐米（bortezomib）、卡非佐米（carfilzomib）；免疫调节剂，包括沙利度胺（thalidomide）、来那度胺（lenalidomide）、泊马度胺（pomalidomide）；化疗药物，包括多柔比星（doxorubicin）、马法兰（melphalan）、环磷酰胺（cyclophosphamide）；糖皮质激素，包括地塞米松（dexamethasone）、泼尼松（prednisone）等。

淋巴瘤（lymphoma）是一种因淋巴组织内淋巴细胞恶性增生而形成的恶性肿瘤，包括霍奇金淋巴瘤（Hodgkin lymphoma，HL）和非霍奇金淋巴瘤（non-Hodgkin lymphoma，NHL）两大类型。霍奇金淋巴瘤少见，主要原发于淋巴结，好发于颈部和锁骨上浅表淋巴结，以及纵隔、腹膜后等处淋巴结。非霍奇金淋巴瘤较多见，可发生于全身任何部位，最常见于淋巴结、扁桃体、脾脏及骨髓。

淋巴瘤通常特征为淋巴结肿大、发热、消瘦、盗汗等，也会因纵隔淋巴结肿大融合成块而导致压迫症状,如压迫食管导致吞咽困难,压迫气管导致咳嗽、胸闷、呼吸困难等。虽然淋巴瘤的确切原因不明,但一般认为与感染、免疫、环境因素和遗传有关。淋巴瘤的早期症状包括无痛性淋巴结肿大及不明原因发热。淋巴结肿大可发生于头颈部、锁骨上、腋窝、腹股沟等部位,如邻近器官受到压迫,会出现相应症状。

淋巴瘤根据病程可分为Ⅰ期(Stage Ⅰ)、Ⅱ期、Ⅲ期和Ⅳ期,Ⅰ期病情较轻,Ⅳ期最为严重。简单理解,Ⅰ期:单一淋巴结区受累为Ⅰ期,有局灶性单一淋巴结外器官受累(involved)为ⅠE期;Ⅱ期:膈肌同侧的两组或多组淋巴结受累为Ⅱ期,有局灶性单个结外器官及其区域淋巴结受累为ⅡE期;Ⅲ期:膈肌上下淋巴结区都受累为Ⅲ期,有局灶性结外器官受累为ⅢE期,脾脏受累(spleen involved)为ⅢS期,以上条件都满足为ⅢE+S期;Ⅳ期:弥漫性单一或多个结外器官受累,伴或不伴(with or without)相关淋巴结肿大,或孤立性(isolated)结外器官受累伴远处淋巴结肿大者为Ⅳ期,如肝脏或骨髓受累,即使病变局限也为Ⅳ期。

淋巴结的检查包括实验室检查(laboratory/lab tests)、影像学检查和病理学检查,可进行淋巴结活检与穿刺活检,病理检查是诊断的主要依据。

淋巴瘤的治疗包括化疗、放疗、靶向治疗(targeted therapy)及生物免疫治疗等,主要依赖化疗和放疗,具体方案取决于淋巴瘤的类型、分期和预后因素(prognostic factor)。化疗可通过口服、静脉滴注(intravenous drip)或脊柱鞘内注射(intrathecal injection)的方式实现。

霍奇金淋巴瘤可采用ABVD方案,包括多柔比星、博来霉素、长春地辛、达卡巴嗪,2周一次治疗,4周一个疗程(course of treatment)。

非霍奇金淋巴瘤可供选用的方案包括R-CHOP方案,包括利妥昔单抗、环磷酰胺、多柔比星、长春新碱、泼尼松,2周或3周一个疗程。

放疗同样是恶性淋巴瘤的重要治疗手段,主要是通过电离辐射的直接及间接作用损伤肿瘤细胞DNA而达到杀伤肿瘤的目的。治疗过程中,根据患者的病情条件及诊疗条件进行放疗线束、放射野和剂量的选择。

恶性淋巴瘤的其他治疗措施还包括:单克隆抗体,对大部分为B细胞型的非霍奇金淋巴瘤表达CD20,利妥昔单抗(CD20单抗)可促进靶细胞(target cell)的溶解及凋亡;干扰素,其具有抗细胞增殖、抗肿瘤、抗病毒及免疫调节作用;CAR-T细胞免疫治疗,即嵌合抗原受体T细胞免疫疗法,其将患者体内的T细胞激活,使其特异性识别肿瘤细胞,释放大量细胞因子杀灭肿瘤细胞,其对复发难治性B细胞淋巴瘤有效;造血干细胞移植(HSCT),人造血干细胞移植是应用健康或相对健康的造血干细胞取代患者的病态骨髓造血,以恢复正常的免疫功能。

淋巴瘤的预防主要是避免感染和提高免疫力,同时,遗传和环境因素也需要予以关注。在人群普查和早期诊断中,神经学检查、血常规检查、血清乳酸脱氢酶、β2-微球蛋白测定等实验室检查以及影像学检查有助于淋巴瘤的诊断和治疗。充分的检查和及时的诊断能够提高淋巴瘤的治愈率,改善生活质量。

霍奇金淋巴瘤已成为可通过化疗治愈的肿瘤之一,非霍奇金淋巴瘤的预后也有明显改善。

大量长期生存患者的随访结果显示,霍奇金淋巴瘤15年死亡率(mortality)较普通人群高31%,除原发病复发外,第二肿瘤(包括实体瘤和急性髓细胞白血病)占死亡原因的11%~38%。Ⅲ~Ⅳ期霍奇金淋巴瘤国际预后评分(IPS)可帮助判断预后,该评分系统中不良预后因素有:白蛋白<40g/L、血红蛋白<105g/L、男性、年龄≥45岁、Ⅳ期病变、白细胞≥15×10^9/L、淋巴细胞占白细胞比例<8%和(或)计数<0.6×10^9/L。

非霍奇金淋巴瘤是一组异质性的淋巴瘤,目前通常采用国际预后指数(IPI)将预后分为低危、低中危、高中危、高危四类。

年龄大于60岁、分期为Ⅲ期或Ⅳ期、结外病变1处以上、需要卧床或生活需要别人照顾、血清LDH升高是五个预后不良的IPI,医生会根据IPI评分来判断非霍奇金淋巴瘤患者的预后。

至于淋巴瘤的转移(metastasis),非霍奇金淋巴瘤的转移特点为跳跃性播散,且较多累及淋巴结外器官,如骨骼、肺门、纵隔、胃肠道、肝脏等部位,引起相应临床症状。如累及胸部,肺门及纵隔受累最多,可导致肺部淋巴结浸润及胸腔积液,也可侵犯心包及心脏;如累及胃肠道,小肠受累最多,可出现腹痛、腹泻和腹块等类似消化道溃疡、肠结核或脂肪泻的症状;如累及肝脏,可出现肝大、肝痛及黄疸;如累及骨骼,则以胸椎、腰椎最为常见,可表现为骨痛、脊髓压迫症等;如累及皮肤,可表现为皮肤肿块、皮下结节、浸润性斑块及溃疡等。

霍奇金淋巴瘤淋巴结外病变相对少见,且与非霍奇金淋巴瘤相比,前者累及脾(表现为脾大)、肺、胸膜更多见,但较少侵犯胃肠道。

中医治疗(Traditional Chinese Medicine, TCM),或称中西医结合医学(integrative medicine)也被用作现代治疗血液肿瘤的手段,但诊断治疗的理论理念与西医截然不同,中医需要辨别证候,辨证施治,不同的患者可能表现出气虚、阴虚、痰湿、血瘀等不同的证候。中医治疗血液肿瘤,除白血病外,主要在于减轻西医治疗后的不良反应,从免疫力调节及整体改善方面发挥积极辅助治疗作用。

第二节 真实世界口译情境

一、主题会议

血液肿瘤主题的医学会议口译量近年来似乎有限,行业内部分公司会举行定期的学术活动,会有一定的会议口译需求。除外专科会议,白血病、多发性骨髓瘤和恶性淋巴瘤在其他专科会议中也时有提及。近年来的中医会议及中西医结合医学会议都会提及血液肿瘤的中医治疗,或有专门的主题演讲。

二、行业特点

血液肿瘤主题的专科会议,一般演讲内容信息量较大,而且相对其他专科医生,血液肿瘤医生似乎语速更快，而且准备的幻灯片中经常引用国家或国际诊疗指南中的内容，有时会出现大段读幻灯片文字内容的情况。

血液肿瘤的治疗，现在越来越重视循证医学（evidence-based medicine，EBM），以及临床试验（clinical trial）证据，而随着年轻一代医生的成长，医生群体的整体英文水平不断提升，有时会议主办方也会安排专科医生进行翻译甚至是与译员搭档进行同传。

三、口译难点

以血液肿瘤为主题的医学会议口译的难点有以下几点：

一是会出现大量的药名，如上所述，大量的化疗用药、免疫治疗用药、激素的使用会被提及。在会议中，讲者可能会提及一种药物的化学名全称，也可能偶尔提到其商品名，很多药物还有三个字母的简写形式，以及单字母的名字，因此译员须进行较为充分的会前准备，否则会跟不上讲者的语速，出现大量药名漏译的情况。

二是血液肿瘤主题会议的演讲者一般会准备大量内容。主题演讲一般从疾病概述开始，讲治疗的历史演进、当前的治疗实践、不同学术机构制定的分型/分类标准、国内的实际情况、单中心（讲者所在医院）的数据分析、当下这一专科领域内临床研究/试验的概况、当下临床亟待解决的问题、专科未来的发展期待等；而病例汇报者则会从患者现病史开始，讲患者用药史、体格检查（physical examination）、既往治疗、病情分析、诊断与鉴别诊断、治疗方案、预后等。无论是哪种，一般都是信息量巨大，且医生语速一般较快，这就需要译员有一定的综合医学素养，否则在会前不提供材料的情况下，或者会前准备不充分的情况下，译员很难跟上讲者的语速。

除去主题演讲，现在会议一般都会安排讨论与问答环节，一般会前仅能提供此环节的话题或问题，而此时点评/讨论嘉宾发言的内容范围一般不限于讲课课件的范围，虽不是天马行空，但学术水平与表达能力俱佳的嘉宾也能做到旁征博引，滔滔不绝，这就对译员提出了更高的要求，需要其纯粹依赖听力与医学素养进行同传。有时线下会议在讨论或圆桌讨论阶段，出于种种安排，会要求译员走出同传间，进行台上交传，而又因讨论嘉宾的"热情激烈讨论"，导致多位嘉宾发言完成后，再让译员进行"总结式交传"，这就需要译员自己对讨论的话题有清晰的理解、强大扎实的笔记能力、一定的归纳总结能力以及较好的医学素养，否则面对台上台下几十位，甚至上百位的专科医生，极难完成任务。

三是在所有血液肿瘤会议中，现在都讲到各类临床试验及研究，此类内容有独特的表达方式，演讲水平较好的讲者，无论中外，一般都能在介绍各类试验时做到条理清晰、逻辑通畅，保持稳定的节奏；但偶尔遇到部分讲者会使用不规则的表述方式，加之跳跃式地介绍试验内容，此时译员如果 EVS 拉得较长，则很容易控制不好节奏，出现幻灯片已翻页，但还有上一页两三句话未翻完的情况，导致听众看到的幻灯片与听到的同传脱节。

第三节 中英对照篇章及分析

一、英译中

But even, very importantly, what they saw was an improvement in overall survival. This was felt to be about a 13-month improvement in overall survival in patients who received the bortezomib, compared to those who received melphalan and prednisone alone. This study, I think, very clearly showed how bortezomib was beginning to change the landscape in multiple myeloma. Now, one of the things that was appreciated very early in the development of the drug is the particular toxicity of peripheral neuropathy. And peripheral neuropathy has been, continues to be, in a sense, the leading toxicity which limits the use of Bortezomib. So that, for example, in the VISTA study, as you can see here, there was a very high incidence of peripheral neuropathy and neuralgia, and just comparing that to what you saw in the control arm, the MP arm. So this huge difference and note that there was a fair amount of grade three or higher neural toxicity. This is an, of course, unacceptable side effect. And it tended to be cumulative so that the longer you were on the Bortezomib, the more likely this was to happen. In the VISTA study, it turned out that about 1/3 of the patients actually had to discontinue Bortezomib or even the entire regimen, because of toxicity is like this. And this was a higher discontinuation rate than you saw in the MP arm. This was one of the motivating factors that led to the development of ixazomib.（本段内容选自2023年一位欧洲医生的学术演讲，有删改调整。）

◎ **参考译文**：更重要的是我们看到了总生存的提升，大概是13个月的总生存的提升，体现在接受了硼替佐米的患者中，相比于只接受了马法兰和泼尼松的患者。这一研究，我想，也非常清晰地展示了硼替佐米是如何开始改变了多发性骨髓瘤的治疗。在这个药物发展的早期有一个显著的问题，就是周围神经病变的毒性。而周围神经病变一直是居首位的毒性，限制了硼替佐米的使用。比如说，在VISTA研究当中，大家可以看到，周围神经病变和神经痛的发生率非常高，相比于在对照组中看到的，MP组。这里差异巨大，注意到有大量的三级及更高的神经毒性。这就是不可接受的副作用。它还像是累积性的，也就是说你用硼替佐米的时间越长，那就越有这种副作用的风险。在VISTA研究中，结果是大概三分之一的患者都停用硼替佐米，甚至是整个方案，就是因为毒性如此。而且相比于MP组的话，它的终止率也更高。这也促进了伊沙佐米的研发。

◎ **分析**：

1. "landscape"译作"治疗"，其实际意义是"形式、情况、局面"，但在同传过程中，这样的处理也可以接受。近年来，"landscape"一词在医学会议中的使用率有所增加；

2. "things"译作"问题"，同传中可接受，结合后面的具体内容，也是合适的。但在没有听到后面语义时，处理为"点"更为合适。如果是交传，面对懂些中文的国外听众，或是懂些英文的国内听众，译员得当心把"things""finding""observation""topic"之类的词翻译为"问题"，此种情况下还是直译为妙。另外，近些年的会议中，美国及非英语母语的讲者对"things"一词的使用频率有所增加；

（3）"appreciate"未译出，同传时如此处理没有问题，"appreicate"一词，近年来在医学会议中被各国讲者广为使用，但表达的意思仅仅是"看到"，其实此类"大词小义"的现象近年来医学口译中出现得越来越多，典型的除了"appreciate"之外，还有用"insight"替代"idea"等；

（4）"development of drugs"译作"药物发展"，同传中可接受，更妥当的表达为"药物开发"。"药物研发"是"drug R&D"，此处处理为"研发"稍有偏差，但也优于"发展"；

（5）"the more likely this was to happen"译作"那就越有这种副作用的风险"，这里就是典型的人为导致口译复杂化，"副作用"和"风险"原文并未出现，其实此处按照顺句驱动的方法，直接处理为"这就越可能发生"，直译出的效果反而更清晰；

（6）"had to discontinue"译作"都停用"，但细究之下，其实"have to"所想表达出的客观及被迫的感觉并未译出，处理为"都得停用"或"都要停用"更好一些，但是此处仅是就翻译而言，并不影响专业听众对内容的理解和判断；

（7）"discontinuation rate"译作"终止率"，此处正确的翻译是"停药率"，但前者并不影响听众理解，只是表达的专业性欠佳；

（8）"one of the motivating factors"此处简单处理成"促进了"，并不影响理解，细究之下，语义并无实质性不同，同传时如果讲者语速过快，类似的简化处理也不失为一种选择。

It was actually a study of daratumumab. It shows the effect of the addition of daratumumab to a commonly used doublet of Bortezomib-dex in patients who had relapsed and refractory multiple myeloma. If you look on the right hand side, you can see that the addition of daratumumab, which is the upper arm here, led to a very substantial improvement in the progression free survival in these patients compared to the Bortezomib-dex arm. So this establishes the effectiveness of their daratumumab in this space. But why I'm showing you this curve? It's not to talk about daratumumab, but to talk about this, what happens when Bortezomib is discontinued? You can see that the Bortezomib is discontinued about six months into the treatment in this, the study. What happens to the PFS even in the dara arm, the highly effective dara arm, it begins to drop. You can see this inflection point. In the control arm, it goes so fast. It may be a little harder to appreciate, but this is the point that's significant. When you stop the proteasome inhibition, you are actually now giving a treatment to the patient which is inferior to that. It's if you could have continued the proteasome inhibitor, in which case the curve might have looked something more like this.

◎ **参考译文**：这个研究的对象其实是达雷木单抗,它展示了达雷木单抗的效果,加入达雷木单抗,在常用的硼替佐米和地塞米松双药中加入,那是用这个方案来治疗具有复发性、难治性、多发性的骨髓瘤。在右边这个图,上边的这一组是加入了达雷木单抗,大大增加了无进展生存,相比于硼替佐米和地塞米松组。所以说明了达雷木单抗的有效性。但是看到这个曲线,我并不是想跟大家说达雷木单抗,而是想说停用硼替佐米会发生什么,大概在治疗6个月的时候停用了,那对PFS的影响,是受到了很大的影响,即使是在达雷木组,它开始下降了。大家可以看到这个拐点,在对照组中,其速度很快。你在停止使用蛋白酶体抑制的时候,实际上为患者提供的治疗效果就变差了,所以如果我们继续使用蛋白酶体抑制剂的话,它的曲线就会是像这样一样。

◎ **分析**：

1. "addition"一词,是之后补充译出的,一句分成了三句,可能是一时难以组织好语言表达,按照顺句驱动法,此处可处理为"其显示了将达雷木单抗加入到常用的硼替佐米与地塞米松的双药联合的效果",需要译员能将"effect"放到最后;

2. "If you look at on the right hand side",此处if不译出并无影响;

3. "arm"一词译作"组",这是正确的译法,但也有一些专业人士、网络信息以及一些出版物将其直接译作"臂",例如"单臂试验"。这种"硬核式"的处理近些年来也时有见到;

4. "But why I'm showing you this curve?"处理为"但是看到这个曲线",在同传的情况下也可勉强接受;

5. "dara arm"译作"达雷木组",此处反映出了此主题下的另一个特点,即有些讲者有时会使用药名简称,译员要能及时反应;

6. "It may be a little harder to appreciate, but this is the point that's significant." 此句未译出,可能是译员未跟上讲者节奏,也可能是EVS拉长之后导致一句脱落。此处的"appreciate"意思是"看到",近年来,越来越多的国外讲者使用"appreciate"一词,但仅仅表达"看到"的意思。

So chemically, these two are very similar. But we've seen that the release from the proteasome is much faster for Ixazomib than for bortezomib. In the oral administration, we've talked about as well. So these combined with the lower incidence of peripheral neuropathy, allow us to administer Ixazomib for a prolonged period of time. In some of our clinical trials, as we'll talk about, it's given continuously to progression and in others it's given for about two years. Both of these drugs do cause thrombocytopenia. This is a class effect of this type of drug. They can be given with hepatic impairment and renal impairment. And for Ixazomib, it requires a small dose adjustment. And with that being said, I don't want to spend much time on this, but I'll just point out a couple of highlights. The half-life of this drug in the blood is 9.5 days. Oral bioavailability is quite good. You can see over half of the drug is readily absorbed in the stomach so that this allows us to do the oral administration. However, it has to be given on an empty stomach because food can interfere with the absorption of the drug. We looked at different tumor types and found that the PK for Ixazomib was very similar across tumor types so that there's no different dosing that's needed for different tumors. In clinical trials, in Asian patients, in China and Japan and others, we have found that the starting dose for the drug is the same as in Western patients, so we don't need to adjust it based on where your patient lives or where they come from.

◎ **参考译文**：它们的化学结构是很相似的。但是，蛋白酶体的释放，伊沙佐米是要比硼替佐米快的，然后我们也说了关于口服的方式。所以，这些加上周围神经病变较低的发生率，这样我们就可以延长使用伊沙佐米的时间，有一些临床试验持续使用直到病情进展，而有些临床试验当中持续使用2年。这两种药物，都会引发血小板减少症，这是一个这种类型药物的类效应。它们还可能会引发肝损伤、肾损伤。对于伊沙佐米，需要调整剂量。讲到这里，我就不在这上面多花时间了，我来指出几个重点。这一药物的半衰期在血液中是9.5天，口服生物利用度非常好。可以看到超过一半的药物在胃内可以很容易地被吸收，这样我们就可以进行口服给药。但是呢，必须要空腹给药，因为食物会影响药物的吸收。我们还看了不同的肿瘤类型，发现伊沙佐米的药代动力学是很类似的，对于不同的肿瘤类型都是如此，所以不同的肿瘤不需要不同的剂量。在临床试验中，在亚洲患者中，在中国、日本以及其他地区，我们发现初始剂量和西方患者是一样的，所以我们不需要再进行调整，无须根据患者在哪里或者患者来自哪里而进行调整。

◎ **分析**：

1. "This is a class effect of this type of drug."译作"这是一个这种类型药物的类效应。"此处想讨论的是不定冠词"a"是否要译出。很多时候，不定冠词的使用更多是出于语法而非语义上的需求，如果英文表达并非"one of"或"a specific"之类的话，中文翻译不一定非要译出"一个"，此处处理为"这是此类药物的类效应"，显然更符合中文表达习惯；

2. "They can be given with hepatic impairment and renal impairment."译作"它们还可能会引发肝损伤、肾损伤。"这是一句错译，此处真正意思是"它们可以在肝损伤和肾损伤时给药/使用。"此处讲者应该是非英语母语讲者，因为表达稍显奇怪；而译员也许是对自己听到的内容有所怀疑，进行了意思和语气上的调整，但最后还是导致了错译，因为"用药导致肝损/肾损"的逻辑，对于稍微有些医学翻译经验的译员而言，要比"肝损/肾损的时候可以继续用药"更加合乎逻辑。但在医学同传中，译员还是应坚持直译，不应该自行调整；

3. "bioavailability"译作"生物利用度"，药理学上指服用的药物中能到达体循环的剂量部分，是评价药物制剂质量的重要指标。按此定义，静脉给药的药物的生物利用度为100%，而当药物以其他方式给药时，如口服，其生物利用度因不完全吸收及首过效应而下降；

4. "administration"此处译作"给药"；

5. "However, it has to be given on an empty stomach because food can interfere with the absorption of the drug."一句中，可以明显感受到讲者为非英语母语者，对于此类讲者，同传时的原则应该是顺句驱动、不纠结语法以及基于医学常识和素养进行判断。

So that being said, the MM 2 study then, as I've mentioned, it's newly diagnosed patients who are not candidates for stem cell transplant. They are randomized to receive either ixazomib with lenalidomide and dexamethasone or placebo with lenalidomide and dexamethasone. At the time the study was designed, there was concern about the prolonged administration of both PIs and IMiDs. So at cycle 18, these patients had a dose reduction. The dexamethasone was stopped and the dose of lenalidomide was reduced to a maintenance dose. If you were in the placebo arm, similarly, the placebo, excuse me, the lenalidomide was dropped to this maintenance dose and dexamethasone was discontinued. What we found in this study, interestingly, was, as you can see, this is progression free survival. There was a really a measurable improvement in progression free survival of about 13 months. So it was it seems to be real. It's rather impressive. Unfortunately, this did not lead to a statistical significance here. You can see that the P value is 0.07. Despite this nice improvement, we found that it did not reach the success for the primary endpoint. And so we were not able to register this drug in a frontline combination because of that. But nonetheless, you can see the clinical effect, the clinical benefit that was seen in this.

◎ **参考译文**：尽管如此，说到MM2研究，就像我说的，它是新诊断的患者，不适合干细胞移植的。他们随机分为接受伊沙佐米加来那度胺和地塞米松，或安慰剂加来那度胺和地塞米松。在最开始设计试验的时候，担心PI和IMiDs的延长给药。所以在第18个周期之后，这些患者就降低剂量了，地塞米松就停了，来那度胺也减量到了维持剂量。要是在对照组也是类似的，安慰剂，抱歉，来那度胺也降到维持剂量，地塞米松停药。在这个研究里我们发现，很有趣，这个是无进展生存。PFS有显著提升，大概延长了13个月，看起来是真实的。还是很令人印象深刻的。不幸的是，这里并没有统计学差异，可以看到P值是0.07。虽然有不错的提升，但我们发现其并未达到主要终点的成功，所以我们没有办法在前线联合中注册这个药物，原因正在于此。尽管如此，还是可以看到临床疗效，临床获益可以在这里看到。

◎ **分析**：

1. 同传中，译员在翻译"MM 2 study"时，可跟读"MM"，"2"可以读"two"也可以读"二"，并无特别要求；

2. "either ixazomib with lenalidomide and dexamethasone"译作"伊沙佐米加来那度胺和地塞米松"，此处的"with"和"and"需要用不同的词，读音轻重最好也能够有所变化，突出研究药物是伊沙佐米，而此处的"either"不一定要译出；

3. "If you were in the placebo arm"译作"要是在对照组"，在此语境下不影响理解，但最后能译作"要是在安慰剂组"；

4. "progression free survival"同传时直接缩略译为"PFS",此处不影响听众理解;

5. "It's rather impressive"译作"还是很令人印象深刻的"。近年来,在医学会议中"impressive"一词的使用频率较高,大多数译员会将其译作"令/让人印象深刻",这样翻译腔较重,最近国内不少医生在中文发言时,也会直接说"印象深刻""令人印象非常深刻",也许是受此影响,"impressive"也可处理为"引人注目"或"出色"。

This is the last study I want to present. It's the same type of study. It's a single agent, ixazomib vs placebo in patients who have completed their primary therapy for frontline myeloma, but have not had a stem cell transplant. Again, these patients are treated for up to two years with either and ixazomib or placebo. And here we saw actually a rather substantial benefit improvement and progression free survival in these patients, and near doubling, it went from 9 months to 17 months. This was quite a favorable improvement in progressions free survival. And this was very significant. What we find from this also is that discontinuation is due to toxicity were relatively low, they were 12% vs 5% of placebo. A number of these patients were able to complete the two years of prescribed therapy that were being done there. Again, I'm going to pass on this. Just to show you the toxicity profile. Again, you see that they're relatively similar between the ixazomib group and the placebo group. However, we still see higher incidence of GI toxicities, nausea, vomiting, diarrhea, and, of course, a higher incidence of rash. Peripheral neuropathy was a little higher. You can see the background rate in placebo is 10.9, 19.5, but most of these were low grade and did not result in discontinuation of the drug.

◎ **参考译文**:这个是我想展示的最后一个研究,它也是同类型的研究。是单药,是伊沙佐米对比安慰剂用于那些已经完成了骨髓瘤前线治疗,但是没有接受干细胞移植的患者。这些患者接受伊沙佐米或者是安慰剂的治疗,时间最多两年。这里我们看到相当明显的获益改善,以及无进展生存,这些患者几乎翻了一番,从9到17个月。这是相当不错的无进展生存的改善,非常显著。我们从这里也能发现,因为毒性的停药也比较低,是12%对比5%。这些患者中的很多人都能够完成两年的治疗。我跳过这里,给大家看一下毒性。可以看到伊沙佐米组和安慰剂组相对类似。但我们还是能看到比较高的胃肠道毒性,恶心、呕吐、腹泻,还有当然,高发生率的皮疹。周围神经病也是高了一点儿。可以看到安慰剂组的背景率是10.9、19.5,但大多数是低级别,并不会导致停药。

◎ **分析**:

1. "primary therapy for frontline myeloma"此处译作"骨髓瘤前线治疗",其实此处大概率是讲者的口误,讲者想表达的应该是"frontline therapy for primary myeloma",此类口误虽不多见,但偶尔也会见到,交传时译员可以与讲者进行确认,但同传时显然不具备这一条件,只能是依靠译员的医学素养与判断;

2. "discontinuation"是医学口译中的常见词,译作"停药";

3. "background rate"译作"背景率",指一定时间范围内某个具体事件在群体中自然发生的频率。

Allogeneic hematopoietic cell transplantation, allo-HCT, is an intensive and curative treatment for various hematologic malignancies and hematopoietic dysfunctions. Chronic graft-versus-host disease (GVHD) is one of the major complications after allo-HCT. In previous studies, the incidence of chronic GVHD has been reported to be 15% to 50%, and chronic GVHD has been shown to have a detrimental effect on the quality of life, functional status, and survival outcomes. Previous studies have reported that recipient age, donor age, peripheral blood grafts, unrelated donor, female donor-male recipient combination, HLA disparity, in-vivo T-cell depletion, and post-transplantation cyclophosphamide were associated with the risk for chronic GVHD. Several studies have also reported that previous acute GVHD was an independent risk factor for chronic GVHD. For example, one of the largest studies conducted by the K group that analyzed only patients who underwent myeloablative conditioning regimens showed that only grade 3 to 4 acute GVHD, but not mild acute GVHD, increased the subsequent risk for chronic GVHD. However, several characteristics of acute GVHD, including the severity and involvement of specific organs, could potentially affect the subsequent risk for chronic GVHD differently in modern GVHD prophylaxis. In this nationwide, retrospective study, we examined the influence of acute GVHD on chronic GVHD according to the acute GVHD profile. An increased understanding of the association between clinical acute and chronic GVHD would contribute to elucidating the underlying pathophysiology of chronic GVHD and help to identify potential candidates for early intervention for chronic GVHD.(本段内容来自网络,有删改调整。)

◎ **参考译文**:异基因造血细胞移植,allo-HCT,是各种血液系统恶性肿瘤和造血功能障碍的一种强化及治愈性治疗。慢性移植物抗宿主病,GVHD,是allo-HCT后的主要并发症之一。在既往的研究中,慢性GVHD的发病率报道为15%至50%,并已证实慢性GVHD对生活质量、功能状态以及生存结局都有不利的影响。既往研究报告称,接受者年龄、供者年龄、外周血移植物、无关供者、女性供者—男性受者的组合、HLA差异、体内T细胞去除,以及移植后环磷酰胺与慢性GVHD风险相关。一些研究还报告称,先前的急性GVHD是慢性GVHD的独立危险因素。例如,由K小组进行的一项最大的研究仅分析了接受骨髓清除性预处理方案的患者,显示只有3到4级急性GVHD,而非轻度急性GVHD,会增加随后慢性GVHD的风险。然而,急性GVHD的几个特征,包括严重度和特定器官的受累,可能会影响随后慢性GVHD的风险,这是现代GVHD的预防。在这项全国性的回顾性研究当中,我们根据急性GVHD特征检查了急性GVHD对慢性GVHD的影响。加深对临床急性和慢性GVHD间关联的了解将有助于阐明慢性GVHD的潜在病理生理学,并有助于确定慢性GVHD早期干预的潜在患者。

◎ **分析**：

1."detrimental effect"译作"不利影响"，"detrimental"一词之前会议使用不多，但最近几年使用频率有所增加；

2."unrelated donor"译作"无关供者"，即无血缘关系供者。

This study elucidated the close association between acute and chronic GVHD. In this large Korean cohort, baseline characteristics, including recipient's age, donor type, sex mismatch, PB, and the use of in vivo T-cell depletion, were associated with the risk for chronic GVHD that requires systemic steroids, which is consistent with previous studies. The risk for chronic GVHD that requires systemic steroids increased with each increase in GVHD grade among grade 0, 1, and 2 to 4 in the BM/PB cohort, and these findings were also confirmed in the UCB cohort. Moreover, we found that the risk for severe chronic GVHD, as assessed by the NIH criteria, was significantly higher among those with grade 3 to 4 acute GVHD, indicating a strong association between the severity of acute and chronic GVHD.

◎ **参考译文**：这一研究阐明了急性和慢性GVHD间的密切关联。在这个大型韩国队列中，基线特征，包括接受者年龄、供者类型、性别不匹配、PB以及体内T细胞去除的使用，都与慢性GVHD风险相关，其需要全身性类固醇治疗，这与先前的研究一致。需要全身性类固醇治疗的慢性GVHD风险会增加，这是随着0、1和2到4级的GVHD等级的增加而增加的，是BM/PB队列，这些发现也在UCB队列中得到证实。此外，我们发现，根据NIH标准评估的严重慢性GVHD风险在3至4级急性GVHD患者中显著较高，这表明急性和慢性GVHD的严重程度之间存在很强的相关性。

◎ **分析**：

1."sex mismatch"此处译作"不匹配"，而不能译作"错配"，这两种译法在两个语境下表达完全不同的意思；

2."The risk for chronic GVHD that requires systemic steroids increased with each increase in GVHD grade among grade 0, 1, and 2 to 4 in the BM/PB cohort"用顺句驱动法处理为"需要全身性类固醇治疗的慢性GVHD风险会增加，这是随着0、1和2到4级的GVHD等级的增加而增加的，是BM/PB队列"，同传情况下这种处理可以接受，可以与"在BM/PB队列中，0、1和2到4级的GVHD等级的增加，需要全身性类固醇治疗的慢性GVHD风险就会增加"进行比较，后者若非译员提前拿到讲稿，在同传时基本无法实现。

Severe chronic GVHD remains one of the most morbid complications after allo-HCT. Specifically, lung chronic GVHD, often referred to as bronchiolitis obliterans syndrome, is one of the most devastating subtypes of chronic GVHD. Although several treatment options have become available for chronic GVHD, long-term survival remains unsatisfactory. In particular, it is challenging to ameliorate organ dysfunction after the involved organs of chronic GVHD progress to fibrosis. Therefore, early interventions before progression to fibrosis are potential treatment strategies for chronic GVHD. Notably, the subsequent risk for severe chronic GVHD increased commensurately with the severity of acute GVHD, whereas the adjustment for the grade of acute GVHD showed no remarkable influence on other risk factors of chronic GVHD. Furthermore, we found that previous severe acute GVHD exhibited a notable adverse impact on survival outcomes among patients who developed chronic GVHD that required systemic steroids. This was not shown in the previous studies, which did not account for the severity of previous acute GVHD. Although a history of acute GVHD alone is not a sufficient trigger to initiate early interventions, the inclusion of a history of acute GVHD could enhance the predictive accuracy of models for chronic GVHD that include baseline characteristics, eg, PB or sex mismatch, and potential biomarkers. Therefore, these findings might help to identify potential candidates who could benefit from early treatment interventions.

◎ **参考译文**：严重慢性GVHD仍然是异基因造血干细胞移植后最严重的并发症之一。具体而言，肺慢性GVHD，通常被称为闭塞性细支气管炎综合征，是慢性GVHD最具破坏性的亚型之一。尽管慢性GVHD已有多种治疗方案，但长期生存率仍然并不令人满意。尤其是很难改善器官功能障碍，在慢性GVHD受累器官进展到纤维化后很难改善。因此，在进展为纤维化之前进行早期干预是慢性GVHD可能的治疗策略。值得注意的是，随后发生严重慢性GVHD的风险与急性GVHD的严重程度呈比例增加，而对急性GVHD等级的调整对慢性GVHD的其他风险因素没有显著影响。此外，我们发现先前的严重急性GVHD对生存结果表现出明显的不利影响，是对于患有需要全身性类固醇治疗的慢性GVHD患者而言的。之前的研究没有发现这一点，之前的研究并未考虑先前急性GVHD的严重程度。虽然仅凭急性GVHD病史不足以启动早期干预，但纳入急性GVHD的病史可以提升慢性GVHD模型的预测准确性，包括基线特征，例如PB或性别不匹配，以及潜在的生物标志物。因此，这些发现可能有助于确定能够从早期治疗干预中获益的潜在患者。

◎ **分析**：

1. "most morbid complications"译作"最严重的并发症"，"morbid"一词指"病态的、疾病的"，"morbid complications"在医学会议中比较少见，同传时将其处理为"严重"，符合此时的语境，也符合中文表达习惯；

2. "most devastating subtypes"译作"最具破坏性的亚型"，非常准确，"devastating"一词，同传时如译不出"破坏性的"，也可简单处理为"严重/可怕的"；

3. "it is challenging to ameliorate"此处处理为"很难改善"，"challenging"一词在近年的医学会议中出现率较高，没有必要每次都译作"具/很有挑战性"，只有在合适的语境下如此翻译才不会显得突兀。

二、中译英

同样，这个 OS 也进行了一个亚组分析。这个亚组分析，首先我们还是来看遗传学改变的高危亚组。这个 OS 的分析上面看到了高危组的患者呢，经过伊沙佐米的联合治疗以后，它的 OS 是要优于它的对照组的，也就是说从这个高危亚组分析来看，OS 是获益的，是有统计学差异的。所以把所有的亚组分析罗列在一起来看呢，还是有一部分亚组的患者，是从通过伊沙佐米的治疗后，获得一个比较好的 OS 的。从遗传学以及 ISS 分期是三期的患者，或者说在之前呢，实际接受过多线治疗的，就是二线或者三线治疗的这部分患者，应该说是特别难治的。这部分患者呢，依然是可以从伊沙佐米组的治疗以后获得一个比较好的 OS。也就是说从这个森林图上面我们也可以看到，阴影部分这个患者呢，是可以获得一个 OS 上面的获益的。也就是说整体的 OS 没有差异，但是如果我们进一步进行亚组分析的话，还是可以看到部分患者是从伊沙佐米治疗的 OS 上面获益的。那为什么会出现这样一个结果呢？（本段内容选自 2023 年一位中国医生的学术演讲，有删改调整。）

◎ **参考译文**：Similarly, a subgroup analysis was conducted for OS. In this subgroup analysis, we first look at the high-risk subgroup with genetic changes. In the OS analysis, for high-risk group patients, after ixazomib combination treatment, their OS is better than that of the control group. In other words, from the high-risk subgroup analysis, OS is beneficial and there is a statistical difference. So if we list all the subgroup analyses together, there is still a part of the patients in the subgroup, after ixazomib treatment, they obtained a better OS. Patients with genetic and ISS staged Ⅲ, or those who have actually received multiple lines of treatment before, that is, second-line or third-line treatment patients, and some patients who are typical refractory, can still obtain a better OS after treatment with ixazomib. In other words, from the forest map, we can also see that the patients in the shaded part can benefit from OS. That is to say, there is no difference in overall OS, but if we conduct further subgroup analysis, we can still see that some patients benefit from ixazomib treatment in terms of OS. Why does such a result occur?

◎ **分析**：

1. 此段中的中文讲者发言未作大幅调整，有时逻辑并不是非常清晰，需要译员拉长 EVS，根据自己的医学素养和常识进行口译；

2. "亚组分析"译作"subgroup analysis"，亚组分析是一个基础概念，指在各种研究和试验中，根据研究对象的某种具体特征，例如性别、年龄、基线状态、疾病严重程度等，将一个研究/试验组中的受试者分为不同的亚组，进行亚组间的比较。

那么中位随访，这个文章发表的时候，我们是 13、10.3 个月。那么对于所有患者来讲呢，ORR 是 95.3%。就是做一个全口服的方案在一线应用，那么在包含两成高危患者的情况下，我们的ORR是 95.3%。那么 VGPR 以上的这个比例是 65.9%，就是三分之二的患者取得了 VGPR 或者更好的这样的一个疗效。那么到反应的时间是 30 天。因为伊沙佐米，它是这个一个月吃三颗。那么也就是说吃第四颗药之前呢，这个病人已经获得了反应。中位的 PFS 呢，由于它是一线的，这个研究它还没有达到。那从这个结果上来看，虽然它没有跟其他的这个 PI 类药物做头对头的研究，应该说符合我们对一线骨髓瘤患者，在一线里面用三药的这个其他的蛋白酶体这些疗效的认知，也就是说虽然是口服，但是呢，并不像我们说一定要比注射类的差，甚至起效的时间也不短，也不长。

◎ **参考译文**：What about the median follow-up, when the paper was published, they were 13, 10.3 months. For all patients, the ORR is 95.3%, which meant an all-oral regimen was developed and used in the first line. In the case of 20% of high-risk patients, our ORR was 95.3%. The proportion of VGPR and above was 65.9%, which meant that two-thirds of patients achieved VGPR or better effects. What about the response time, it was 30 days, because ixazomib is taken three tablets a month. That is to say, before taking the fourth tablet, the patient had already responded. As for the median PFS, because it has not reached the first-line study, judging from the result, although it has not been studied head-to-head with other PI drugs, regarding first line myeloma patients, using three drugs in the first line, other proteasome, it is consistent with our understanding of the efficacy. That is to say, although it is oral, it is not necessarily worse than the injectables, and the time it takes to be effective, it's neither short nor long.

◎ **分析**：

1. "文章"译作"paper"，医学会议中的"文章"指论文，直接译作 paper 即可；

2. "中位"只能译作"median"，应注意与"平均""均值"等区分开，现在的研究中，中位值的应用多于平均值。

我记得在 2016 年去美国 MD Anderson 的时候，他们 2015 年其实是批了四种新药，当时四种多发性骨髓瘤的新药，有的是新的适应证，比如说这个卡非佐米啊，它是有新的适应证。关于前面我们对这个疾病的认知，目前对于它的治疗模式，大家这个图虽然看过好多遍。从我们特别早的时候，10 年前，15 年前可能就看这张图，但现在呢，它一线、二线、三线治疗的时间在拉长。而且呢，它的每一线治疗的药物在不断地更新。那么就刚才我提到这个，我们看 2015 年，包括帕比司他，包括 CD38 单抗和 CS1 单抗。那么之后的话，你看包括 XPO1 的抑制剂，新的 CD38 单抗，包括免疫治疗的一系列的药物，包括我们熟知的 CAR-T 跟 BiTE……那么免疫治疗逐渐成为一个新的领域，而不是说单纯的那个管线的问题，它是一个领域。

◎ **参考译文**：I remember that when I went to MD Anderson in the United States in 2016, they actually approved in 2015, four new drugs. At that time, four new drugs for multiple myeloma, some of which had new indications, such as carfilzomib, it had new indications. Regarding our previous understanding of this disease, and its current treatment model, although everyone has seen this picture many times, since very early, 10 years ago, 15 years ago, you might have seen this picture, but now, its first-line, second-line, and third-line treatment time is getting longer. Moreover, the drugs for each line of treatment are constantly being updated. As I mentioned earlier, in 2015, there were panobinostat, CD38 monoclonal antibody and CS1 monoclonal antibody. After that, there were XPO1 inhibitors, new CD38 monoclonal antibodies, and a series of immunotherapy drugs, including the well-known CAR-T and BiTE. Immunotherapy has gradually become a new field, not just a pipeline issue. It is a field.

◎ 分析：

1. "MD Anderson"指的是"得克萨斯大学安德森癌症中心"，是世界级的癌症诊疗机构，集癌症治疗、研究、教育和预防于一身，在业内有顶级的影响力，口译时译员无须翻译，直接跟读"MD Anderson"即可；

2. "CAR-T"指"嵌合抗原受体T细胞免疫疗法"，全称是Chimeric Antigen Receptor T-Cell Immunotherapy，是一种新型的肿瘤精准免疫靶向疗法。口译时译员无须译出，直接跟读"CAR-T"即可。

那四药的联合呢，在于适合移植的病人当中，那么45例病人，可以看到他6个周期的D-IRD之后，在移植之后再进行四个周期的巩固，然后再用R来维持。那么45例当中，有43例都完成自体这个巩固治疗，那么它的ORR高达100%。所以这个里面也体现了不光是耐受，就是安全性好，它的疗效也体现出了Dara和IMiDs跟PI药物这三类基石性药物它的联合，它发挥出来的稳定的作用。它的中位随访大概有两年的时间，那么其中95.2%的人还没有进展，就是这个几乎只有5%的人在两年之内发生了进展，而且他的MRD阴性率也是非常高的，那如果按照10的-5的灵敏度的话，会高达50%。而这个就是刚才这个四药联合，在于不适合移植的病人当中，我们看一下，他的这个诱导治疗都是12个周期的，来那度胺、伊沙佐米、Dara这样的一个D-IRD的吧，然后A组病人呢，是进行来那度胺的单药维持。B组呢，是进行一个三药维持。

◎ 参考译文：The combination of the four drugs is in the patients who are suitable for transplantation. Well, 45 patients, after 6 cycles of D-IRD, after transplantation, they have four cycles of consolidation, and then use R to maintain. Among the 45 cases, 43 completed autologous consolidation treatment, and its ORR was as high as 100%. So this also reflects not only tolerance, but good safety. Its efficacy also reflects Dara, IMiDs and PI drugs, the combination of these three cornerstone drugs, and its stable effect. Its median follow-up is about two years, and 95.2% of them have not progressed. That is only nearly 5% of them have progressed within these two years, and its MRD negative rate is also very high. If it is based on the sensitivity of 10 to the −5, it would be as high as 50%. And this, it is the four-drug combination mentioned earlier. For patients who are not suitable for transplantation, let's take a look. The induction therapy is 12 cycles, lenalidomide, ixazomib, Dara, such a D-IRD. Then, patients in group A are maintained with lenalidomide alone, and patients in group B are maintained with three drugs.

◎ 分析：

1. "巩固治疗"译作"consolidation treatment"或"consolidation therapy"，有时也会见到"intensification treatment"的用法，但后者对应的是"强化治疗"，翻译时应注意鉴别；

2. "10 的-5"指"十的负五次方"，即 10^{-5}，此处译作了"10 to the -5"，也可以译作"10 to the power of -5"；

3. "诱导治疗"译作"induction treatment"或"induction therapy"。

而且其中的亚组分析，我注意到他的年龄，如果只是年龄脆弱的话，大概有 50% 人是在 80 岁以上。因为 80 岁以上的直接就是 frail，他器官功能可能还挺好，如果单纯只是因为年龄的话，那么它的 PFS 可以达到——如果没记错，应该是 20 个月左右，所以它耐受性还是非常好的。从整体的这个安全性来看，有大于等于三级的。这个血液学毒性呢，有 20 名病人，非血液学毒性的话，有 48 名，最主要还是血液学跟胃肠道反应，还有感染等。总体来说，对高龄的和虚弱的病人来说，这个是可以接受的。那还有生活质量的评分，可以看到他的生活质量的评分其实是在不断改善的，尤其是 9 个疗程之后，是不断改善的。

◎ 参考译文：And in its subgroup analysis, I noticed his age, if it is just age frailty, about 50% of the people are over 80 years old, because people over 80 years old are frail, because their organ function may be quite good. If it is simply because of age, then its PFS can reach, if I remember correctly, it should be about 20 months, so its tolerability is still very good. In terms of the overall safety, there are grade three and above events. Regarding hematology toxicity, there are 20 patients, as for non-hematology toxicity, there are 48 patients. The main ones are hematological and gastrointestinal reactions, as well as infections and others. I think overall, for such elderly patients, frail patients, this is acceptable. There is also a quality-of-life score. We could see that the quality of life score has been actually improving, especially after 9 courses of treatment, it has been improving.

◎ 分析：

1. "器官功能可能还挺好"译作"organ function may be quite good"，其实应该译作"organ function might still be good"，"quite"和"still"意义完全不同；

2. "那么整体的这个安全性来看，有大于等于三级的"一句中，句末没有说出是"不良事件"，"安全性"和"不良事件"是医学口译中的基础概念，译员应至少补出"event"，否则用"ones"或其他方式翻译难度较大，也说不清楚；

3. "血液学跟胃肠道反应"译作"hematological and gastrointestinal reactions"，首先是"血液学"译作英文，名词形式或形容词形式在实际同传时都可接受，不必非要拘泥于词性。而"胃肠道反应"在英文中可直接表达为"GI reactions"，所有讲英语的听众都能理解，从而节省时间。

第四节　补充练习

一、中译英

中药的砒霜是一个混合物，它的主要成分是三氧化二砷，但同时还有其他杂质。后来学者发现，砒霜里面的三氧化二砷是治疗起作用的主要成分。中医里有"以毒攻毒"这样的理论。肿瘤是一个"毒"，我们又用"毒"的东西来治疗，所以时间久了，就被认为是"以毒攻毒"的一个典型范例。但是有一个事情要搞清楚，并不是说砒霜或者砷剂对所有的肿瘤都有效。到目前为止，在所有的癌种中，它只对急性早幼粒细胞白血病的治疗是有效的。我们还没有突破到可以有效治疗其他的肿瘤。因此，我认为不能因为这一个病种，我们就将肿瘤治疗和中医"以毒攻毒"的说法联系起来。这是一种误解。"以毒攻毒"是中医的一个重要理论，但在没有充分依据的情况下贸然在其他肿瘤的治疗中"以毒攻毒"，也是危险的，所以要分清其中的区别，尊重客观、尊重事实、理性对待。

一个中药，说它有效，那么它的有效成分到底是什么？一定要搞清楚。现在往往在这个问题上不少人不理解，认为中药就是中药，不应该把它研究分析得那么细。果真是这样吗？很多人知道屠呦呦研究员关于青蒿素的研究。青蒿素就是有效成分，而不是整株草做药。青蒿素的研究过程又是怎样的呢？原来，以前在我国一些疟疾多发地区，当地的老百姓染病后会用中药青蒿来治。怎么治呢？他们把青蒿的汁液绞出来喝，发现效果不错。这就是中医药研究的第一步：首先要确信有效。这种治疗经验被古代的中医记录下来。屠呦呦研究员关注到相关记载后就对青蒿进行了研究。一开始，她用的是传统中医药常用的水煎的方法，发现好像没有效果。再拿中医书来反复看，发现不对，当时记载老百姓用的是新鲜青蒿挤出来的汁。她就怀疑是高温煎煮的时候把有效成分破坏了，于是改用了乙醚低温提取。后来的结果大家都知道了，我们国家的医药科技工作者终于研发出了青蒿素，并且弄清楚了青蒿素的化学结构。

中医药研究的第二步：寻找到它的有效成分，甚至进一步弄清楚它的作用机制。我认为，现在我们的中医药研究就应该走这样的路。我们在研究动脉粥样硬化过程中发现，中医的理论中没有"动脉粥样硬化"这个概念。但是中医师通过对动脉粥样硬化患者的辨证，会发现一些中医的证候，比如血瘀等。我们从西医的角度就会思考，像血瘀这类概念，从物质的角度来讲究竟是什么东西？我们要将中医理论中的这些概念具体化。会不会是胆固醇？因为胆固醇摄入过度，会在血管壁上沉积，进而阻塞血管，导致动脉粥样硬化。中医是怎么治疗这个病呢？就是采用活血化瘀的方法。这当中常用到一味药，就是生蒲黄。那么，生蒲黄的有效成分又是什么呢？具体起什么作用呢？我们就研究这个问题。人为什么会产生动脉粥样硬化？主要是饮食中胆固醇含量太高了。我们就开始做动物实验：把兔子分为两组，一组兔子喂食大量的高胆固醇食物蛋黄，另一组不吃蛋黄。对比后发现，吃了蛋黄的兔子跟不吃的兔子就有了区别，前者的血管斑块就很明显，不吃的就没有。这样，我们就在动物身上造成了食饵性动脉粥样硬化。接着，我们进一步研究，生蒲黄能起什么作用？我们就跟药物研究所一起合作研究，发现生蒲黄的所有成分，并从中找到对抑制动脉粥样硬化有作用的成分。相关研究结论发表在国外学术期刊后，也得到了国外同行的认可。

◎ **参考译文**：Arsenic in traditional Chinese medicine is a mixture. Its main component is arsenic trioxide, but there are also other impurities. Later, scholars discovered that arsenic trioxide in arsenic is the main component that works in treatment. In traditional Chinese medicine, there is a theory called "fighting poison with poison". Tumor is a "poison", and we use "poisonous" things to treat it, so over time, it is considered a typical example of "fighting poison with poison". But there is one thing to make clear, it does not mean that arsenic or arsenic agents are effective for all tumors. So far, among all types of cancer, it is only effective for the treatment of acute promyelocytic leukemia. We have not yet made a breakthrough to effectively treat other tumors. Therefore, I think we cannot link tumor treatment with the traditional Chinese medicine saying of "fighting poison with poison" just because of this disease. This is a misunderstanding. "Fighting poison with poison" is an important theory of traditional Chinese medicine, but it is also dangerous to rashly "fight poison with poison" in the treatment of other tumors without sufficient basis, so we must distinguish the difference, respect objectivity, respect facts, and treat it rationally.

A Chinese medicine is said to be effective, so what is its active ingredient? We must find out. Now, many people often do not understand this issue and think that Chinese medicine is Chinese medicine and should not be studied and analyzed in such detail. Is this really the case? Many people know about the research of artemisinin by researcher Tu Youyou. Artemisinin is the active ingredient, not the whole plant. What is the research process of artemisinin? It turns out that in some malaria-prone areas in my country, local people would use the Chinese medicine artemisia annua to treat the disease. How to treat it? They squeezed out the juice of artemisia annua and drank it, and found that the effect was good. This is the first step in the research of Chinese medicine: first, you must be sure that it is effective. This treatment experience was recorded by ancient Chinese medicine practitioners. After paying attention to the relevant records, researcher Tu Youyou conducted research on artemisia annua. At first, she used the water decoction method commonly used in traditional Chinese medicine, and found that it seemed to have no effect. She took the Chinese medicine book and read it repeatedly and found that it was wrong. At that time, it was recorded that the people used the juice squeezed from fresh artemisia annua. She suspected that the active ingredients were destroyed during the high-temperature decoction, so she switched to low-temperature extraction with ether. Everyone knows the results that followed. Our country's medical and technological workers finally developed artemisinin and figured out its chemical structure.

The second step of TCM research is to find its effective ingredients and even further figure out its mechanism of action. I think that this is the path that our TCM research should take now. In the process of studying atherosclerosis, we found that there is no concept of "atherosclerosis" in TCM theory. However, TCM physicians will find some TCM syndromes, such as blood stasis, through the differentiation of atherosclerosis patients. From the perspective of Western medicine, we will think about what concepts like blood stasis are from a material perspective. We need to concretize these concepts in TCM theory. Could it be cholesterol? Because excessive cholesterol intake will deposit on the blood vessel wall, blocking the blood vessels and causing atherosclerosis. How does TCM treat this disease? It uses the method of promoting blood circulation and removing blood stasis. Among them, one medicine is often used, which is raw pollen. So, what is the effective ingredient of raw pollen? What is its specific role? Let's study this question. Why do people develop atherosclerosis? It is mainly because the cholesterol content in the diet is too high. We started to do animal experiments: the rabbits were divided into two groups, one group of rabbits was fed a large amount of high-cholesterol food egg yolk, and the other group did not eat egg yolk. After comparison, we found that there was a difference between rabbits that ate egg yolks and those that did not. The former had obvious vascular plaques, while the latter did not. In this way, we caused dietary atherosclerosis in animals. Then, we further studied what effect raw pollen can have? We worked with the Institute of Pharmacology to discover all the components of raw pollen and found the components that can inhibit atherosclerosis. After the relevant research conclusions were published in foreign academic journals, they were also recognized by foreign peers.

二、英译中

Chemotherapy is the use of certain kinds of drugs that destroy or control the growth of cancer cells. These drugs can be taken by mouth or given in a vein or a muscle. They enter the bloodstream and reach almost all areas of the body. At one time, chemo was often part of the main treatment for multiple myeloma. As newer types of drugs have become available in recent years, chemo has become less important in treating myeloma, although it is still used in some situations. Chemo drugs that can be used to treat multiple myeloma include: Cyclophosphamide, Etoposide, Doxorubicin, Liposomal doxorubicin, Melphalan, Bendamustine. Often one of these drugs is combined with other types of drugs like corticosteroids and immunomodulating drugs. If a stem cell transplant is planned, most doctors avoid using certain chemo drugs, like melphalan, that can damage bone marrow.

Chemo drugs kill cancer cells but also can damage normal cells. They are given carefully to avoid or reduce the side effects of chemotherapy. These side effects depend on the type and dose of drugs given and how long they are taken. Common side effects of chemo include: hair loss, mouth sores, loss of appetite, nausea and vomiting, diarrhea or constipation. Chemotherapy often leads to low blood counts, which can cause: an increased risk of serious infection (from having too few white blood cells), easy bruising or bleeding (from having too few blood platelets), feeling tired or short of breath (from having too few red blood cells), most side effects go away after treatment is finished. Along with these short-term side effects, some chemo drugs can permanently damage certain organs such as the heart or kidneys. The possible risks of these drugs are carefully balanced against their benefits, and the function of these organs is carefully monitored during treatment. If serious organ damage occurs, the drug that caused it is stopped and sometimes replaced with another.

Corticosteroids, such as dexamethasone and prednisone, are an important part of the treatment of multiple myeloma. They can be used alone or combined with other drugs as a part of treatment. Corticosteroids are also used to help decrease the nausea and vomiting that chemo might cause. Common side effects of these drugs include: high blood sugar, increased appetite and weight gain, problems sleeping, changes in mood, some people become irritable or "hyper". When used for a long time, corticosteroids also suppress the immune system. This increases the risk of serious infections. Steroids can also weaken bones.

The way immunomodulatory drugs (IMiDs) affect the immune system isn't entirely clear, but these drugs are often helpful in treating multiple myeloma. These drugs are taken daily as pills, with breaks from treatment on certain days each month. These drugs might cause severe birth defects when taken during pregnancy, so they can only be obtained through a special program run by the drug company that makes them. Because these drugs can increase the risk of serious blood clots, they are often given along with aspirin or a blood thinner.

Proteasome inhibitors work by stopping enzyme complexes (proteasomes) in cells from breaking down proteins important for controlling cell division. They appear to affect tumor cells more than normal cells, but they are not without side effects. Bortezomib was the first of this type of drug to be approved, and it's often used to treat multiple myeloma. It may be especially helpful in treating myeloma patients with kidney problems. It's injected into a vein (IV) or under the skin, once or twice a week. Carfilzomib is a newer proteasome inhibitor that can be used to treat multiple myeloma in patients who have already been treated with other drugs that didn't work. It's given as an injection into a vein (IV), often in a 4-week cycle. To prevent problems like allergic reactions during the infusion, the steroid drug dexamethasone is often given before each dose in the first cycle. Ixazomib is a proteasome inhibitor that is a capsule taken by mouth, typically once a week for 3 weeks, followed by a week off. This drug is usually given after other drugs have been tried.

◎ **参考译文**：化疗是使用某些药物来破坏或控制癌细胞的生长。这些药物可以口服、静脉或肌肉注射。它们进入血液，到达身体的几乎所有部位。化疗曾经是多发性骨髓瘤的主要治疗方法。随着近年来新药的出现，化疗在治疗骨髓瘤方面的重要性已降低，尽管在某些情况下仍会使用化疗。可用于治疗多发性骨髓瘤的化疗药物包括：环磷酰胺、依托泊苷、阿霉素、脂质体阿霉素、美法仑、苯达莫司汀。通常，这些药物中的一种会与其他类型的药物，例如皮质类固醇和免疫调节药物，结合使用。如果计划进行干细胞移植，大多数医生会避免使用某些可能损害骨髓的化疗药物，例如美法仑。

化疗药物可以杀死癌细胞，但也会损害正常细胞。为了避免或减少化疗的副作用，必须谨慎使用化疗药物。这些副作用取决于所用药物的类型、剂量以及服药时间。化疗的常见副作用包括：脱发、口腔溃疡、食欲不振、恶心呕吐、腹泻或便秘。化疗通常会导致血细胞计数降低，从而导致：严重感染风险增加（白细胞太少）、容易瘀伤或出血（血小板太少）、感到疲倦或呼吸急促（红细胞太少）。大多数副作用在治疗结束后会消失。除了这些短期副作用外，一些化疗药物还会对某些器官造成永久性损害，例如心脏或肾脏。这些药物的潜在风险和益处需要经过仔细权衡，并且在治疗期间会仔细监测这些器官的功能。如果发生严重的器官损伤，则应停止使用导致器官损伤的药物，有时还会用另一种药物代替。

皮质类固醇，如地塞米松和泼尼松，是多发性骨髓瘤治疗的重要组成部分。它们可以单独使用，也可以与其他药物联合使用作为治疗的一部分。皮质类固醇还用于帮助减少化疗可能引起的恶心和呕吐。这些药物的常见副作用包括：高血糖、食欲增加和体重增加、睡眠问题、情绪变化，有些人变得易怒或"亢奋"。长期使用皮质类固醇也会抑制免疫系统。这会增加严重感染的风险。类固醇还会削弱骨骼强度。

免疫调节药物（IMiD）影响免疫系统的方式尚不完全清楚，但这些药物通常有助于治疗多发性骨髓瘤。这些药物以药丸的形式每日服用，每月的某些天暂停治疗。这些药物在怀孕期间服用可能会导致严重的出生缺陷，因此只能通过生产这些药物的制药公司运行的特殊计划获得。由于这些药物会增加严重血栓的风险，因此它们通常与阿司匹林或血液稀释剂一起服用。

蛋白酶体抑制剂的作用原理是阻止细胞中的酶复合物（蛋白酶体）分解对控制细胞分裂至关重要的蛋白质。它们似乎对肿瘤细胞的影响大于对正常细胞的影响，但并非没有副作用。硼替佐米是第一种获批的此类药物，常用于治疗多发性骨髓瘤。它可能对治疗有肾脏疾病的骨髓瘤患者特别有用。它每周一次或两次注射到静脉（IV）或皮下。卡非佐米是一种较新的蛋白酶体抑制剂，可用于治疗已接受其他药物治疗但无效的多发性骨髓瘤患者。它以静脉（IV）注射的方式给药，通常以四周为一个周期。为了防止输液期间出现过敏反应等问题，通常在第一个周期的每次给药前给予类固醇药物地塞米松。伊沙佐米是一种蛋白酶体抑制剂，是一种口服胶囊，通常每周一次，持续三周，然后停药一周。通常在尝试过其他药物之后才给予此药。

第十单元 实体肿瘤

第一节 实体肿瘤口译知识点

癌症（cancer）是一种疾病，指的是遍布体内的细胞不受控制地分裂（division）。当实体组织（如：器官、肌肉或骨骼）里出现癌细胞增长时，可称其为肿瘤（tumor），后者或可从血液及淋巴系统扩散到周围的组织中。癌症治疗旨在消除这些异常细胞，或减缓、阻止癌细胞的扩散。

实体肿瘤（solid tumors）分为两大类：恶性（malignant，具有致癌性）肿瘤和良性（benign，不具有致癌性）肿瘤。具有致癌性的肿瘤可以侵入到身体内周围组织中，且随着这些肿瘤的生长，有些癌细胞或许还会跑到身体的其他部位，以形成其他的"继发性"肿瘤（secondary tumor），后者也被称为转移（瘤）（metastasis）。

实体恶性肿瘤包括癌（carcinoma）和肉瘤（sarcoma）。癌是来源于上皮组织的恶性肿瘤，例如肺腺癌起源于支气管黏膜上皮；肉瘤是来源于间叶组织（mesenchymal tissue）的恶性肿瘤，例如纤维组织的纤维肉瘤（fibrosarcoma）、骨肉瘤（osteosarcoma）等。癌的发病率远高于肉瘤，肉瘤发病率较低，部分肉瘤主要见于年轻人及儿童，部分肉瘤多见于中老年人。

良性肿瘤不会在身体内扩散或游离。大多数良性肿瘤都不具有致命性，但部分脑肿瘤仍可引发炎症或因占位压迫周围组织出现症状。医生可通过活检（biopsy）来判断一个肿瘤为良性或是恶性。

面对实体恶性肿瘤，有如下疗法可供选择，例如：放疗（radiation）、化疗（chemotherapy）、免疫疗法（immunotherapy）和/或手术（surgical treatment）去除（或部分去除）肿瘤。

下面介绍几种口译中常遇到的实体恶性肿瘤，以及临床肿瘤学中几个重要概念。

肺癌（lung cancer）

肺癌是当异常细胞在肺部以不受控制的方式生长时开始的一种癌症，是严重的健康问题，可导致严重的伤害和死亡。肺癌的症状包括咳嗽、痰中带血或咯血、喘鸣、胸痛、呼吸急促、声嘶、发热等。

最常见的肺癌类型是非小细胞癌（non-small cell lung cancer，NSCLC）和小细胞癌（small cell lung cancer，SCLC）。非小细胞癌更常见且生长缓慢，而小细胞癌不太常见，但常常生长迅速。

肺癌是一个重大的公共卫生问题,在全球造成大量死亡。国际癌症研究机构(IARC)对癌症发病率和死亡率的 GLOBOCAN(全球癌症观察站)2020 年估计显示,肺癌仍然是癌症死亡的主要原因,2020 年估计造成 180 万人死亡(18%)。

根据组织病理学分类,小细胞肺癌约占肺癌总发生率的 15%,因癌细胞呈类圆形或梭形、细胞浆少、体积小而得名。小细胞肺癌患者多为男性,与吸烟密切相关,是肺癌中恶性度最高的一种,小细胞肺癌增殖快、早期广泛转移,大部分患者在发现时即已出现全身转移,患者常因肺门肿块和纵隔肿大淋巴结引起的咳嗽和呼吸困难等。

小细胞肺癌分为局限期(limited-stage small cell lung cancer)和广泛期(extensive-stage small cell lung cancer)两个主要阶段。局限期是指肿瘤局限在单侧肺(unilateral lung)或可能转移到了附近的淋巴结,尚未转移到对侧肺或肺以外的部位,一个放射野的根治性放疗。广泛期是指肿瘤已经转移到双侧肺和胸腔,可能已经转移到了肺周围或肺以外的其他部位(如肝、脑、骨等)。

非小细胞肺癌约占肺癌总发生率的 85%,主要分为鳞状细胞癌、腺癌、大细胞癌。非小细胞肺癌分为Ⅰ期、Ⅱ期、Ⅲ期、Ⅳ期。Ⅰ期为早期,指肿瘤位于肺组织中,尚未发生转移。Ⅱ期属于中期,指癌细胞已经转移到了肺门附近的淋巴结。Ⅲ期属于中晚期,指癌细胞已经进一步转移到纵隔或肺外淋巴结。Ⅳ期属于晚期,指肿瘤出现胸膜转移、胸腔积液或全身多处转移,如肝、脑、骨等。

肺癌一般需要与肺结核、肺炎、肺脓肿、肺良性肿瘤等相鉴别。

肺癌的治疗包括手术治疗、化疗、靶向治疗、免疫治疗、内科治疗、中医治疗等。

乳腺癌(breast cancer)

乳腺癌是乳腺上皮细胞在各种致癌因子的作用下出现的增殖失控。早期常表现为乳房肿块、乳头溢液、腋窝淋巴结肿大等症状,晚期可出现远处转移,导致多器官病变,威胁患者生命。乳腺癌发病率居女性恶性肿瘤之首,男性也可罹患乳腺癌,但较为少见。随着医学科技的不断发展,乳腺癌亦称为实体肿瘤中疗效最佳的肿瘤之一。

乳腺癌包括非浸润性癌、浸润癌、浸润性非特殊癌等。

乳腺癌早期症状常为乳房肿块、乳房皮肤异常、乳头溢液、乳头或乳晕异常等局部症状。到了中晚期,乳腺癌患者可能会出现恶病质(cachexy)表现,可出现消瘦、乏力、贫血、发热等症状。患者可能会出现肺及胸膜转移,肺转移为乳腺癌的常见情况,患者可出现咳嗽、呼吸困难、咯血、胸痛等症状;胸膜转移可表现为咳嗽、疲乏、呼吸困难、胸痛等。患者也可能出现骨转移,常为脊柱、肋骨、骨盆及长骨,患者可出现骨痛、高钙血症等症状。还有可能出现肝转移、脑转移等,导致相应症状。

乳腺癌临床分期,根据 TNM 分期,乳腺癌可分为 0~Ⅳ期。乳腺癌需要与乳腺纤维腺瘤(fibroadenoma of breast)、乳腺增生(breast hyperplasia)、浆细胞性乳腺炎等疾病相鉴别。

乳腺癌的治疗包括手术治疗、化疗、辅助治疗、内分泌治疗、靶向治疗、放疗及中医治疗等。

胃癌(gastric cancer)

胃癌即胃部的癌症，癌细胞来源于胃的黏膜上皮细胞，最常见的病理类型为胃腺癌。早期胃癌术后的5年生存率(five-year survival rate)可达90.9%~100%，而晚期胃癌尚缺乏有效的治疗方式。

全球范围内胃癌发病率在恶性肿瘤中排名第五，死亡率排第三，男性发病率为女性的两倍以上，而东亚地区发病率高于全球，我国2019年的数据显示胃癌发病率(incidence rate)和死亡率(mortality rate)位于所有恶性肿瘤的第二位和第三位，高于世界平均水平。

胃癌临床分期也是根据TNM分期分为0~Ⅳ期，分期越晚，预后越差。

大部分胃癌早期患者无症状(asymptomatic)，少数患者可有轻微不适，例如饱胀不适、消化不良等，不易引起重视；进展期可能会出现上腹痛、体重下降等情况；晚期患者可能出现贫血、消瘦等症状。

胃癌应与胃炎(gastritis)、胃溃疡(gastric ulcer)、胃淋巴瘤、胃良性肿瘤相鉴别。

胃癌患者获得根治的唯一可行的方法就是手术，早期患者可获根治，进展期患者可接受手术治疗，联合围手术期化疗、放疗、生物靶向治疗等进行综合治疗，以延长生存并改善患者的生活质量(quality of life，QoL)。

下面介绍肿瘤主题会议中常讲到的概念。

临床试验(clinical trial)：指任何在人体(患者或健康志愿者)进行药物/治疗的系统性研究，以证实或揭示试验药物/治疗方法的作用、不良反应及/或试验药物的吸收、分布、代谢和排泄，目的是确定试验药物的疗效与安全性。有些国家也将参加临床试验的人员称作"志愿者"，国内一般称之为"受试者"。精心设计及实施的临床试验，是提高人类健康及寻找新的治疗药物和方法的最快、最安全的途径。

结局(outcome)：指研究或试验中患者或受试者(subject)可能出现的一种结果，也就是某种疾病或某种状态下，接受特定治疗后最终的健康状态。

终点(endpoint)：用于测量结局的指标(indicator，measure)称为"终点"，临床试验中常提到主要终点(primary endpoint)与次要终点(second endpoint)。临床试验的主要终点和次要终点是用于评价药物疗效/治疗和安全性的重要指标。

总生存期(overall survival，OS)：指从随机化(randomization)开始到因各种原因导致患者死亡之间的时间。OS是评估治疗干预对患者生存时间的影响的重要指标。

无疾病生存期(disease free survival，DFS)：指从随机化开始到出现肿瘤复发或由任何原因引起死亡之间的时间。DFS可用于早期诊断的癌症患者，评估治疗对预防疾病复发的效果。

无进展生存期(progression free survival，PFS)：指从随机化开始(或单组试验中的治疗开始)至肿瘤进展或任何原因导致死亡(以先发生者为准)的时间。当受试者生存期延长而难以将OS用作试验的主要终点时，DFS、PFS可用作重要的终点指标。

客观缓解率（objective response rate，ORR）、完全缓解（complete response/remission，CR）、部分缓解（partial response/remission，PR）。ORR 指按照公认的缓解评价标准，肿瘤体积缩小达到预先规定值并能维持最低时限要求的患者比例。CR 指肿瘤靶病灶（target lesion）消失，无新病灶出现，且肿瘤标志物（tumor marker）正常，持续至少四周。部分缓解指肿瘤靶病灶最大径之和减少超过 30%，持续至少四周。

疾病进展时间（time to progression，TTP）：指从随机化至出现肿瘤客观进展的时间，不包括死亡。

TNM 分期，国际抗癌联盟（International Union Against Cancer，法语缩写为 UICC）提出了专门用于在癌症治疗过程中确定肿瘤病变范围的分期方法。TNM 三个字母分别代表不同的含义。T 表示原发肿瘤大小和范围，有 T1、T2、T3、T4 四个等级，数字越大表示肿瘤的体积和侵犯的范围越大；同时还有 Tis 和 T0 两种，分别表示肿瘤只到上皮层（原位癌）、所检查的部位没有发现肿瘤病灶。N 代表区域淋巴结，反映与肿瘤有关的淋巴结转移情况，有 N0、N1、N2、N3 四种。N0 表示未发现淋巴结受侵犯，数字越大则表示局部淋巴结转移越多。如果淋巴结转移情况无法确定就用 Nx 表示。M 表示远处转移情况，M0 表示没转移，M1 则表示有转移。在此基础上，用 TNM 三个指标的组合划分出不同的时期。

第二节　真实世界口译情境

一、主题会议

医学会议口译译员会遇到大量以实体肿瘤为主题的会议。由于人口的老龄化，全球实体肿瘤患者大量增加，肿瘤的化疗药物及免疫治疗药物研发是药物研发领域的热点，因此出现了大量的此类主题的会议，包括每年各类学术组织的年会、跨国药企与各类学会/协会共同组织的大量学术研讨会、专门的研发咨询会议、某一临床试验相关的定期研究者会议、欧美大会的在线直播，林林总总，不一而足。

会议的主题多为某一具体肿瘤的综合治疗，前些年以化疗为主，也有部分以放疗为主题的会议，专业性更强。近年来，免疫治疗主题的会议越来越多，会议中对肿瘤外科手术治疗的讨论较少，也少有专门以肿瘤外科治疗为主题的会议，可能是因为最近几十年，现代肿瘤外科的发展已经渐趋完善，但随着近十几年腔镜手术与机器人手术的发展，以及各类手术机器人在国内医院装机量的不断上升，也出现了以腔镜肿瘤手术、机器人肿瘤手术为主题的会议，这些会议也会侧重器械设备的使用，重点并非完全放在肿瘤手术本身。

近年来，在以肺癌为主题的会议中，外科方面更偏重精准有限的手术治疗，手术范围从肺切除术（pneumonectomy），到肺叶切除术（pulmonary lobectomy），再到肺段切除术（segmentectomy）；手术方式也从开放手术（open surgery）到电视辅助胸腔镜手术（video-assisted thoracoscopic surgery，VATS），努力控制手术范围，减小对患者的手术创伤(surgical trauma)。而在综合治疗方面,则更加注重辅助化疗(adjuvant chemotherapy)、靶向治疗与免疫治疗(immunotherapy)等的综合运用与比较。

关于以乳腺癌为主题的会议,除了上述类似内容外,还有一类以乳腺癌术后乳房重建为主题的会议。近年来,随着患者对生活质量的不断增加以及理念的转变,部分此类会议也需要会议翻译。

二、行业特点

实体肿瘤的综合治疗,与血液肿瘤有很多类似之处,无论是放疗、化疗还是免疫治疗,现在临床更加注重或遵从循证医学证据与各类指南的推荐,因而常规肿瘤治疗在会议中少有讨论,会议中更多讨论的是尚无定论的治疗方式以及各类最新的临床试验与研究,欧美部分权威级别的肿瘤大会更是成为了肿瘤治疗领域的风向标,每年都会有大量新的临床试验研究结果在这些大会上公布,成为肿瘤界的盛事。

随着人工智能(artificial intelligence,AI)的发展,现在部分会议也会讲到 AI 辅助病理读片、影像判读以及治疗决策,也会提到将大数据(big data)用于肿瘤治疗方案的制定等内容。

三、口译难点

实体肿瘤主题的会议口译有以下几个难点:

一是大量的药名,包括化学名、商品名、简写形式及不规则表达方式,这一点与血液肿瘤很相似;另外在肿瘤病理分型时经常讲到分子病理,会涉及众多基因名称、检测方法的名称,这些内容往往中英混杂在一起,译员必须有一定的积累或做好会前准备。

二是在涉及肿瘤外科治疗内容时,很多时候讲者会准备一些手术视频,在演讲时一边播放视频一边解说,此部分内容对于译员来说挑战不小,难度主要在于手术器械的名称、手术涉及的解剖名称、手术具体操作步骤及讲者的思路。

遇到此类内容,哪怕做了充分的译前准备,译员如果在此领域的口译经验不足,口译时也很容易出现"外行感"的情况,即译员所使用的语言词汇及表述方式与这一领域专科医生所使用的词汇及表达方式风格迥异,很可能译员翻译准确,听众也都能听懂,但听众却感觉是"外行在翻译",导致听众对口译内容的不信任。而中国幅员辽阔、人口众多,不同医院、不同地区、不同"流派"医生之间的表述方式及风格也存在一定差异,这就对译员提出了更微妙的要求,在这一点上似乎只能靠译员本身的背景,以及循序渐进,慢慢积累相关经验,如果译员强行模仿,恐有东施效颦之风险。

三是译员对于缩略语的掌握程度及实际运用经验,在肿瘤综合治疗主题的会议口译中,缩略语大量存在,如 OS、PFS、CR、PR、ITT 等,这些缩略语在讲者解读/分析各类试验研究时使用频率很高,此时无论是同传还是交传,译员如果经验丰富,则不必拘泥于准确的对应关系,即不必每次都将讲者所说的"总生存"译作"overall survival",可简化为 OS;对于讲者所说的"PR",也不必次次跟读,可以适时展开为"部分应答/缓解"。由于中文和英文差异过大,很多时候译员对这些内容进行准确的对应翻译不一定能够达到最佳的同传效果,例如英文为"CR only exists in a small part of patients",此时如果译作"CR只存在于一小部分患者中",虽然完全正确,但表达效果就不及"只有一小部分患者能做到完全应答/缓解"。译员如果拥有足够的经验,能够适时进行简化与展开调整,其同传流畅度与效果会有所提升。

第三节　中英对照篇章及分析

一、英译中

I will talk a little bit more about pleural mesothelioma. So, it's a very fatal cancer with a very low survival rates which is induced by exposure to historical asbestos, fiber or asbestos fibers in the past. Why is it so fatal? It's because it's a very long latency periods between the first exposure to the fibers and the diagnosis of the disease. And treatment options currently are chemotherapy, consisting of platinum-salts combined with pemetrexed and recently new the immuno-oncology, it was approved combining ipilimumab with nivolumab, which has really nice results. However, there's a very low disease control rate, so only 20% of the patients really react to this treatment. So, there's a lack in improving and selecting these patients out who will respond to certain treatments or not in order to improve the survival rates and in that way, we try to identify markers of companion diagnostic biomarkers and exhale breath to do so. Now exhale breath contains volatile organic compounds and these arise from the different metabolism, and change in metabolism that happens when a mesothelioma is developing after asbestos, exposure. So, by inhaling asbestos, you induce, for instance, a lot of necrosis, you induce oxidative stress and this liberates these oxide and these volatile compounds, and since these volatile come into the breath, we can detect them in the exhale breath.(本段内容选自2023年一位美国医生的学术演讲,有删改调整。)

◎ **参考译文:** 我来稍微谈一谈胸膜间皮瘤。这是一种非常致命的癌症,生存率非常低,是由既往暴露于石棉、纤维或石棉纤维引起的。为什么它如此致命?是因为它有一个很长的潜伏期,从第一次纤维暴露到疾病诊断间的潜伏期。而治疗方案目前是化疗,包括铂盐与培美曲塞的联合治疗,以及最近新的免疫肿瘤学,该疗法已获批准,将伊匹单抗与纳武单抗联合,效果非常好。然而,这种疗法的疾病控制率非常低,只有20%的患者对这种疗法有应答。因此,在改善和选出对特定治疗有应答或没有应答的患者方面存在不足,目的是提高生存率,以这样的方法,我们想识别伴随诊断生物标志物的标记,以及通过呼气来做到这一点。呼出的气体中含有挥发性有机化合物,这些化合物来自不同的代谢,而代谢的变化是发生在石棉暴露后间皮瘤进展时。因此,吸入石棉会导致大量坏死,会导致氧化应激,而这会释放出这些氧化物和挥发性化合物,而由于这些挥发性化合物会进入呼吸,我们可以在呼出的气体中检测到它们。

◎ 分析：

1. "exposure"在医学口译中多译作"暴露"，此处也可处理为"接触"，但不如"暴露"准确客观；

2. "react"译作"应答"，而非"反应"，更符合中文的表达习惯；

3. "metabolism"译作"代谢"即可，无须译作"新陈代谢"。

But today I'd like to focus on using it to try to see who or who will not respond to a certain treatment. Why is that? Because in the past one of the group of CB also investigated this use, using a kind of a sensor, it's an electronic nose which can really smell the compounds in exhale breath. But the downside was that this does not allow to identify the compounds that are present in the breath and this's linked to the pathways that are associated with the type of response. So our goal was to identify these compounds that differ between these profiles and see whether or not responders after treatments can be differentiated from non-responders after treatment. And afterwards if we can use this breathprint to predict the response earlier on. So it just was a little bit of a feasibility study included 15 patients with mesothelioma, and every three months they come for their follow-up, and they get a CT scan, and they get a breath sampling. So the CT scan is done scored as according to the MRIs criteria as a stable disease or a progressive disease. And we use a technique called multi-capillary column-ion mobility spectrometry to sample the exhale breath according to protocol we have used in the past.

◎ 参考译文：但今天我想重点讲一下用它来看谁对特定治疗有应答，谁没有应答。为什么会如此？因为过去CB团队中的一个人也研究过这种用法，使用一种传感器，是个电子鼻，它可以闻到呼气中的化合物。但缺点是，这无法识别呼吸中存在的化合物，而这是与通路相关，这又与反应类型有关。所以我们的目标是识别这些特征间存在差异的化合物，看看应答者在治疗后是否能与无应答者鉴别开来。然后就是我们是否能用这个呼吸印记来提前预测应答。这只是一项可行性研究，入组了15名间皮瘤患者，他们每三个月来随访一次，进行CT扫描，并进行呼吸采样。CT扫描进行评分，根据核磁的标准，分为稳定疾病或进展性疾病。我们使用一种技术，叫作多毛细管柱离子迁移谱的技术，对呼出气体进行采样，按照我们过去使用的方案进行采样。

◎ 分析：

1. "can be differentiated from"译作"鉴别开来"，医学中"鉴别诊断"是一个基础概念，此处译作"鉴别"更好一些；

2. "breathprint"译作"呼吸印记"，指人呼出的气体中所含的独特化学物质组合，可用于疾病检测及个体识别，也可译作"呼吸指纹"；

3. "MRIs"可以直接跟读，也可以译作"核磁"；

4. "to sample the exhale breath according to protocol we have used in the past"按照顺句驱动法处理为"对呼出气体进行采样，按照我们过去使用的方案进行采样"，虽稍有

重复，但在同传时这样处理减轻了译员的压力。

So looking after treatment, we see that most of our groups were nicely matched. But most of our patients contains or are getting the chemotherapy but they could differentiate all of our groups with an acceptable accuracy. We were very happy to see that after treatment differentiate between the two. And we have found here six of the volatiles which are listed over here who were the drivers of the differences between the two groups. Now after treatment this was the response so we looked also if we apply this model on beforehand in a predictive setting, can we predict response and non-response based on the previous measurements. And we get a likely results, so we have a really nice discrimination based on the previous breath sample to differentiate responders to non-responders before the treatment has started. And nice to see it was also based upon these six volatiles presented over here. So we have seen in this preliminary study that exhale breath really can be promising and predicting a treatment outcome of mesothelioma patients based upon certain volatiles which we now will be further validated in a larger population. We will also define the VOC-profile for each treatment because most of our patients get now chemotherapy so it was not powered enough to differentiate between the chemotherapy and then the immunotherapy patients so we will elaborate more on that.

◎ 参考译文：再看治疗后，我们发现大多数的组都匹配得很好。但是我们的大多数患者都接受过或正在接受化疗，但他们能够区分我们所有的组，准确度可以接受。我们很高兴看到治疗后能够区分两者。我们在这里发现了六种挥发性物质，列在了这里，它们是导致两组之间差异的驱动因素。现在这是治疗后的应答，我们也看了如果我们事先将此模型应用到预测设置中，我们能否预测应答和无应答呢，根据之前的测量结果。我们得到了可能的结果，我们得到了很好的区分，是根据之前的呼吸样本得到了很好的区分，能鉴别有应答者和无应答者，在治疗开始之前就可以鉴别开来。很高兴看到也是基于这六种挥发物质，都展示在这里。我们在这项初步研究中也看到了，呼出气体确实很有希望，可以预测间皮瘤患者的治疗结局，根据特定挥发物质进行预测，这些物质我们现在会在更大的人群中进行验证。我们还会为每种治疗定义 VOC 特性，因为我们大多数患者现在都接受化疗，所以它不足以区分化疗患者和之后免疫治疗的患者，我们会详细说明这一点。

◎ 分析：

1. "discrimination"译作"区分"，这个用法在近年来的会议中不多见，遇到时译员应及时反应，不要"下意识翻译"；

2. "profile"一词，此处处理为了"特性"，在医学口译中，很多时候"profile"一词不必译出，而在此语境中，译员需要灵活处理。

What we are going to present today are the two-year follow-up data of A monotherapy in patients with metastatic or advanced UKLP-mutated non-small cell lung cancer patients. These are results from the GOOST-1 trial. So the A is a covalent inhibitor of UKLP, and recently it received approval, accelerated approval by the US FDA for the treatment of pre-treated UKLP non-small cell lung cancer patients based on the results of the Phase 2 Cohort A from GOOST-1 trial. In this cohort, 116 patients were treated without aggressive at a dose of 600 milligrams BID and at a response rate of 42.9% and a median duration of response of a 8.5 months. Today we're going to present the results of a two-year outcomes of 132 patients enrolled in the Phase 1 dose escalation, dose expansion cohorts as well as the Phase 2 Cohort A of GOOST-1 trial. Again, all the 132 patients were treated with a dose of 600 milligrams BID and the median follow-up of this analysis is 26.9 months. The median survival of these 132 patients treated with A was 14.1 months. The one-year survival rate was 52.8 percent and the two-year survival rate was 31.3%. The median progression-free survival in this patient population was 6.9 months with one-year progression-free survival rate of 35% and two-year progression-free survival of 13.9%. The overall response rate was 43%, and the median duration of response was 12.4 months.

◎ **参考译文**：今天我们要介绍的是 A 药单药治疗转移性或晚期 UKLP 突变非小细胞肺癌患者的两年随访数据。这些是 GOOST-1 试验的结果。A 药是一种 UKLP 共价抑制剂，最近该药获批，是美国 FDA 的加速批准，用于接受过治疗的 UKLP 非小细胞肺癌患者的治疗，这是基于 GOOST-1 试验Ⅱ期队列 A 的结果。在这个队列中，116 位患者接受了治疗，剂量不高，600 毫克 BID，应答率为 42.9%，中位应答持续时间为 8.5 个月。今天，我们会展示一个两年的结果，132 位患者，入组到Ⅰ期剂量爬坡及扩展队列，以及Ⅱ期队列 A 中，是 GOOST-1 试验。所有者 132 位患者都接受 600 毫克 BID 剂量的治疗，该分析的中位随访期为 26.9 个月。接受 A 药治疗的这 132 位患者的中位生存期为 14.1 个月。一年生存率为 52.8%，两年生存率为 31.3%。该患者群体的中位无进展生存期为 6.9 个月，一年无进展生存率为 35%，两年无进展生存率为 13.9%。总体应答率为 43%，中位应答持续时间为 12.4 个月。

◎ **分析**：

1. "What we are going to present today are the two-year follow-up data of A monotherapy in patients with metastatic or advanced UKLP-mutated non-small cell lung cancer patients."这一句不一定要使用顺句驱动法，"two-year follow-up data"是医学口译中很常见的表达，记忆相对容易，可以之后译出；

2. "Phase 2"译作"Ⅱ期"，读音"二期"，在讲临床试验时，"phase"只能译作"期"；

3. "In this cohort, 116 patients were treated without aggressive at a dose of 600 milligrams BID"此句处理为"在这个队列中，116 位患者接受了治疗，剂量不高，600 毫克 BID"，口语表达很多时候语法并不完整，译员须根据常识和积累加以调整翻译，此处"BID"指给药频率"每日两次"，此处跟读即可，无须译出；

4. "response rate"此处译作"应答率"，也有人会说"反应率"，更多的人会说"缓解率",但英文中"缓解率"有其对应说法,即"remission rate"。

  Benefit was also assessed in different subsets. Efficacy was observed in subsets based on presence of co-mutations at baseline in the tumor. And the median survival range from 5.7 months among patients with KEAP1m co-mutated tumors, and it was 18.7 months among patients with TP53 co-mutated tumors. Efficacy was also observed among patients with baseline CNS metastases, at a median survival of 14.7 months and a median progression free survival of 6.9 months. The swimmer plot represents the duration of therapy among the 55 responders. Dose modification defined as any dose interruption or any dose reduction did not appear to impact efficacy with A in that 33 of the responding patients who received the drug for more than one year and 12 patients who received the drug more than 12 years, all required dose modification. In addition, among patients who underwent dose modification the two-year survival rate was 32%. No new safety signals were identified with this two-year follow-up. Importantly, even with the long-term follow-up, none of the 12 patients who started the drug within 30 days of immunotherapy developed Grade 3 or greater hepatotoxicity, and only one patient discontinued the drug due to grade 3 hepatotoxicity. In addition, among patients who had received the drug for one year or longer, none of the patients develop new onset treatment related AEs after one year. Rather very few patients develop new onset treatment related AEs after one year, and most of these were GI toxicities, fatigue or elevation in blood serum creatinine levels.

  ◎ **参考译文**:也对不同子集中获益进行了评估。在子集中观察了疗效,根据的是基线时肿瘤中存在的共突变。KEAP1m 共突变肿瘤患者的中位生存期为 5.7 个月,而 TP53 共突变肿瘤患者的中位生存期为 18.7 个月。在基线 CNS 转移患者中也观察了疗效,中位生存期为 14.7 个月,中位无进展生存期为 6.9 个月。泳道图反映了 55 名有应答者的治疗持续时间。剂量调整定义为任何剂量的中断或任何剂量的减少,其似乎不会影响到 A 药的疗效,在应答患者中,有 33 名接受该药物超过一年,有 12 名患者接受该药物超过 12 年,都需要调整剂量。此外,在接受剂量调整的患者中,两年生存率为 32%。这项两年的随访中未发现任何新的安全信号。重要的是,即使进行了长期随访,12 位患者中也没有一人在免疫治疗后 30 天内开始使用该药物后,出现 3 级及以上的肝中毒,只有一位患者因 3 级肝毒性而停药。此外,在接受该药物一年或更长时间的患者中,没有一人在一年后出现新的治疗相关不良反应。而很少有患者在一年后出现新的治疗相关不良反应,其中大部分是胃肠道毒性、疲劳或血清肌酐水平升高。

  ◎ **分析**:

  1. "CNS"意为"中枢神经系统",口译时直接跟读即可;

  2. "The swimmer plot"译作"泳道图",泳道图最常用于展示肿瘤研究中的评估结果;

  3. "AEs"意为"adverse events",译作"不良事件",是医学口译中的基础概念,遇到时可以跟读，但因为其为双元音字母，还是建议译员译为"不良事件"，以方便听众理解；

4. "GI"指"gastrointestinal"，译作"胃肠（道）"，口译时一般都要译出，可译作"胃肠道"。国内习惯说"胃肠道毒性"而非"GI 毒性"。

So words matter is not just a catchphrase, it's a simple yet profound when talking about lung cancer. There we go. So recognizing the urgency to combat stigma and to promote patient respect and dignity, the IASLC language guide was created. It was a collaborative effort between IASLC Patient Advocates, the National Lung Cancer Roundtable Stigma Task Group and others from different organizations and disciplines. On the left side, you'll see the four principles. Now the guide isn't an exhaustive list of dos and don'ts or rules. It's not meant to call anybody out, rather it's meant to call people in to help with raising awareness and promoting inclusion when we talk about lung cancer. And so this guide was approved unanimously by the IASLC board in May of 2021 and so what our study did was we analyze presentations from World Conference 2022, just one year after the guide was implemented or published to assess the adoption of non-stigmatizing language within the first year, and also to see if there were any correlations with presenter characteristics. Now we focused on the term smoker, because it was the first word in the list of stigmatizing language in the guide. So we searched for its usage in the slide presentations and we also explored presenter backgrounds. And when looking at the results, we used two different types of analysis, yielding consistent data. So we were happy to see that and we'll talk a little bit more about the data within the oral abstract session.（本段内容选自 2022 年一位美国医生的演讲，有删改调整。）

◎ **参考译文**：言语很重要不止是一句口号，在说到肺癌的时候，它既简单又深刻。就是这样。所以认识到对抗病耻感、促进患者尊重和尊严的紧迫性，IASLC 用语指南便应运而生。它是 IASLC 患者倡导者委员会、国家肺癌圆桌病耻感工作组和来自不同组织和学科的其他人员共同努力的成果。在左边，你会看到四项原则。现在，该指南并不是一份面面俱到的清单，或是注意事项。它并不是要点名批评任何人，而是要号召人们在我们讲到肺癌时帮助提高认识和促进包容。而这一指南也在 2021 年 5 月获得了 IASLC 董事会的一致批准，因此我们的研究是分析 2022 年世界大会的演讲，即指南实施或发布后的一年，以评估第一年内非污名化语言的使用情况，同样探索是否与演讲者特点存在任何关联。现在我们关注吸烟者这个词，因为它是指南中污名化语言清单中的第一个词。所以我们在幻灯片演示中搜索了它的使用，我们也了解了演讲者的背景。在看结果的时候，我们用了两种不同类型的分析，得出了一致的数据。所以我们很高兴能看到这一点，我们会在口头摘要环节中讲一些数据。

◎ **分析**：

1. "stigma"译作"病耻感"，比"耻辱"更准确；

2. "stigmatizing language"译作"污名化语言"，此处与"stigma"的主体不同，stigma

指特定疾病患者的感受，故译作"病耻感"，而"stigmatizing language"指他人在讲到特定疾病患者时所用的词汇和语言，译作"污名化语言"，指的是他人对一类人群的描述，而非该人群的自我描述。

We categorize the nine distinct interventions we identified into three broad categories here. And it really shows that interventions typically provided information or instruction or reference material to individuals affected by respiratory disease stigma, which we deemed educational interventions; or perhaps guided behavior change often via group programs in the behavioral interventions I've described here; or finally provided formal psychotherapeutic intervention such as to improve mood, coping skills and thought patterns. One intervention was directed oncology care providers, and one targeted family members and supporters, in addition to higher risk individuals. So across this, the study is included in the systematic review, most of the identified stigma-reducing interventions were aimed at reducing feelings of self-blame and shame, or implementing strategies to deal with stigma arising in interpersonal interactions. Most included interventions reported achieving reductions in stigma with similar effects observed for remote and digital intervention delivery compared to traditional in-person and face-to-face modes, which does show promise in increasing accessibility for patients with co-morbidities or loss of function related to respiratory disease. These findings also highlight that we need to further develop and evaluate stigma reducing interventions in diverse social cultural contexts and importantly in partnership with those affected by smoking related diseases.

◎ **参考译文**：我们分类了九种不同的干预方式，并把它们分成了三大类。这里显示，干预措施通常提供信息、指导或参考材料，提供给那些有呼吸疾病病耻感的患者，我们认为是教育干预；或者可能是引导行为改变，通常是通过团队项目，用于行为干预，我在此处已有描述；或者最终提供正式的心理治疗干预，例如改善情绪、应对技巧和思维模式。一种干预是给到肿瘤医护人员，一种以家庭成员和支持者为目标，还有就是高风险个体。这项研究也被纳入系统性回顾，大多数所确定的病耻感减低干预，其目的都是减低自我责备和羞愧感，或者实施策略以处理在人际交往中遇到的病耻感。大多数纳入的干预都报告了病耻感的降低，效果是差不多的，远程及数字干预，相比于传统当面、面对面模式，效果相差无几，这就显示能提高可及性，惠及患者，他们可能有共病、功能丧失，这些都与呼吸疾病相关。这些发现同样也强调了我们要进一步制定并评估病耻感减低干预，在不同的社会文化背景下进行，重要的是，与受吸烟相关疾病影响的患者合作。

◎ **分析**：

1. "in addition to"此处译作"还有就是"，此处进行意义调整后译出，顺利完成这一句话；

2. "systematic review"可译作"系统综述"或"系统性回顾"；

3. 本段倒数第二句较长,同传时只能使用顺句驱动的方法处理为许多短句。

So the presentations we heard today address several areas that are really important to patients. Obviously, one of them is treatment. We always like to hear about treatment options that allow us to live longer, especially if you get to stop treatment. But it's also important to have treatment options that while they don't allow us to live as long as others that they still allow us to be around for things that are important, especially for those patients who have difficult to treat lung cancers or that don't have many good treatment options yet like KRAS non-small cell lung cancer and mesothelioma. But there are other things that are in here too lung cancer diagnosis and treatment can be very invasive and take over your life. And to have that all happen and then have the treatment not work is incredibly disappointing and has a huge impact on the patients and their families, so being able to find biomarkers that, one, help you determine which treatment is more likely to work and two, are non-invasive, is huge. It's also important that we find effective ways to help patients deal with the stigma. I've experienced it myself. It's amazing how easily it comes up my very first breakfast conversation here at this conference when one of the people at the next table found out I had lung cancers but "oh you're a smoker." It's everywhere and it doesn't matter. The patient should be able to get treatment regardless of what their background is.

◎ **参考译文**:今天我们听到的演讲涉及的几个领域,对患者来说都非常重要。显然,其中一个就是治疗。我们通常都喜欢听到有治疗方法能让我们活得更久,尤其是在要停止治疗的时候。但同样也很重要的是,我们有治疗选择,虽然这些治疗选择不能让我们活得像其他人那样长,但还是能多给我们一段时间处理重要事情,尤其是对于难以治疗的肺癌患者而言,或者是压根没有好的治疗方法,比如说KRAS非小细胞癌或者是间皮瘤。但是,还有其他方面,肺癌的诊断和治疗可能有创性很强,从此占据整个生活。发生这一切,治疗也不管用,这会非常令人失望,对患者及家属来说影响巨大,所以要能找到生物标记物,一是它能帮助决定哪种治疗更有可能起效;二是无创性,这非常重要。同样重要的是,我们找到有效的方式来帮助患者处理病耻感。我自己曾经经历过。令人惊讶的是,很容易它就出现在了我的第一场早餐对话中了,就在本场会议上,一个人在旁桌,听到我有肺癌,但是说出了"噢,你抽烟。"这种情况到处都是,已经不重要了。患者应该能得到治疗,不管他们的背景如何。

◎ **分析**:
1. "address"一词,此处译作"涉及",一般来说,医学口译中但凡涉及"address"一词,从来不表示"地址"的意思,大多用作动词,表示"解决"或"演讲";
2. "KRAS"跟读即可,一般读音是"K-rus";
3. "invasive"此处译作"有创性",也可译作"创伤性"。

It's also important to realize that just increasing the overall survival is not the only thing that's important to patients. The study for small cell lung cancer did give us longer overall survival. And it's not just overall survival that's important, quality of life is important too. And it needs to be the patient who makes the decision about which one matters most. If somebody just wants to live long enough to see their child get married, living for a few more months even if you're not particularly comfortable may be worth it. For someone else living a few more months if they're miserable might not be worth it, and you need to ask the patient and get their opinion on what's important to them. Being able to find which of these treatments is going to make a big difference and has the best chance of being a good treatment is also huge. And while we those of us with oncogene-driven lung cancers do have a biomarker that allows us to know which treatments are likely to work. There's a large percentage of lung cancer patients who don't have that. Anything we can find that helps move that needle is wonderful and a test that doesn't require getting a needle stuck in your arm or getting cut open is a wonderful option.

◎ **参考译文**：同样重要的就是要意识到，只延长总生存时间并不是唯一对患者重要的事情。对小细胞肺癌的研究确实给到我们更长的总生存时间。但并不是只有总生存时间才重要，生活质量同样重要。而且应该是患者自己来决定哪一个更为重要。如果有些人只想要活到看见他们的孩子结婚，多活几个月，尽管他们可能不舒服，你可能觉得不一定值。对于有些人而言，多活几个月，但是他们很痛苦，可能不值得，而你要问患者，了解他们的想法，了解对于他们来说什么重要。能找到哪个治疗能够带来巨大的改变，而且最有可能成为一个好的治疗方案，也非常重要。对于我们这些致癌基因导致的肺癌，我们有生物标志物，能够让我们知道哪种治疗可能有效。有很大一部分肺癌患者他们没有标志物。任何我们能发现的，能有助于推动前进的都很好，一个检测不需要胳膊扎针，也不要做切口，就是很好的选择。

◎ **分析**：

1. "There's a large percentage of lung cancer patients who don't have that."处理为"有很大一部分肺癌患者他们没有标志物。"此处的"that"译作"标志物"，比"那个""那一点"明确得多，且更便于听众理解，在医学口译中，"it""this""that"之类的代词，可根据上下文灵活处理，以方便听众理解；

2. "move that needle"此处译作"前进"。

二、中译英

全身治疗是提高肝癌疗效的最重要的方法。国内大多数肝癌患者在确诊时已处于进展期或晚期，肿瘤细胞在肝外存在广泛转移，肿瘤从早期局部发展为晚期全身的状态，因此，手术、放疗、介入等局部治疗手段难以满足临床治疗的需求；这就需要系统的全身治疗，即药物治疗来实现肿瘤治疗并提高疗效。最近，卫健委发布了《原发性肝癌诊疗规范（2019年版）》，该规范针对系统治疗进行了更新。近年来，肝癌的系统治疗取得了突破性的进展，治疗药物不再是单一的抗血管生成的靶向药物索拉非尼。继瑞戈非尼奠定了索拉非尼治疗进展后的二线治疗地位后，2018年公布的全球多中心Ⅲ期临床研究REFLECT结果确立了仑伐替尼在肝癌一线治疗中的地位。目前，仑伐替尼一线治疗不可切除肝细胞癌被国内外指南一致推荐。自此，肝癌的抗肿瘤靶向治疗有了更多选择。（本段内容选自2024年对三位国内专家的采访，有删改调整。）

◎ **参考译文**：Systemic treatment is the most important method to improve the efficacy of liver cancer. Most liver cancer patients in China are already in the progressive or advanced stage when diagnosed, and tumor cells have extensive metastasis outside the liver. The tumor develops from early local to late systemic state. Therefore, surgery, radiotherapy, intervention and other local treatment methods are difficult to meet the needs of clinical treatment; this requires systemic treatment, that is, drug therapy to achieve tumor treatment and improve the efficacy. Recently, the National Health Commission issued the "Guidelines for the Diagnosis and Treatment of Primary Liver Cancer (2019 Edition)", which has updated the systemic treatment. In recent years, breakthrough progress has been made in the systemic treatment of liver cancer, and the therapeutic drug is no longer a single anti-angiogenic targeted drug sorafenib. After regorafenib established the second-line treatment for the progression after sorafenib treatment, the results of the global multicenter phase Ⅲ clinical study REFLECT published in 2018 established the position of lenvatinib in the first-line treatment of liver cancer. At present, lenvatinib is unanimously recommended by domestic and foreign guidelines as a first-line treatment for unresectable hepatocellular carcinoma. Since then, there are more options for targeted anti-tumor treatment of liver cancer.

◎ **分析**：

1. "晚期"此处译作"advanced stage"，也可处理为"late stage"或"terminal stage"，但在讲"terminal"时，注意与"终末期"相区别；

2. "系统的全身治疗"译作"systemic treatment"；

3. "2018年公布的全球多中心Ⅲ期临床研究REFLECT结果确立了"译作"the results of the global multicenter phase Ⅲ clinical study REFLECT published in 2018 established"，其实在听到"2018年公布的全球多中心"时，译员就可以开始译出"the results"了，因为后面必然讲的是××研究/试验结果，这就是预测先说的具体应用，当然，这需要译员具有一定的经验。

近两年来的癌症治疗中，免疫检查点抑制剂已获得美国FDA批准，可用于治疗十多种恶性肿瘤。基于CheckMate-040和KEYNOTE-224研究，纳武利尤单抗和帕博利珠单抗获批用于晚期肝癌的二线治疗。2019年美国临床肿瘤学会年会公布了KEYNOTE-240研究结果，进一步巩固了帕博利珠单抗的二线治疗地位。但免疫单药治疗肝细胞癌的有效率仅为20%左右。鉴于单药治疗效果有限，晚期肝细胞癌的联合治疗是近年来临床研究的热点话题。仑伐替尼是各指南推荐的HCC一线治疗手段,帕博利珠单抗则在肝癌二线治疗中获得成功。仑伐替尼联合帕博利珠单抗对于治疗不可切除的HCC患者的Ⅰb期研究,KEYNOTE-524,初步结果显示,ORR为44.8%,优于REFLECT试验的仑伐替尼组,是24.1%;联合治疗组的中位OS为20.4个月,中位PFS为9.7个月。

◎ **参考译文**:In the past two years, regarding cancer treatment, immune checkpoint inhibitor has been approved by the US FDA for the treatment of more than ten types of malignant tumors. Based on the CheckMate-040 and KEYNOTE-224 studies, nivolumab and pembrolizumab were approved for the second-line treatment of advanced liver cancer. In 2019, American Society of Clinical Oncology annual meeting published the results of the KEYNOTE-240 study, further consolidating the second-line treatment status of pembrolizumab. However, the effectiveness rate of immunotherapy alone in the treatment of hepatocellular carcinoma is only about 20%. Given the limited effect of monotherapy, combination therapy for advanced hepatocellular carcinoma has been a hot topic in clinical research in recent years. Lenvatinib is the first-line treatment for HCC recommended by various guidelines, while pembrolizumab has been successful in the second-line treatment of liver cancer. Lenvatinib combined with pembrolizumab for the treatment of patients with unresectable HCC, the preliminary results of the phase Ib study, KEYNOTE-524, showed that the ORR was 44.8%, which was better than the lenvatinib group in the REFLECT trial, it's 24.1%; the median OS of the combination treatment group was 20.4 months, and the median PFS was 9.7 months.

◎ **分析**:

1. "美国临床肿瘤学会"英文是"American Society of Clinical Oncology",缩写为ASCO。其成立于1964年,是现今全球范围内领先的肿瘤专业学术组织,在肿瘤主题的医学会议上经常会被提及;

2. "肝细胞癌"译作"hepatocellular carcinoma",也常缩写为HCC。

肝癌表现出的时间和空间上的高度异质性使得制定精准治疗策略变得困难重重。肝癌的发生与进展涉及多个信号通路的改变,每个癌细胞平均有30余个突变,其中部分可能为驱动基因。目前尚无法确定同一患者的每个癌细胞的驱动因子是否相同。当前的测序技术虽证实了原发及复发肿瘤的突变明显不同,但是肝癌的增殖和耐药机制会发生变异,这为找到固定的药物靶点带来挑战;因此,目前的精准医学还很难对肝癌进行分子病理水平的精准诊断和治疗,也就无法促进肝癌液体活检技术的应用和分子靶向药物的研发。

◎ **参考译文**:The high temporal and spatial heterogeneity of liver cancer makes it difficult to develop precise treatment strategies. The occurrence and progression of liver cancer involve changes in multiple signaling pathways, and each cancer cell has an average of more than 30 mutations, some of which might be driver genes. It is currently impossible to determine whether the driver factors of each cancer cell in the same patient are the same. Although current sequencing technology has confirmed that the mutations in primary and recurrent tumors are significantly different, the proliferation and resistance mechanisms of liver cancer will mutate, which poses a challenge to finding fixed drug targets; therefore, it is still difficult for current precision medicine to accurately diagnose and treat liver cancer at the molecular pathology level, and it is impossible to promote the use of liquid biopsy technology for liver cancer and the development of molecular targeted drugs.

◎ 分析：

1. "测序"译作"sequencing"，只有此一种译法；

2. "液体活检"译作"liquid biopsy"，指在体液样本中提取分子标志物进行检测分析；

3. "研发"可译作"R&D"，即"research and development"，但也可简单处理为"development"。

新辅助治疗的目标，第一是提高肿瘤根治性切除率；第二是更早根除术前无法检测到的微转移，从而提高整体的治疗效果；第三是在肿瘤尚存的情况下，提前了解药物治疗的敏感性，为后续治疗和全程管理过程中的药物选择提供重要信息。术后辅助治疗的目标是消灭手术后体内仍残留的癌细胞。传统的治疗药物是化疗，但是既往研究显示NSCLC 辅助化疗仅可提升约5%的5年生存率。在靶向治疗和免疫治疗等全身性治疗药物在晚期患者治疗中发挥重大作用后，其也正在向新辅助治疗推进。目前，围手术期免疫治疗的模式包括单纯的新辅助免疫治疗、术前新辅助+术后辅助免疫治疗、术后辅助免疫治疗。就预期疗效而言，期待疗效包括使肿瘤缩小、提高手术切除率以及根治性切除率。在肿瘤缩小后，外科手术做得更小，从而减小对患者的创伤和痛苦，患者更好地恢复，以更好的身体状况接受后续治疗、改善生活质量、最终转化为更好地生存。目前，NSCLC 围手术免疫治疗已获得了非常好的结果，希望 NSCLC 新辅助靶向治疗领域也能够产生很好的结果，期待最新一系列试验数据的发布，从而为临床医生提供更多的手段来进行更为有效的综合治疗。

◎ 参考译文：The goals of neoadjuvant therapy are, first, to increase the radical resection rate of tumors; second, to eradicate micro-metastases that cannot be detected before surgery, thereby improving the overall treatment effect; third, to understand the sensitivity of drug treatment in advance when the tumor is still present, and to provide important information for drug selection during subsequent treatment and full management. The goal of postoperative adjuvant therapy is to eliminate cancer cells that remain in the body after surgery. The traditional treatment drug is chemotherapy, but previous studies have shown that adjuvant chemotherapy for NSCLC can only increase the 5-year survival rate by about 5%. After targeted therapy, immunotherapy and other systemic therapeutic drugs have played a major role in the treatment of advanced patients, they are also moving towards neoadjuvant therapy. At present, the perioperative immunotherapy modes include simple neoadjuvant immunotherapy, pre-op neoadjuvant + post-op adjuvant immunotherapy, and post-op adjuvant immunotherapy. In terms of expected efficacy, the expected efficacy includes shrinking the tumor, increasing the surgical resection rate and radical resection rate, and making the surgical operation smaller after the tumor is reduced, thereby reducing the trauma and pain to the patient, and the patient recovers better, receiving follow-up treatment in a better condition, improving the quality of life, and ultimately translating into better survival. Currently, perioperative immunotherapy for NSCLC has achieved very good results. It is hoped that the field of neoadjuvant targeted therapy for NSCLC can also produce good results, the latest series of trial data will be released, to provide clinicians with more means to carry out more effective comprehensive treatments.

◎ 分析：

1. "新辅助治疗"译作"neoadjuvant therapy"，指患者在手术或者接受其他治疗前，接受药物或其他方式进行预处理，对于许多原本无手术条件或风险过高的患者来说，新辅助治疗使得手术成为可能或风险降低，新辅助治疗是近年来肿瘤会议的基础概念；

2. "肿瘤缩小"此处译作"shrinking the tumor"，也可译作"tumor shrinkage"。

术前新辅助免疫治疗是Ⅱ～Ⅲ期 NSCLC 患者的重要治疗方式，在 EGFR 突变阴性，尤其是 PD-L1 表达阳性的 NSCLC 患者中能带来显著获益。但 NSCLC 新辅助免疫治疗尚有诸多问题有待解答，需要进一步地探索。对于接受手术治疗的 NSCLC 患者，在术前如果进行了新辅助免疫治疗，是否有必要再进一步接受免疫维持治疗？目前尚无高级别的术后免疫维持和不采用免疫维持的头对头比较证据，这一领域有待进一步研究。这一问题可包括两种极端的情况：其一，术前新辅助免疫治疗非常好，达到了病理学完全缓解，再进行免疫维持治疗是否意味治疗过度？我们在临床试验中看到一些事实，似乎 pCR 患者在手术切除后还存在一定的复发转移风险，有必要进行后续治疗。其二，如果术前新辅助治疗并没有获得效果，术后免疫维持治疗是否还需要？这一问题目前尚无答案，也是诸多医生关注的话题。

◎ 参考译文：Preoperative neoadjuvant immunotherapy is an important treatment for patients with stage Ⅱ～Ⅲ NSCLC, for EGFR mutation-negative, especially those with PD-L1 positive expression, for these patients, it can bring significant benefits. However, there are still many questions to be answered in neoadjuvant immunotherapy for NSCLC, which need further exploration. For NSCLC patients who undergo surgical treatment, if they have received neoadjuvant immunotherapy before surgery, is it necessary to receive further immune maintenance therapy? There is currently no high-level head-to-head comparative evidence between postoperative immune maintenance and non-immune maintenance, and this area needs further research. This issue may include two extreme situations: first, if the preoperative neoadjuvant immunotherapy is very good and achieves pathological complete remission, does the subsequent immune maintenance therapy mean excessive treatment? We have seen some facts in clinical trials that it seems that pCR patients still have a certain risk of recurrence and metastasis after surgical resection, and it is necessary to undergo follow-up treatment. Secondly, if the preoperative neoadjuvant therapy does not achieve results, is postoperative immune maintenance therapy still necessary? This question has no answer yet, and it is also a topic of concern for many doctors.

◎ 分析：

1. "治疗过度"此处译作"excessive treatment"，也可翻译为"overtreatment"；

2. "pCR"即前文提及的"pathological complete remission"，意为"病理学完全缓解"。在肿瘤主题的医学会议中，不少中文演讲者为了方便，会夹杂大量英文缩略语、药名、试验名等，同传时译员应注意区分。

第三种模式是先行手术治疗，在术后再进行免疫联合化疗的辅助治疗。辅助免疫治疗的一个适应证是较早期的 NSCLC 患者，例如 Ib 期。临床医生希望较早期的 NSCLC 患者能够更好地接受局部物理治疗，在此基础上判断术后是否需要药物治疗。因为更早期的 NSCLC 患者手术切除大部分病灶不太困难，而且任何药物治疗都有一定的毒副作用，所以并不希望新辅助治疗的药物影响手术。在一些免疫治疗临床试验中，一小部分患者最终并未接受手术。此外，PD-L1 检测可能因为肿瘤异质性而结果不准确，对手术切除的肿瘤标本进行标志物检测，检测结果会更加精准，也能更好地指导术后治疗策略，也有可能发现术前未检测到的基因突变，进而确认术后靶向治疗的药物选择，而且临床上大多数患者术前并不做基因检测。所以，对于更早期的 NSCLC 患者，先做手术，术后再进行生物标志物检测，此种模式可精准指导术后辅助治疗的选择。而 NSCLC 围手术免疫治疗模式，对于不同分期的患者，不同身体条件的患者，不同地区的患者，治疗模式的选择会有所不同。更为重要的是，临床医生应从提高安全性和有效性的角度出发，为患者选择获益最大的治疗模式，最终目的是让患者获得更好的生存。

◎ 参考译文：The third model is to perform surgical treatment first, and then after surgery, perform immunotherapy combined with chemotherapy as adjuvant therapy. One indication for adjuvant immunotherapy is patients with earlier NSCLC, such as stage Ib. Clinicians hope that patients with early stage NSCLC can better accept local physical therapy, and on this basis, they can determine whether they need drug treatment after surgery. Because for early stage NSCLC patients, surgical removal of most lesions is not very difficult, and any drug treatment has certain toxic side effects, it is not hoped that the neoadjuvant therapy drugs will affect the surgery. In some immunotherapy clinical trials, a small number of patients did not eventually undergo surgery. In addition, PD-L1 testing may be inaccurate due to tumor heterogeneity. Marker testing of surgically removed tumor specimens will have more accurate test results and better guide postoperative treatment strategies. It is also possible to discover gene mutations that were not detected before surgery, and then confirm the drug selection for postoperative targeted therapy. In clinical practice, most patients do not undergo genetic testing before surgery. Therefore, for patients with earlier stage NSCLC, surgery first, and biomarker testing after surgery. This model can accurately guide the choice of postoperative adjuvant therapy. The choice of perioperative immunotherapy for NSCLC, for patients at different stages, with different physical conditions, and in different regions, will be different. More importantly, clinicians, in order to improve safety and effectiveness, should choose the treatment model that will benefit patients the most, with the ultimate goal of allowing patients to achieve better survival.

◎ 分析：

1. "肿瘤异质性"译作"tumor heterogeneity"，指肿瘤在分裂增殖及生长过程中，肿瘤病灶处细胞在分子生物学及基因方面发生改变，从而使肿瘤的生长速度、侵袭能力（invasion）、对治疗物的敏感性等方面产生差异。肿瘤异质性是实体肿瘤领域中最基础的概念之一；

2. "先做手术，术后再进行生物标志物检测"此处译作"surgery first, and biomarker testing after surgery"，在同传的情况下此种译法可接受。

围术期胃癌治疗是一个重要议题。得益于免疫治疗在围手术期的广泛应用，我们积累了大量临床数据，包括双免药物治疗和ADC药物等，这些信息都对围术期治疗策略产生了深远影响。随着免疫治疗时代的来临，局部进展期胃癌在围手术期接受免疫治疗后，获得PCR的患者的比例显著上升。在RESOLVE研究中，试验组在引入免疫治疗后，PCR率由原来的5%提升至20%。面对PCR患者的增多，胃肠外科医生要深入思考未来手术策略的调整。以食管胃结合部的局部进展期胃癌为例，经过新辅助免疫化疗后，部分患者能够达到完全缓解，且复查胃镜时，肉眼下病灶消失，活检结果为阴性。对于这类患者，术后大概率也是阴性结果。由于当前缺乏直接证据支持，我们难以简单采用直肠癌的观望等待策略。根据当前指南，手术治疗仍是推荐方案。然而，从我们中心的经验来看，即使手术，我们也会倾向于有意识地缩小胃切除范围，以最大限度地保留胃的功能。同样，在淋巴清扫范围上，我们也在有意识地缩小范围，尽管这方面的证据尚显不足，但也引起了广泛关注。

◎ 参考译文：Perioperative treatment of gastric cancer is an important issue. Thanks to the widespread use of immunotherapy in the perioperative period, we have accumulated a large amount of clinical data, including dual-immune drug therapy and ADC drugs, which have had a profound impact on perioperative treatment strategies. As the era of immunotherapy has come, locally advanced gastric cancer, during the perioperative period, after receiving immunotherapy, the proportion of patients who achieve PCR has increased significantly. In the RESOLVE study, after the introduction of immunotherapy in the trial group, the PCR rate increased from 5% to 20%. Faced with the increase in PCR patients, gastrointestinal surgeons should think deeply about the adjustment of future surgical strategies. For example, the locally advanced gastric cancer at the esophageal-gastric junction, after neoadjuvant immunochemotherapy, some patients can achieve complete remission, and when reexamining with the gastroscopy, the lesions disappear under the naked eye and the biopsy results are negative. For such patients, the postoperative result is also likely to be negative. Due to the lack of direct evidence support, it is difficult for us to simply adopt the wait-and-watch strategy from rectal cancer. According to current guidelines, surgical treatment is still the recommended option. However, from the experience of our center, even if surgery is performed, we tend to consciously reduce the range of gastrectomy to maximize the preservation of gastric function. Similarly, we are consciously reducing the scope of lymph node dissection, although the evidence in this regard is still insufficient, but is has attracted widespread attention.

◎ 分析：

1. "观望等待"即"等待观察策略"，译作"wait and watch"，指对于新辅助治疗后，原发病灶达到 cCR 的直肠癌患者，通过密切的随访及观察，其可免除手术的策略；

2. "淋巴清扫"译作"lymph node dissection"。

晚期胃癌的治疗，特别是在创新药物治疗方面，近期也取得了显著的进展，例如，国产双抗药物 AK-104 在美国 AACR 上展示了出色的Ⅲ期临床研究数据，其疗效和安全性都令人印象深刻。AK-104 的独特之处在于，它将抗 PD-1 单抗与抗 CTLA-4 单抗合二为一，从而在避免抗 CTLA-4 药物可能带来的毒副作用的同时，显著提高了治疗效果。值得注意的是，对于那些 CPS<1 的患者，传统的抗 PD-1 单抗治疗效果有限，但 AK-104 在这类患者中也展现出了有效性，这为晚期胃癌的治疗提供了新的可能性。另外，ADC 药物，即抗体偶联药物，也展现了显著的进步。传统的曲妥珠单抗主要对 HER2/3+或 FISH 阳性的胃癌患者有效，但这类患者仅占胃癌患者总数的约 8%。ADC 药物的引入极大地扩展了胃癌治疗范围，即使对于 HER2+甚至 FISH 阴性的患者也显示出疗效。除上述药物外，针对 Claudin 18.2 靶点的 ADC 药物等的探索也为临床医生提供了大量的有利数据。这些进展有望推动 ADC 药物从后线治疗逐渐扩展到围手术期的治疗策略中。

◎ 参考译文：The treatment of advanced gastric cancer, especially in the field of innovative drug therapy, has also made significant progress recently. For example, the domestic bispecific antibody AK-104 showed excellent Phase Ⅲ clinical research data at the AACR in the United States, with impressive efficacy and safety. The unique feature of AK-104 is that it combines anti-PD-1 monoclonal antibody and anti-CTLA-4 monoclonal antibody into one, thereby significantly avoiding the possible toxic side effects of anti-CTLA-4 drugs, while improving the therapeutic effect significantly. It is worth noting that for patients with CPS <1, traditional anti-PD-1 monoclonal antibody treatment has limited effect, but AK-104 has also shown effectiveness in such patients, which provides new possibilities for the treatment of advanced gastric cancer. In addition, ADC drugs, antibody-drug conjugates, have also shown significant progress. Traditional trastuzumab is mainly effective for patients with HER2/3+ or FISH-positive gastric cancer, but such patients only account for about 8% of the total number of gastric cancer patients. The introduction of ADC drugs has greatly expanded the scope of gastric cancer treatment, showing efficacy even for patients with HER2+ or even FISH-negative. In addition to the above drugs, the exploration of ADC drugs targeting Claudin 18.2 has also provided clinicians with a large amount of favorable data. These advances are expected to promote the gradual expansion of ADC drugs from late-line treatment to perioperative treatment strategies.

◎ 分析：

1. 关于"令人印象深刻"的译法，近年来，随着"impressive"一词在医学会议中的广泛应用，加之大多数译员选择将其译作"令人印象深刻"，而非"引人瞩目"或"出色"，导致不少有国际交流经验的国内医生在中文发言时也频繁使用"令/让人印象深刻"等表达；

2. "单抗"指"单克隆抗体"，译作"monoclonal antibody"，缩写为"mAb"。

第四节　补充练习

一、中译英

近年来，胃癌治疗领域取得了显著的进步，尤其是在免疫治疗方面。RESOLVE 研究在 2023 年 ESMO 大会上公布的五年随访结果为我们提供了强有力的证据，证实围手术期 SOX 围手术期治疗能够显著提高局部进展期胃癌患者的无病生存率和总生存率，这奠定了中国胃癌围手术期治疗模式的基石。近年来免疫治疗的快速发展，尤其是 CHECKMATE-649 研究，已经奠定了胃癌晚期一线标准治疗模式的基础。现在，无论是 NCCN、ESMO 还是中国的 CSCO、CACA 指南，都推荐免疫联合化疗作为晚期胃癌的标准治疗模式。

鉴于中国胃癌的特殊性，我国局部进展期胃癌占到 70% 以上，晚期胃癌也占到 20%，所以我国胃癌患者绝大部分都需要综合治疗。中国学者近年来进行了大量围手术期免疫治疗的探索性研究，例如，Ⅲ期随机对照研究——DRAGON-IV 研究，采用靶-免-化联合治疗围手术期胃癌，其近期结果显示靶-免-化治疗组的 PCR 率达到了 18%，比对照组提高了 13%。实际上，许多单臂Ⅱ期研究也采用了免疫围手术期化疗，并观察到了较高的 PCR 率，通常在 20% 左右，最高可达 30%，与放疗结合后，PCR 率可提升至 40%。在 HER2 阳性胃癌的治疗中，沈琳院长牵头的Ⅱ期对照研究初步结果显示，靶-免-化新辅助治疗组的 PCR 率达到了 38%，而对照组仅为 14%，几乎提高了三倍。

所以我觉得这些研究成果都充分证明，胃癌治疗已经全面进入免疫治疗时代，并展现出巨大的潜力和希望。

C-HIPEC是一项具有中国特色的技术，其背后是腹腔热灌注化疗理念，然而，关于其机制的深入研究却相对匮乏。我们通过自己的基础研究发现，热疗与化疗、放疗结合能够显著增强化疗和放疗的敏感度。为了满足这一技术的需求，国内相关厂家研发了热灌注设备。其中，温控是热灌注技术的关键参数。热灌注的温度要高于正常体温37℃，而我们经过研究发现，当温度控制在43℃时，既能有效杀灭肿瘤细胞，又不损伤正常组织，因为肿瘤细胞对热的耐受性较正常组织低，而如果温度超过43℃，就可能导致正常组织细胞的损伤。在这方面，我们国内的腹腔热灌注设备展现出了卓越的温控性能，其温度控制精度达到了正负0.1℃，确保了热灌注治疗的安全性和有效性。这种技术主要应用于腹腔、胸腔、心包或膀胱等空腔脏器内的原发性肿瘤以及继发性腹腔、胸膜转移瘤治疗，尤其在预防方面发挥着重要作用。

◎ **参考译文**：In recent years, significant progress has been made in the field of gastric cancer treatment, especially in immunotherapy. The five-year follow-up results of the RESOLVE study published at the 2023 ESMO Congress provide us with strong evidence that perioperative SOX perioperative treatment can significantly improve the disease-free survival and overall survival of patients with locally advanced gastric cancer, which lays the foundation for the perioperative treatment model of gastric cancer in China. The rapid progress of immunotherapy in recent years, especially the CHECKMATE-649 study, has laid the foundation for the first-line standard treatment model for advanced gastric cancer. Now, whether it is NCCN, ESMO or China's CSCO and CACA guidelines, immunotherapy combined with chemotherapy is recommended as the standard treatment model for advanced gastric cancer.

Given the particularity of gastric cancer in China, more than 70% of locally advanced gastric cancer and 20% of advanced gastric cancer in my country, so most of the gastric cancer patients in my country need comprehensive treatment. In recent years, Chinese scholars have conducted a large number of exploratory studies on perioperative immunotherapy. For example, the DRAGON-IV study, a phase III randomized controlled study, used a combination of target-immune-chemotherapy to treat perioperative gastric cancer. Its recent results showed that the PCR rate of the target-immune-chemotherapy group reached 18%, an increase of 13% over the control group. In fact, many single-arm phase II studies also used immunotherapy perioperative chemotherapy and observed a higher PCR rate, usually around 20%, up to 30%. When combined with radiotherapy, the PCR rate can be increased to 40%. In the treatment of HER2-positive gastric cancer, the preliminary results of the phase II controlled study led by Dean Shen Lin showed that the PCR rate of the target-immune-chemotherapy neoadjuvant treatment group reached 38%, while the control group was only 14%, almost three times higher. So I think these research results fully prove that gastric cancer treatment has fully entered the era of immunotherapy and has shown great potential and hope.

C-HIPEC is a technology with Chinese characteristics, with the concept of intraperitoneal hyperthermic perfusion chemotherapy. However, in-depth research on its mechanism is relatively scarce. Through our own basic research, we found that the combination of hyperthermia with chemotherapy and radiotherapy can significantly enhance the sensitivity of chemotherapy and radiotherapy. In order to meet the needs of this technology, domestic manufacturers have developed hyperthermic perfusion equipment. Among them, temperature control is a key parameter of hyperthermic perfusion technology. The temperature of hyperthermic perfusion is higher than the normal body temperature of 37 degrees Celsius. After research, we found that when the temperature is controlled at 43 degrees Celsius, it can effectively kill tumor cells without damaging normal tissues, because tumor cells have lower tolerance to heat than normal tissues, and if the temperature exceeds 43 degrees Celsius, it may cause damage to normal tissue cells. In this regard, our domestic intraperitoneal hyperthermic perfusion equipment has demonstrated excellent temperature control performance, and its temperature control accuracy has reached plus or minus 0.1 degrees Celsius, ensuring the safety and effectiveness of hyperthermic perfusion therapy. This technology is mainly used to treat primary tumors in hollow organs such as the abdomen, chest, pericardium or bladder, as well as secondary abdominal and pleural metastases, and plays an important role in prevention.

二、英译中

The primary barrier for consideration of solid-organ transplantation (SOT) in patients with pre-transplant malignancy (PTM) is the concern that immunosuppression amplifies the risk of cancer recurrence, potentially impacting post-transplant mortality. While it is clear that immunosuppression administered to SOT recipients is associated with an increased likelihood of de novo cancer, clinical evidence on the safety of immunosuppression in the circumstance of PTM is limited.

The most utilized guidelines for the selection of patients with PTM for SOT were extrapolated from recommendations made for potential renal transplant recipients. In most cases, a minimum of two years between cancer treatment and SOT was advised. Two-year waiting times were recommended even for cancers with extremely low or zero risk of recurrence, such as ductal carcinoma in situ of the breast. For cancers at increased risk of recurrence, even longer wait times of two to five or greater than five years were recommended, with little or no supporting data. Historical data on transplant recipients with PTM obtained from the Israel Penn International Transplant Tumor Registry reported a 21% overall risk of cancer recurrence following SOT, and higher rates in certain, high-risk malignancies. This information formed the basis for previous recommendations.

Contemporary, population-based studies have reported lower cancer recurrence rates than the original registry provided, although poorer outcomes persist in those with PTM. Recent studies also have indicated a higher incidence of all-cause mortality in SOT recipients with PTM than those without, but the cause of mortality is not entirely linked to recurrence of the cancer. However, despite these increased risks, overall patient survival may still be superior to what would be anticipated without transplantation and may approach acceptable transplant-specific outcomes. In addition, newer therapies may improve outcomes for recurrences.

◎ **参考译文**：对于移植前恶性肿瘤（PTM）患者来说，考虑进行实体器官移植（SOT）的主要障碍是担心免疫抑制会增加癌症复发的风险，从而可能影响移植后的死亡率。虽然很明显，对 SOT 接受者实施免疫抑制与新发癌症的可能性增加有关，但关于在 PTM 情况下免疫抑制安全性的临床证据有限。

用于选择 PTM 患者进行 SOT 的最常用指南是从针对潜在肾移植接受者的建议中推断出来的。在大多数情况下，建议癌症治疗和 SOT 之间至少间隔两年。即使对于复发风险极低或为零的癌症，例如乳腺导管原位癌，也建议等待两年。对于复发风险较高的癌症，建议等待时间更长，为两到五年或超过五年，但几乎没有或根本没有支持数据。以色列宾夕法尼亚国际移植肿瘤登记处获得的 PTM 移植接受者的历史数据显示，SOT 后癌症复发的总体风险为 21%，某些高风险恶性肿瘤的复发率更高。这些信息构成了先前建议的基础。

当代基于人群的研究报告显示，癌症复发率低于原始登记处提供的数据，尽管 PTM 患者的预后仍然较差。最近的研究还表明，患有 PTM 的 SOT 接受者的全因死亡率高于未患有 PTM 的接受者，但死亡原因并不完全与癌症复发有关。然而，尽管这些风险增加，但总体患者生存率仍可能优于未接受移植的预期生存率，并且可能接近可接受的移植特异性结果。此外，较新的疗法可能会改善复发的结果。

第十一单元　骨科与运动医学

第一节　骨科与运动医学口译知识点

骨科（orthopedics department）属于外科的一个分支，主要是诊治骨骼、肌肉系统疾病的科室，常见的骨科疾病包括骨折、软组织损伤、关节损伤、脱位、骨肿瘤等。随着现代医学的发展，学科的划分也越来越细致，三甲医院的骨科继续细分亚专科（subspecialty），可分为创伤外科/创伤骨科、关节外科、脊柱外科、手足外科（手外科/足踝外科）、运动医学科等。以下简单介绍医学会议口译中涉及的骨科知识。

骨科中的创伤（trauma）是骨科的基础。骨科创伤指由外力作用于骨骼和相关组织而导致的损伤，可能的创伤机制包括意外事故、运动损伤、跌倒、坠伤或其他暴力行为。常见的骨科创伤包括骨折、脱位及软组织损伤。

骨折（fracture）是最常见的创伤，指骨骼断裂，影像学定义为骨连续性的破坏。根据创伤情况，骨折可分为：开放性骨折（open fracture），指骨折端刺破皮肤，形成开放性伤口；闭合性骨折（closed fracture），指骨骼断裂，但未穿破皮肤；稳定性骨折，指骨折端仍然对齐，不易移动；不稳定性骨折，指骨折端无法保持对齐，容易移动。

骨折需要通过复位（reduction）以将断裂的骨折端重新对齐，以及通过固定（fixation），即使用石膏、金属螺钉或钢板等器械固定骨骼来治疗。创伤手术最多的就是切开复位内固定术（open reduction and internal fixation，ORIF），通过切口（incision），暴露（expose）骨折端（fracture end），在复位后，使用钢板螺钉（plate and screw）加以固定。骨折康复期间，患者需要进行物理治疗（physical therapy）和康复锻炼（rehabilitation exercise），以有助于骨骼功能的恢复。

医学会议中常见的骨折部位有四肢长骨骨折（long bone fracture），例如肱骨（humerus）骨折、尺骨（ulna）桡骨（radius）骨折、股骨（femur）骨折、胫骨（tibia）骨折、髋臼（acetabulum）骨折及骨盆（pelvis）骨折。而肋骨（rib）骨折不属于骨科诊疗范围，临床上属于胸外科（thoracic surgery）的诊疗范围，近年来也有此主题的会议。

脱位（dislocation）指人体关节遭受外力作用，使得构成关节的骨组织关节面脱离正常位置，从而导致功能障碍。常见的有肩关节脱位，其他关节也可脱位，脱位也可与骨折一同出现，也可单独发生。单独发生的脱位主要靠手法复位（manual reduction）治疗，即通过推、拿、按、压等手法使骨折部位恢复到原有解剖位置，如患者关节周围肌肉较为发达，单纯手法复位难以实现时，也可通过麻醉使周围肌肉松弛后进行手法复位。当今的医学会议口译中，没有专门以脱位为主题的会议，但脱位在骨科及运动医学会议中属于基础概念，无处不在。

关节外科会议中主要涉及的内容包括人工髋关节置换（hip replacement/arthroplasty）、人工膝关节置换（knee replacement/arthroplasty）、人工肩关节置换（shoulder replacement/arthroplasty）等。

髋关节置换术包括全髋置换与半髋置换，早期只置换人工股骨头，俗称"半髋置换术"。全髋置换术（total hip replacement/arthroplasty，THR/THA）是通过手术的方式，将病变的骨组织与病变组织去除，在准备好髋臼侧与股骨侧后，将人工假体（prosthesis），包含股骨部分（femoral component）和髋臼（acetabular component）部分，利用或不利用骨水泥（bone cement）和螺丝钉固定在准备好的骨质上，以取代病变的关节，重建患者髋关节的正常功能。全髋置换的手术适应证包括髋关节骨性关节炎（osteoarthritis，OA）、骨头坏死（femoral head necrosis，FHN）、股骨颈骨折（femoral neck fracture）、类风湿性关节炎（rheumatoid arthritis，RA）、创伤性关节炎（traumatic arthritis，TA）、良性和恶性骨肿瘤等。人工假体的材质随着科技发展有各类合金、陶瓷等。

膝关节置换术包括单髁置换术（unicompartmental knee arthroplasty，UKA）以及全膝关节置换术（total knee replacement/arthroplasty，TKR/TKA）。UKA与TKA的治疗理念有所不同，患者人群也有所不同，但不同环境下手术适应证有时会有所重叠。膝关节置换术在手术操作方法学上与髋关节置换术类似，也是通过手术的方法，将病变的骨组织与病变组织去除，在准备好股骨侧与胫骨侧后，将人工假体，包含股骨部分和胫骨部分（tibial tray）固定在准备好的骨质上，以取代病变的关节，至于髌骨（patella）表面是否放置髌骨假体，主要取决于假体系统、患者具体情况以及手术医生的选择。膝关节置换会涉及的一些基础词汇，包括膝关节内的前交叉韧带（anterior cruciate ligament，ACL）、后交叉韧带（posterior cruciate ligament，PCL）、内侧副韧带（medial collateral ligament，MCL）、外侧副韧带（lateral collateral ligament，LCL）、髌骨轨迹（patellar tracking）。还包括一些概念，比如保留后交叉韧带的CR（cruciate retaining，CR）假体与后稳定PS（posterior stabilized，PS）假体，CR假体可以保留后交叉韧带，从而保留本体感觉，而PS假体则切除后交叉韧带，从而导致关节本体感觉缺失；以及在截骨（osteotomy，bone cut）完成后所形成的屈/伸膝间隙（flexion/extension gap）、软组织平衡（soft tissue balance）等。

肩关节置换术包括全肩关节置换（total shoulder arthroplasty，TSA）与反向肩关节置换术（reverse shoulder arthroplasty，RSA）两种。其手术整体概念与髋关节置换类似，但解剖名称、具体手术步骤、注意事项等全然不同。未来几年，肩关节置换术或有较快发展。

脊柱外科会议中主要涉及的内容有各类颈椎手术（cervical surgery）、腰椎手术（lumbar surgery）以及侧弯矫形手术（scoliosis correction surgery）。

颈椎手术主要用于治疗各种颈椎病（cervical spondylosis），手术入路（surgical approach）主要包括前方入路（anterior approach）与后方入路（posterior approach）。手术主

要包括减压(decompression)和重建(reconstruction)稳定两个部分,前路手术可切除突出的(herniated)椎间盘、大部分椎体和肥厚骨化的后纵韧带(posterior longitudinal ligament, PLL),从而解除神经根(nerve root)的压迫。重建稳定包括融合与非融合技术,而后路手术包括进行椎管扩大、椎板成形术(laminoplasty)和椎板切除加固定融合术。通过扩大椎管的有效面积从而解除压迫。涉及的主要解剖结构和概念包括:颈椎(从第一颈椎到第七颈椎,C1~C7,简称为C)、椎间盘(intervertebral disc)、椎管(spinal canal)、椎间孔(intervertebral foramen)、脊髓(spinal cord)、前凸与后凸(lordosis/kyphosis)、椎板切除(laminectomy)、减压(decompression)、固定(fixation)、融合(fusion)、椎弓根螺钉(pedicle screw)等。

腰椎手术主要用于治疗各种腰椎病(lumbar spondylosis),手术入路主要包括前入路、后入路及侧方入路(lateral approach)。涉及的主要解剖结构和概念包括:腰椎,从第一腰椎到第五腰椎(L1~L5),简称为L;骶椎,成人骶椎融合成骶骨,称为Sacrum;终板(endplate);腰椎滑脱(lumbar spondylolisthesis)等。

而侧弯矫形手术主要用于治疗各类脊柱侧弯,手术主要为后方入路。涉及的内容更多,包括患者的心肺功能(cardio-pulmonary function)、下肢关节力线(lower limb alignment)、截骨(osteotomy)等。

脊柱外科会议中会涉及大量的解剖名称以及手术器械与器械名称,译员应做好会前准备。

近年来,随着生活水平的提升、大众健康意识的提升以及技术的发展,运动医学也有了长足的进步,运动医学会议口译主要涉及肩袖损伤的治疗、膝关节韧带的重建等。

肩袖损伤(rotator cuff injury)会引发肩周疼痛、肩关节功能障碍。肩袖由肩胛下肌(subscapularis)、冈上肌(supraspinatus)、冈下肌(infraspinatus)和小圆肌(teres minor)的肌腱(tendon)组成,其包裹了肩关节的前方、上方及后方,围绕着肩关节,形成了像"袖套"一样的结构。在这些软组织损伤时,即为肩袖损伤。而对于肩袖损伤的治疗,现在多以关节镜手术为主,在肩关节周围皮肤处做四个左右的小切口,将关节镜(arthroscope)进入关节内,从其他切口进入特殊手术器械与器材进行缝合修补。

第二节 真实世界口译情境

一、主题会议

骨科的各个亚专科中,关节(joint)、脊柱(spine)、创伤(trauma)所使用的内植物较多,近年来随着运动医学的发展,以及器械公司不断的产品研发,运动医学所使用的器械、生物制品也越来越多,因而这四个亚专科的医学口译会议也越来越多。

脊柱主题会议主要是颈椎(cervical spine)、腰椎(lumbar spine)与畸形矫正(deformity correction);关节主题会议主要是髋关节(hip joint)、膝关节(knee joint)损伤与置换,未来随着技术与器械的进步,相信与肩关节置换(shoulder replacement)相关的会议也会越来越多；创伤主题会议主要是四肢长骨骨折与复杂髋臼骨盆骨折的诊疗；运动医学主题会议主要是膝关节韧带重建与肩关节肩袖(rotator cuff)的治疗。

近年来，随着政策的调整以及带量采购(volume-based procurement, VBP)政策的出台，骨科会议的量和内容发生了显著的改变。

二、行业特点

随着科技的发展，影像学水平的进步与发展也是日新月异，这在骨科及运动医学领域尤为明显，无论术前、术中、术后，诊断治疗随访，各类影像学检查(X线、CT及MRI)无处不在。因此译员须对运动系统(骨骼、肌肉)的影像学有一定了解，这样才能在口译过程中应对自如，更好地跟上讲者的思路。

而会议中讨论得最多的，除了各类手术的技术细节外，还包括不同国家的医生所持的不同临床思路，以及各个国家大量的临床试验结果的解读与讨论。

三、口译难点

骨科与运动医学口译难点众多。

第一，骨科与运动医学有别于其他临床专科，有很多本专业独有的理念与操作，而这些理念与操作又是会议发言与讨论时逻辑背后的基础，不大会有讲者专门就这些基础理念与操作展开专门论述与讨论，例如骨科创伤领域的"张力带技术""关节内骨折的解剖复位"，关节领域的"软组织平衡"，脊柱领域的"责任节段"，运动医学中的"阶梯治疗"等。这些概念之于医生，就如同语法之于口译员，译员间互相交流口译工作经验时，不会专门讨论英语语法。而如果口译员对这些理念与操作没有基本的理解，就很难理解讲者的讲话逻辑，此时只能单纯依赖听力与同传技能，就会导致同传难度明显增加，这一点在会议讨论环节的同传中表现得尤为明显，而此时同传高级技能之一的"预测先说"则根本无从谈起。

第二，骨科与运动医学主题的医学会议口译中，存在大量的专业名词与专业术语，而且很多专业术语并非讨论的重点，而是作为沟通过程中的基础表达，讨论的重点在于新技术、新器械的使用方法与选择，以及不同治疗方式间优劣势的平衡与取舍。这就要求译员在没有太多反应时间的情况下，对大量的相关专业术语要做到随口译出，很多时候没有太多反应的时间。这样的要求，对于不熟悉本领域的译员来说，需要极长的会前准备时间，而且最好还能做到像考前押题一样进行高效精准的会前准备，否则就是事倍功半。举一个创伤主题会议的简单例子："患者高坠伤伴重物砸伤，多处骨折合并骨盆'开书样'损伤，X线检查提示：右侧肩锁关节脱位，右侧肱骨螺旋形骨折，右侧尺骨鹰嘴骨折，右侧髋臼及左侧髂骨翼骨折，耻骨联合间隙增宽。"短短七八十个字，提到了"肩锁关节""肱骨螺旋形""尺骨鹰嘴""髋臼""髂骨翼""耻骨联合"等六个相对不常见专业术语，而对于"高坠伤""骨折""骨盆""开书样"等表达，不同译员的词汇积累不同，或许也需要提前准备。掌握并译出这些名词只是一个难点，而真正的难点是在基本情况介绍之后，就要开始讨论治疗方案与具体方法，其中可能涉及多种骨科内固定、术式与治疗理念，而且要兼顾患者的基础疾病与术者所在医院的医疗条件，包括医疗设备、器械准备情况等。而更难的一点在于，有时候因为各种原因，译员很可能会前无法提前拿到讲者的材料。

第三，此主题会议口译量的减少以及会议主题难度的增加。前些年，在骨科与运动医学领域，还有不少会议内容相对基础，以上文提到的全膝关节置换主题为例，前些年的会议主题相对简单，包括全膝手术适应证选择、手术患者选择、围手术期管理、初次手术的手术操作技术、围绕某一款假体的具体培训、学习与讨论等。而经过近20年的发展，国内医生在以上各个主题方面已经有了长足的进步，并积累了大量病例经验与数据，而在近年VBP实施之后，相关的医学会议口译数量与主题发生了明显的改变。仍以全膝关节置换主题举例，现在不仅会议口译数量有所减少，且主题也变得更加细致，从医学角度讲，诊疗难度明显提升；从口译角度讲，译员理解的难度有所上升，译员必须有较好的基础，方能有更好的理解。例如全膝置换翻修手术（TKA revision）、全膝置换后感染的管理、复杂骨缺损的全膝置换、机器人辅助全膝置换手术、人工智能在全膝置换中的应用等。较为理想的医学口译员成长模式，仍以全膝关节置换主题为例，应该是从基础主题会议口译开始，先接触假体与工具培训口译，再经历适应证及手术患者选择，积累一定的手术操作与问答讨论的口译经验后，再逐步细化到难度较大的话题，例如翻修手术、感染管理，到现在的机器人手术，最后参与手术直播的同传。而口译形式也最好是从交传开始，因为交传要求译语更加准确清晰，译员对内容理解必须全面，对译员的心理素质也是极好的锻炼，经过一定量的交传后，译员会对此主题有一定的理解与积累，再开始同传，才能逐渐成熟，并保证一定水平的翻译质量，就如同外科医生讲的学习曲线（learning curve）一样。但近年来随着各类医学口译会议数量的相对减少，会议内容难度的提升，主办方对口译工作的不理解以及对会议效率的要求，口译活动中交传比例相对较小，新手译员很难再经历上述的完整过程，所接触到的也多为会议同传。这就需要会前高效且充分地准备，以及会议中搭档的密切配合。

第四，这一点在运动医学表现得相对明显，就是与之前一些章节主题中的难点类似，在运动医学领域中，也有不少术式、内植物乃至手术器械，都是直接使用英文，译员需要提前熟悉或有一定经验，才能在同传时及时判断哪些需要翻译，哪些内容跟读即可。另外运动医学有一个难点，就是很多运动医学主题的口译活动都与关节镜相关，常见有膝关节镜、肩关节镜以及髋关节镜，关节镜下的术野与常规开放手术和内镜手术的视野又不相同，译员最好能有一定的了解，否则较难跟上讲者的逻辑，只能依靠听力与同传技能进行翻译，而且关节镜下手术涉及多根缝线的反复操作，此时EVS应尽量短，太长会导致画面与同传声音脱节。

第三节 中英对照篇章及分析

一、英译中

I've been given the task of talking about management of chronic PJI and I would like to perhaps start by going through some basics and then we will discuss some of the treatment options. Obviously, chronic PJI or PJI overall is a very challenging condition. We have been dealing with this problem for a long time, and our solutions are still not so great leading to morbidity and mortality amongst for our patients. Definition of PJI is something we first need to all be on the same page, definition of chronic PJI has been described by the international consensus meeting. And then there was a 2018 diagnosis, which assigns specific scores to each one of the tests being used for diagnosis. And then these scores are added together. If the score is greater than six patients definitely infected, if score is three or less, patient is definitely not infected. Score of four and five is indeterminate, and patient would require further additional tests. The threshold for all the parameters that we use for diagnosis has been described, CRP 10, D-dimer, the ESR of 30, cell count 3,000 and others. We do have some of those parameters that we rely on for diagnosis of chronic PJI. Patient having a sinus tract, that has drainage and obviously is also infected. （本段内容选自2023年一位美国医生的学术演讲，有删改调整。）

◎ **参考译文**：给我的任务是讲慢性PJI的管理。我想也许先从一些比较基础的内容开始，然后我们会做一些治疗的选择。显然，慢性PJI或者是PJI是很有挑战性的一种情况。我们一直都在解决这个问题，而我们的解决方案仍然不是很好，导致发病率和死亡率在我们的患者中仍然存在。关于PJI的定义我们首先需要达成一致。慢性PJI的定义在国际共识会议上已经有所描述，然后还有2018年的诊断，上面有明确的用于诊断各项检查的分数，这些分数是相加在一起的。如果分数大于6，那患者肯定是感染了；如果分数小于等于3，患者肯定就没感染。4分、5分不确定，患者需要进一步的额外检查。所有指标的阈值，我们用于诊断的都有描述，包括CRP10、D-dimer、ERS30、细胞计数3000，还有其他的指标。我们还有一些诊断所需的指标，用于诊断慢性PJI。患者有窦道，有引流的患者，显然也是有感染。

◎ **分析**：

1. 大多数会议主办方会前至少会给出会议日程，因而"management of chronic PJI"可以预先获知；

2. "basics"译作"基础的内容"，补充了"内容"两字，听起来更符合中文表达习惯；

3. "condition"译作"情况"，其实condition在医学翻译中的不同语境下，可以表达"诊断""病情""疾病"等，译员在无法判定的情况下，译作"情况"是不错的选择；

4. "deal with"译作"解决"，其实译作"处理"更佳，此处更加强调过程而非结果，当然在同传的情况下，译作"解决"也可行；

5. "leading to morbidity and mortality amongst for our patients"译作"导致发病率和死亡率在我们的患者中仍然存在"，这是顺句驱动技巧处理后的结果；

6. "if score is three or less"译作"如果分数小于等于3"，"小于等于"或"大于等于"等表达在医学口译中经常见到，有多种表达方法，此处的方式很简单。

First of all, how do we start treating a patient? First, we need to make sure that the patient is medically optimized. Diabetes, anemia, malnutrition, smoking, all others have been taken care of. Diabetes control is very important. Hemoglobin A1c needs to be less than eight, the fasting glucose needs to be less than 200. And then in recent years, we and others have published papers related to the use of fructosamine, which is a faster serological test for diabetes, basically glycated protein in the serum. And that has a shorter half-life of 2 weeks, as opposed to hemoglobin A1c that usually takes about 3 months. We do know that glucose variability and hyperglycemia overall influences the outcome of any surgical procedures, particularly two stage exchange arthroplasty. As you will see here, from previous publications. Anemia is another terrible condition that needs to be recognized and optimized prior to surgery if possible. In this observational study, we found that presence of anemia led to a higher cardiovascular complication, infection, and mortality. Malnutrition is another one of those conditions that is under recognized and can be present, either in the obese or even a very thin patients. And it's very important for us to make sure that the patients albumin and hemoglobin is optimized prior to operation. If you look over here in this particular study, low albumin was shown to be one of the strongest predictors of failure of two stage exchange arthroplasty and revision for aseptic reasons.

◎ **参考译文**：首先，我们怎么开始治疗一位患者？首先我们要确保患者的健康情况是好的。糖尿病、贫血、营养不良、吸烟，还有其他的因素都要先处理。糖尿病控制非常重要，糖化血红蛋白要小于8，空腹血糖要小于200。而近几年，我们发表了一些文章，关于果糖胺的使用，它是一种更快的血清学检测，用于检测糖尿病，基本上就是血清当中的糖化蛋白。它的半衰期比较短，是两周，不同于HbA1c，它通常是三个月。我们都知道血糖变异和高血糖，会影响任何手术操作的结果。尤其是对于二期关节置换来说。这之前的文章都有体现。贫血是另一个可怕的情况，要在术前识别并控制改善。在这个观察性研究当中，我们发现贫血导致了更高的心血管并发症，感染率、死亡率也会更高。营养不良是另外一种情况，不太容易识别但会存在，不管是在肥胖甚至是比较瘦的患者中都会发生。所以对我们来说很重要的一点是，要确保患者的白蛋白和血红蛋白在术前能控制得很好。看这里的一项具体研究，较低的白蛋白，显示能够很强地预测到失败，二期关节置换术的失败，以及无菌原因翻修手术的失败。

◎ **分析**：

1. "how do we start"译作"我们怎么开始"，其实此处译作"我们如何开始"更好一些，在学术会议中译员还是应当对口语化的表达作适当调整；

2. "medically optimized"译作"健康情况是好的"，此处可以处理为"内科情况进行过处理"，这里指的是在外科手术之前，对患者的基础/内科疾病(高血压/糖尿病/肾脏病/贫血状态)进行治疗，以期获得最佳的外科手术治疗效果；

3. "less than eight"译作"小于8"，没有问题，但更符合中国医生表达的方式是"控制在8以下"。但对于此类表达，译员须非常熟悉此类主题会议中中国医生发言习惯才能做到；

4. "published papers"译作"发表了一些文章"，"文章"比较符合专业表达，当然也可译作"论文"；

5. "optimized"译作"控制改善"，此处指的是术前升高患者的血红蛋白水平以利于术后恢复，译作"优化"比较生硬，更符合专业表达的处理方式为"加以纠正"；

6. "very thin"译作"比较瘦的"，此处是非常典型的口译错误，属于译员不经意间随口对语义的弱化。当然每个人以及中外学者对于"比较瘦"和"非常瘦"定义不同，此处如此翻译也不会造成听众理解的重大偏差，但如此处理并未如实传递信息。

But one stage exchange is a good operation for patients with good soft tissue coverage, and infection by an organism that has sensitivity to most of the antibiotics. It is not a good operation for patients who have severe soft tissue deficiency or damage, severe bone loss, if they are systemically sick and perhaps not very good for patients with culture negative periprosthetic joint infection. What about the results? Honestly, the results of one stage versus two stage is pretty similar and comparable. I realized that one stage is usually done for patients that are healthier and better hosts. But overall, it looks like the result of one stage and two stage, at least based on retrospective series, is pretty similar. In this study by my good friend, Craig Della-Valle and Bryan Springer, they did call for the need for randomized, controlled comparative trials to determine if a one stage exchange is an option. And if so, for who? Their call was answered by the British and the Swedish investigators who completed the INFORM trial that was published in British Medical Journal recently. All patients with chronic periprosthetic joint infection were randomized to one versus two stage exchange. And the outcome of these patients were evaluated. The primary outcome was WOMAC. And secondary outcome was recurrence of infection, complications, and cost effectiveness. What did they find? I'm sure you've seen the INFORM trial, no difference in the outcome between single stage versus two stage exchange arthroplasty.

◎ **参考译文**：一期置换手术适合患者的软组织包裹好，以及对于大多数抗生素敏感的微生物感染。但不适合的患者包括，有严重的软组织缺失或损伤，严重的骨量丧失，全身性疾病，以及PJI培养阴性。那结果呢？诚实地说，一期二期的结果非常相似且具有可比性。我知道一期通常是身体更健康的患者。但总体而言，看起来一期和二期的结果，至少基于回顾性的队列，是非常类似的。在这个研究当中，我的朋友 Craig 和 Bryan，他们呼吁需要随机对照比较实验，以决定一期手术是不是一个选择，应该为谁而做。英国和瑞典的研究者回应了这项呼吁，他们完成了 INFORM 试验，最近在《英国医学杂志》上发表了。所有慢性假体周围关节感染的患者，被随机分组到一期和二期翻修手术，最后评估这些患者的结局。主要结局是 WOMAC，次要结局是感染复发、并发症以及成本效益。他们发现了什么呢？我相信大家都看过 INFORM 试验了，没有区别，就一期和二期关节翻修手术的结局，是没有区别的。

◎ 分析：

1."coverage"译作"包裹"，此处译作"覆盖"更为妥当；

2."It is not a good operation for patients who"译作"不适合的患者包括"，此处的处理非常灵活，避免了长定语的使用；

3."systemically sick"译作"全身性疾病"而非"系统性生病"，更符合此主题的专业表达；

4."periprosthetic joint infection"同传时直接处理成"PJI"而非"假体周围关节感染"，可能是因为译员来不及或一时语塞，但没有关系，PJI 是本次会议主题，并不影响听众理解。但如果讲者未使用缩略语，不建议译员图方便使用缩略语；

5."versus"此处未译出，没有问题，语言表达通顺，不影响听众理解，切勿直接译作"vs."；

6."better hosts"此处未译出，意思是"更好的宿主骨"，但对于"宿主骨"三字，译员如果没有此领域的翻译经验，一般无法译出。此处"better hosts"未译出，也可接受，并不影响听众对语义的理解；

7."trials"此处译作"实验"，应该译作"试验"，临床医学会议中，"试验"一词的使用居多，译员口译时应注意发音；

8."And if so"此处未译出，最好能够补出来"如果是的话"，这样逻辑更加通顺，但此处未译出并不影响理解；

9."British Medical Journal"是"英国医学杂志"，这是著名的四大综合性医学期刊之一，此处翻译正确，但在同传压力较大，或者语速跟不上的情况下，也可灵活处理为"BMJ"，国内大多数医生能够理解；

10." no difference in the outcome between single stage versus two stage exchange arthroplasty."译作"没有区别，就一期和二期关节翻修手术的结局，是没有区别的。"此处的同传处理，进行了适当重复，避免了译员将 EVS 拉得过长或者使用预测先说的策略，前者会加重译员的短时记忆负担，后者有一定风险。同传的时候，译员可以进行适当重复。另外，此处的"区别"最好译为"差异"，使表达更正式。

But how do you do one stage or two stage? First, we have to make sure we place the incision in the right place. Second, we have to perform extensive debridement. Debridement starts from superficial tissues, opening up the joint and removing a whole synovial membrane, almost like doing a tumor prosthesis. We can't just get … and remove some of those so-called infected tissues. We must remove large amounts of the synovial fluid. Then we also have to explant, which includes taking very good care to remove the implants without bone loss. We need to make sure that we work around the implants with use of appropriate instruments, including saw, osteotome, etc. To be able to remove those implants without much bone loss, then we need to do further debridement and reaming of the intramedullary canal. We also need to do chemical debridement, which in my hands include four solutions, 4% CHG scrubs, those things that we use our hands to wash. I use Dakin solution, which is 0.125% hypochlorite, half a percent hydrogen peroxide. And then I finish up by using half a percent, a povidone-iodine irrigation solution. I change to a new setup, and then I start the reimplantation. This procedure basically takes time. One needs to be meticulous, one needs to make sure that the dirty instruments are removed.

◎ **参考译文**：那怎么做一期或者是二期的手术呢？首先我们要确保切口的位置是准确的。第二，我们要做大范围的清创，清创要从浅表组织开始，打开关节，然后去除整个滑膜，几乎就像做一个肿瘤型的假体。我们不能只清除部分所谓的感染组织。我们必须要去除大量的滑液。然后我们还要取假体，一定要很小心地取出植入物，不要造成骨损失。也要确保我们在植入物周围使用合适的器械，包括骨锯、骨刀等，这样就能够把这些植入物移出而不损伤骨头。然后我们需要做进一步的清创，以及扩髓。我们也要做一些化学清创，有四个选择，4%的 CHG scrub，我们用手来洗。我也用 Dakin 溶液，就是 0.125%的次氯酸盐，0.5%的双氧水。然后我用 0.5%的聚维碘酮灌洗液来收尾。我换了一套新的配置，然后开始再植入。这个过程需要一些时间，首先需要很小心仔细，第二要确保受污染的器械都撤出来了。

◎ **分析**：

1. "right"译作"准确"，此处最好译作"正确"。医学口译中，"正确""准确""精准"三个词意义不同，最好不要轻易互换；

2. "to perform extensive debridement"译作"要做大范围的清创"，此处最好译作"要进行广泛清创"，后者在此语境下更为准确，语言表达的学术性也更强；

3. "remove"译作"移出"，此处最好译作"取出"；

4. "without much bone loss"译作"不损伤骨头"，可调整为"而没有很多骨损失"；

5. "need to do chemical debridement"译作"我们也要做一些化学清创"，此处的"一些"可能是译员的填补，对于语义和语气都没有帮助，最好去掉；

6. "solution"译作"选择"，但此处讲者其实指代的是"溶液"。译员翻译至此，如果无法确定，可暂时处理为"方法"；或暂时拉长 EVS，稍等后续内容即可确认。想直接快速译出"溶液"，译员需要有一定经验；

7. "in my hands"未译出，可处理为"在我这里"；

8. "setup"译作"配置"，但此处具体指的是"手术台铺巾、手术衣及手术器械"。如此翻译实际是过度翻译，而且这里可以将 setup 省略，处理为"然后我换一套新的"，这是感染翻修手术的常规操作，听众都能理解，而"配置"一词可能会让听众误解；

9. "procedure"译作"过程"，应译作"操作"；

10. "dirty"此处译作"受污染的"，可以直接译作"脏/脏的"，这样的表述也符合此主题的语言表达习惯。

What about the length of antimicrobial treatment? It's been shown that at least a minimum of six weeks of antibiotic treatment is needed, whether that needs to be antimicrobial treatment intravenously, orally, probably doesn't matter. In one of the studies related to acute infections, the use of 12 weeks of antimicrobial was shown to be superior to 6 weeks. Two stage exchanges also similar principles, incision, initial debridement. I usually use a dynamic spacers that I make myself. And that includes knowing which antibiotics to add, how much of those to mix together, and then fashioning the dynamic spacer to try to place it in the joint before leaving. Now, the type of spacers we use appears to influence the outcome to some extent. I personally prefer to use the dynamic or the articulating spacers, because that is so much better. But occasionally, we have used static spacers in patients who have massive bone loss, when they don't have the collateral ligaments, etc. If I want to rest the soft tissues, I also use a static spacers. The type of antibiotics we add to cement is critical, as we've seen from the works of Dr Buchholz, showing that antibiotic does elude from the cement, not all of it, but some does. Some antibiotics are heat stable, some are not. It's very important to add antibiotics that are available in powder form. They have wide antibacterial spectrum. They elude from PMMA. They are active for a long period of time. They have thermal stability, low serum protein binding, and do not influence the mechanical strength.

◎ **参考译文**：那抗菌治疗的时长呢？在这里可以看出来，至少需要六周的抗菌治疗，不管是静脉注射或者是口服都没关系。在一个关于严重感染的研究中，使用十二周的抗生素，显示优于六周。二期翻修手术的原则、切口、初次清创都是类似的。我通常都会用一个动态垫片，是我自己做的。这包括知道要加什么抗生素，多少混在一起，然后塑形，把它放到关节里面，最后再关上。现在我们用的垫片种类，似乎在某种程度上会影响结局。我个人比较喜欢用活动型或成关节的垫片，因为效果会更好。但是偶尔我们也会用静态的，如果患者有大量的骨损失，或者是没有侧副韧带的话。如果我想保留软组织，我也会用静态的。我们在骨水泥里加入的抗生素也很重要，Dr Buchholz 的研究表明，有些抗生素会从骨水泥里释放出来，不是全部的，但会有一些。有些抗生素具备热稳定性，有些不具备。所以很重要的是加入抗生素，能呈粉末状的，有较宽的抗菌谱，能从 PMMA 中释放，能保持较长的活跃时间，具有热稳定性，血清蛋白结合低，又不会影响机械强度。

◎ 分析：

1. "What about the length of antimicrobial treatment?"译作"那抗菌治疗的时长呢？"可处理为"抗生素要用多久？"更符合此主题的语言表达习惯；

2. "intravenously"译作"静脉注射"，其实译作"静脉给药"更为合适；

3. "dynamic spacer"译作"动态垫片"，此处应译作"活动占位器"。此处需要译员对此领域有一定经验；

4. "antibiotic does elude from the cement"译作"有些抗生素会从骨水泥里释放出来"，此处"有些"二字可能会使听众产生困惑，应该去掉；

5. "that are available in powder form"译作"能呈粉末状的"，此处处理为"有粉剂形式的抗生素"更合适些，前者虽然不影响听众理解，但其语言的专业性稍逊一等；

6. "active"译作"活跃"，此处译作"活性"更合适一些。

Since the introduction of the reverse shoulder arthroplasty, RSA, indications for its use have continued to expand. The early results of RSA in elderly, low-demand patients with cuff tear arthropathy demonstrated reliable improvements in pain, range of motion, and overall functional status. Studies have since shown that RSA can also be used to successfully manage proximal humerus fractures, fracture sequelae, arthroplasty in the setting of glenoid bone deficiency, particularly biconcave glenoids, and even revision arthroplasty. The potential role of the RSA to manage painful osteoarthritis of the shoulder in the elderly patient with an intact rotator cuff but limited preoperative motion is not yet clear. Professor LK reported on the experience from the National Arthroplasty Register, which included RSAs treating cuff tear arthropathy as well as glenohumeral osteoarthritis but did not analyze outcomes by indication. Other small studies have reported predictably good outcomes and implant survivorship after RSA to manage glenoid deficiencies in the setting of an intact rotator cuff. RSA is less dependent on a functional rotator cuff and generally produces reliable clinical results; however, RSA has been described in some studies as having a higher rate of complications and less functional improvements when compared with TSA, and long-term clinical survivorship is still largely unknown.（本段内容选自2023年一篇学术论文，有删改调整。）

◎ 参考译文：自反肩关节置换术，RSA，推出以来，其适应证便持续扩大。RSA用于老年、要求低且有肩袖撕裂关节病患者的早期结果显示，RSA可有效改善疼痛、活动度以及整体功能状态。此后的研究显示，RSA还可用于成功管理肱骨近端骨折、骨折后遗症、关节盂骨缺损情况下的关节成形术，尤其是双凹关节盂，甚至是关节置换翻修。RSA在管理肩关节疼痛性骨关节炎的作用，对于老年患者，肩袖完整但术前活动受限的老年患者，其作用尚不清楚。LK教授报告了国家关节置换登记的经验，其中包括了RSA，用于治疗肩袖撕裂关节病以及盂肱骨关节炎，但未按适应证分析结局。其他小型研究报告了可预测的良好结局以及假体生存率，都是在RSA用于管理肩胛盂缺损后，在肩袖完整的情况下获得的。RSA 对功能性肩袖依赖性较小，通常可带来可靠的临床结果；然而，RSA 在一些研究中被描述为并发症率较高，功能改善较少，在将其与 TSA 相比时有以上情况，长期临床生存情况在很大程度上仍然未知。

◎ 分析：

1. "range of motion"译作"活动度"，指关节活动度，是骨科运动医学科的基础概念，缩略词为 ROM；

2. "arthropathy"是"关节病"，与"关节炎"（arthritis）不同，口译时译员应予注意；

3. "arthroplasty"译作"关节成形术"，也可以直接译作"关节置换"，国内医生对后者的接受程度更高，即"joint replacement"；

4. "osteoarthritis"译作"骨关节炎"，在口语与书面语中，也经常缩略为"OA"，是骨科关节的基础概念之一；

5. 最后两句在同传的情况下，如果不提供讲稿，需要译员有较好的顺句驱动能力，才能顺利应对；

6. "TSA"为"total shoulder arthroplasty"，即"全肩关节置换术"，而"RSA"为"reverse shoulder arthroplasty"，即"反式肩关节置换术"，简称"反肩"。

Anatomic TSA remains the "benchmark" for reliable and predictable outcomes in the surgical management of glenohumeral osteoarthritis in the setting of an intact rotator cuff. However, indications for RSA are rapidly expanding and could have a role in the surgical management of primary glenohumeral osteoarthritis in select patients. Our study demonstrates that patients over age 70 with a structurally intact rotator cuff but limited preoperative motion can achieve predictable clinical improvement in pain, function, and range of motion after either anatomic TSA or RSA for glenohumeral arthritis. Both complication and revision surgery rates were similar between our RSA and TSA groups; however, the nature of the complications were different. In the anatomic TSA group, most reoperations were related to cuff dysfunction. Revision surgery was performed at a mean of two and a half years after the index operation. Previous studies have demonstrated that secondary rotator cuff dysfunction does occur after anatomic TSA, with one study demonstrating a rate of 16.8% at an average 103.6 months postoperatively. Rotator cuff dysfunction increased with increasing time from surgery and was predictive of worse clinical and radiographic outcome measures.

◎ 参考译文：解剖性 TSA 仍然是手术治疗盂肱骨关节炎时可靠且可预测结果的"基准"，这是对于肩袖完整的情况。然而，RSA 的适应证正在快速扩大，并可能在特定患者的原发性盂肱骨关节炎手术管理中发挥作用。我们的研究表明，70 岁以上的患者，肩袖结构完整但术前活动度受限，能实现疼痛、功能以及活动度可预测的临床改善，这是在解剖性 TSA 或 RSA 治疗盂肱关节炎之后的情况。并发症和翻修手术率是相似的，我们的 RSA 组和 TSA 组间是相似的；但是，并发症的性质不同。在解剖性 TSA 组中，大多数再次手术是与肩袖功能障碍有关。翻修手术是在首次手术后平均两年半的时候进行的。先前的研究表明，继发性肩袖功能障碍确实会在解剖性 TSA 后发生，一项研究表明，平均术后 103.6 个月的比率为 16.8%。肩袖功能障碍随着手术时间的延长而增加，并能预测更差的临床和影像学结局指标。

◎ 分析：

1. "preoperative" 译为 "术前"，口语中常译作 "pre-op"，"术中" 常译作 "intra-op"，"术后" 常译作 "post-op"。近年来 "围手术期" 的概念讲得越来越多，但一般是 "perioperative"，少见用 "peri-op"；

2. "radiographic" 译作 "影像学"，更符合此处语境及表达习惯，不一定非要将其译作 "放射学"；

3. "rotator cuff" 译作 "肩袖"，肩袖是由肩胛下肌（subscapularis）、冈上肌（supraspinatus）、冈下肌（infraspinatus）和小圆肌（teres minor）的腱性部分组成的鞘状结构，是近年来骨科肩关节置换以及运动医学肩袖损伤会议中的基础概念。

Another study found rotator cuff failure to be the most common complication after TSA, with failure occurring in 6% of shoulders, at an average follow-up of just 3 years. In an elderly cohort, baseline muscle health is compromised and the progression of rotator cuff degeneration may be accelerated or more common in these patients after TSA, compromising outcomes or leading to need for revision. The risk of cuff dysfunction in this cohort of patients after TSA at midterm follow-up is a concern and must be considered, especially given the similar outcomes and patient satisfaction rates seen with RSA and TSA. We did have one revision in the RSA group, which was an infection case. Although the complication and revision surgery risks in the RSA group were low, the number of subjects in this group was small and the findings of our study must be interpreted with caution. Although there are concerns about high rates of complications with RSA, studies have demonstrated excellent survivorship of RSA in elderly populations, as high as 91% at 10 years. In fact, in a recent database study from one large single-payer health organization, age over 75 years was associated with a significant decrease in risk of revision after RSA compared with those under 75. Other studies of RSA in glenohumeral arthritis in the setting of an intact rotator cuff have primarily focused on shoulders with significant glenoid bone loss where glenoid fixation was suboptimal. Some scholars came up with a conclusion that RSA was a reliable procedure to manage glenohumeral osteoarthritis in the setting of glenoid bone loss. Our study demonstrates that elderly individuals with primary glenohumeral osteoarthritis and limited forward elevation but an intact rotator cuff can also achieve reliable outcomes with RSA.

◎ 参考译文：另一项研究发现，肩袖失败是 TSA 后最常见的并发症，6% 的肩部发生失败，平均随访仅是 3 年。在一个老年队列中，基线肌肉健康受损，而肩袖退变的进展可能会加速或更为常见，是在这些患者接受 TSA 后出现，影响结局或导致需要翻修。肩袖功能障碍的风险，在这个患者队列中，在 TSA 后中期随访时，值得关注且必须予以考虑，尤其是考虑到结局和患者满意率都相似，RSA 和 TSA 手术后两者均相似。我们在 RSA 组中是有一例翻修，是一例感染病例。尽管 RSA 组的并发症和翻修手术风险较低，但该组的受试者数量较少，因此我们研究结果的解读必须谨慎。尽管有担心 RSA 的并发症率较高，但研究表明，老年人群中 RSA 的生存率很高，10 年时高达 91%。事实上，在最近一家大型单一支付方医疗机构的数据库研究中，75 岁以上人群 RSA 术后翻修风险显著降低，相较于 75 岁以下。其他对于肩袖完整情况下的盂肱关节炎 RSA 的研究主要集中在肩盂骨严重缺失，且肩盂固定不理想。一些学者得出一条结论，RSA 是一种可靠的手术，可用于管理盂肱骨关节炎，对于肩盂骨缺失的情况。我们的研究表明，患有原发性盂肱骨关节炎、前向抬高受限但肩袖完整的老年患者，也可通过 RSA 获得可靠的结局。

◎ 分析：

1. "The risk of cuff dysfunction in this cohort of patients after TSA at midterm follow-up is a concern and must be considered, especially given the similar outcomes and patient satisfaction rates seen with RSA and TSA."这一句很长，译员可用顺句驱动法将其处理成多个短句；

2. "We did have one revision in the RSA group"此句处理成了"我们在 RSA 组中是有一例翻修"，其中的"did"不一定要译作"确实"，同传时译员通过语音和停顿加以强调即可。而"revision"译作"翻修"，在关节置换领域，指代初次关节置换手术后因各种原因进行同一关节的二次手术，更换部分或全部假体。

Elderly patients are at high risk of complications when undergoing shoulder arthroplasty. In one large database study of hemiarthroplasty, RSA, and TSA, patients over 80 years of age had higher hospital mortality, longer length of stay, and more postoperative anemia than those under age 80. Another study demonstrated increased 1-year mortality as well as a higher 90-day readmission rate for those over 75 years undergoing TSA, but not for those over 75 years undergoing RSA. A third study found an increasing risk of hospital readmission, mostly for medical causes, with increasing age after both RSA and TSA. Elderly individuals are at higher risk when undergoing any type of surgery and shoulder arthroplasty too bears increased risk in this cohort. Our results demonstrate a similar rate, but different types of complication between RSA and TSA. In this cohort of elderly patients with limited preoperative motion, the risk of TSA failure due to rotator cuff tear is notable and may be considered a factor when considering recommendations to patients such as those in this cohort. Although RSA is less dependent upon rotator cuff function, previously published rates of complications including instability and stress fracture after RSA should be considered when determining the procedure most likely to provide reliable results.

◎ 参考译文：老年患者进行肩关节置换术时并发症风险很高。在一项关于半关节置换术、RSA 以及 TSA 的大型数据库研究中，80 岁以上患者的住院死亡率更高、住院时间更长、术后贫血更多，相较于80岁以下患者。另一项研究表明，1年死亡率和90天再入院率较高，对于接受TSA的75岁以上患者的而言，但对于75岁以上接受RSA的患者则并非如此。还有第三项研究发现，再入院风险会增加，主要是内科原因，在RSA和TSA术后，随着年龄的增加而再入院增多。老年人在接受任何类型的手术时都面临更高的风险，而肩关节置换术在此队列中的风险也一样高。我们的结果表明，RSA和TSA之间的并发症率相似，但类型不同。在这个老年患者队列中，他们术前活动受限，由于肩袖撕裂导致TSA失败的风险显著，在考虑向此类患者提供建议时，可以将其作为一个因素。尽管RSA对肩袖功能的依赖性较小，之前公布的并发症率，包括不稳定以及和应力性骨折，都是RSA术后的并发症，是要考虑的，在确定哪种术式最有可能提供可靠结果的时候，要考虑以上因素。

◎ 分析：

1. "length of stay"译作"住院时长"，缩写为"LOS"，是医学会议中的一个基础概念；

2. "A third study found an increasing risk of hospital readmission, mostly for medical causes, with increasing age after both RSA and TSA."按照顺句驱动法，译员可将其处理为"还有第三项研究发现，再入院风险会增加，主要是内科原因，在RSA和TSA术后，随着年龄的增加而再入院增多。"其中的"medical cause"很容易被错译为"医疗原因"，这里指的是内科原因，例如心脏、肾脏、呼吸系统的问题等。

二、中译英

在微创脊柱外科技术发展的过程中，从早期的显微镜技术到后来的众多包括胸腔镜、腹腔镜、显微内镜和经皮内镜等一系列内镜技术以外，脊柱的经皮内固定技术可以说是微创脊柱外科技术另一项里程碑式的技术。其被认为是里程碑式的技术，是因为在经皮椎弓根螺钉固定技术出现之前，微创脊柱外科技术仅局限于单纯的减压手术。因为经微创小切口完成脊柱的修复和重建具有极大的难度，因此，最初的所谓微创技术仅能完成单纯减压部分。由于其操作太过单一，适应证局限，在微创脊柱外科技术发展的早期并不被脊柱外科医师所看好。而随着经皮椎弓根螺钉技术的出现，微创脊柱外科技术可完成包括病灶切除、脊柱内固定甚至畸形的矫正，从而真正地开启了微创条件下脊柱外科修复与重建的新时代。微创经皮固定技术早期由国外引入，最开始被认为是非常具有挑战的技术，但之后国内开发的各种技术也逐渐发展起来。因此，现在的经皮椎弓根螺钉固定技术已经成为一个非常普遍的、能被大多数临床医师所掌握的常规技术。（本段内容选自2022年对一位医生的采访，有删改调整。）

◎ **参考译文**：In the process of the development of minimally invasive spine surgery, from the early microscope technology to the subsequent series of endoscopic technologies including thoracoscopy, laparoscopy, microendoscopy and percutaneous endoscopy, the percutaneous internal fixation technology of the spine is another milestone technology of minimally invasive spine surgery. It is considered a milestone technology because before the percutaneous pedicle screw fixation technique, minimally invasive spine surgery was limited to simple decompression surgery. Because it is extremely difficult to complete the repair and reconstruction of the spine through minimally invasive small incisions, the initial so-called minimally invasive technique can only complete the simple decompression part. Because its operation was too simple and its indications were limited, it was not favored by spine surgeons in the early development of minimally invasive spine surgery. With the emergence of percutaneous pedicle screw technique, minimally invasive spine surgery can complete lesion resection, spine internal fixation and even deformity correction, thus truly opening a new era of spine surgical repair and reconstruction with minimally invasive technique. Minimally invasive percutaneous fixation technique was introduced from abroad in the early days and was initially considered a very challenging technique, but then various technologies were gradually developing in China. Therefore, the current percutaneous pedicle screw fixation technique has become a very common routine technique that can be mastered by most clinicians.

◎ 分析：

1. "微创"译作"minimally invasive"，"微创手术"译作"minimally invasive surgery"，缩写为 MIS，是近些年来外科的基础概念之一，随着材料学与技术的发展，现在的手术切口越来越小，越来越多地从传统的大切口开放手术转为各种各样的小切口微创手术；

2. 脊柱外科的三大核心手术技术包括减压（decompression）、固定（fixation），以及融合（fusion）；

3. "椎弓根螺钉"译作"pedicle screw"，口语表达时也有"椎弓根钉"这一省略说法。译员应注意的是，骨科中的"screw"译作"螺钉"，而"nail"是"钉"。

在微创脊柱外科技术的发展过程中，微创的融合技术使得微创脊柱外科从过去的单纯减压，走向了微创减压和脊柱融合的道路，包括各种从早期小切口到后来的包括可扩张通道、微创管道等。当然，这些所谓的微创通道或者微创入路，都需要显微镜或者内镜的辅助才能得以完成。在当前微创融合技术当中，贡献最大、同时也是影响最广且应用最广泛的就是微创下的微创经椎间孔入路腰椎椎间融合，MIS-TLIF 技术。最经典的 MIS-TLIF 技术是在微创的通道下实现神经减压、椎间植骨、椎间融合器植入以及经皮的节段性固定。这一技术从入路设计上避免了传统方法，即在脊柱后方做纵行长切口，广泛剥离肌肉、韧带所带来的入路创伤。

◎ 参考译文：In the development of minimally invasive spine surgery, minimally invasive fusion technique has promoted minimally invasive spine surgery from simple decompression in the past to minimally invasive decompression and spine fusion, including various small incisions in the early days to expandable channels and minimally invasive tubes. Of course, these so-called minimally invasive channels or minimally invasive approaches all require the assistance of microscopes or endoscopes to be completed. Among the current minimally invasive fusion techniques, the one that has made the greatest contribution, also the most influential and widely used is the minimally invasive surgery-transforaminal lumbar interbody fusion, MIS-TLIF technique. The most classic MIS-TLIF technique is to achieve nerve decompression, intervertebral bone grafting, intervertebral cage implantation and percutaneous segmental fixation under minimally invasive channels. This technique avoids the traditional method of making a long longitudinal incision at the back of the spine and widely stripping muscles and ligaments, which causes surgical approach trauma.

◎ 分析：

1. 在翻译"微创"时，译员如果觉得"minimally invasive"音节过多，跟不上节奏的时候，可以使用"MIS"，即"minimally invasive surgery"的缩写，中文是"微创外科"或"微创手术"，可以简化为"微创"，音节少了很多，同传压力明显减小；

2. "MIS-TLIF"读音为"Miss Tea Leaf"；

3. "椎间融合器"译作"intervertebral cage"。

而除了最早发展、目前应用最广的 MIS-TLIF 技术，近年来，腰椎侧前路微创融合技术包括经侧方入路腰椎椎间融合（DLIF）、极外侧入路腰椎椎间融合（XLIF）、前侧入路腰椎椎间融合（ALIF），以及侧前方的斜外侧入路腰椎椎间融合（OLIF），技术也在临床中不断得到推广与使用。腰椎侧方微创融合技术的最大优点就在于其避免了传统腰椎融合过程中对后方稳定结构的破坏。该技术通过患者侧方小切口入路，实现了直接进行椎间盘的切除、椎管减压、椎间撑开复位以及椎间融合，而不干扰后方腰背部软组织和椎管内神经结构。同时，对于需要多节段腰椎融合的病例，传统后路微创技术需要做多个切口，既费时费力，又增加了手术创伤，同时也不美观，而侧方技术完美地避免了这一弊端。随着技术的发展，通过微创方法完成退变性脊柱畸形矫正也将成为现实。现今，经皮内镜辅助下的腰椎融合包括脊柱内镜下腰椎椎间融合技术、Endo-LIF、PT-LIF 技术，以及 PLIF 技术等，都在不断的临床探索和应用中得到了实现。

◎ 参考译文：In addition to the earliest and currently most widely used MIS-TLIF technique, in recent years, minimally invasive lumbar lateroanterior fusion techniques, including direct lateral lumbar interbody fusion, DLIF, extreme lateral interbody fusion, XLIF, anterior lumbar interbody fusion, ALIF, and oblique lumber interbody fusion, OLIF, techniques, have also been continuously promoted and used in clinical practice. The biggest advantage of minimally invasive lumbar lateral fusion is that it avoids the destruction of the posterior stabilizing structure during traditional lumbar fusion. This technique achieves direct discectomy, spinal canal decompression, intervertebral distraction and reduction, and intervertebral fusion through a small lateral incision approach without interfering with the posterior lumbar soft tissue and neural structures in the spinal canal. At the same time, for cases requiring multi-segment lumbar fusion, traditional posterior minimally invasive techniques require multiple incisions, which is time-consuming and labor-intensive, increases surgical trauma, and is not aesthetically pleasing. The lateral technique perfectly avoids this drawback. With the development of technology, correction of degenerative spinal deformity through minimally invasive methods will also become a reality. Today, percutaneous endoscopy assisted lumbar fusion, including endoscopic lumbar interbody fusion, Endo-LIF, PT-LIF, and PLIF, have been realized in continuous clinical exploration and application.

◎ 分析：

1. "手术入路"译作"surgical approach"，"切口"译作"incision"，这两个术语是医学口译的基础词汇；

2. "微创方法"译作"minimally invasive methods"，在同传时，译员如果语速跟不上讲者，完全可以使用"MIS"来应对，"MIS"需要读出三个字母而非读成"miss"，当今微创的概念在所有外科专科领域都已广为医生所接受。

随着科技的发展，民用导航系统已在我们日常生活中得到了广泛的应用，使我们的生活变得非常便捷。同样，导航技术在医学中的应用也极大地推动了医学的进步和发展。特别是数字导航技术的应用，使现代微创脊柱外科技术走上了一个新的发展道路。数字导航技术在临床的应用以光学导航技术为主，通过红外光导航的引导可实现手术器械的示踪。手术室目前常规采用O-ARM联合导航技术来完成各种微创脊柱外科手术。在脊柱外科，导航技术早期主要用于复杂的椎弓根螺钉的植入，包括脊柱畸形的矫正、上颈椎内固定等。现在，其不仅用于椎弓根螺钉的植入，还可以实现手术的全流程导航，包括皮肤切口的设计、术区的显露、病灶的切除及局部的修复与重建。导航技术在脊柱外科已经成为很重要的方法和手段。目前开展的导航引导的颈椎后路内镜技术，由皮肤的定位到手术通道的植入，都可实现导航的全流程引导。在脊柱外科应用中，导航技术不仅提高了手术的精准性，同时还避免了射线对临床医师的伤害，更重要的是，实现了全程的实时手术示踪，具有更加精准便捷的特性。电磁导航是近几年来发展成熟的导航技术，具有其独特的优点。在电磁导航辅助的经皮内镜手术中，可以直接观察到电磁导航下的器械穿刺成形过程。

◎ 参考译文：With the development of science and technology, civil navigation systems have been widely used in our daily lives, making our lives very convenient. Similarly, the application of navigation technology in medicine has greatly promoted the progress and development of medicine. In particular, the use of digital navigation technology has put modern minimally invasive spine surgery on a new development path. The use of digital navigation technology in clinical practice is mainly based on optical navigation technology, and the tracking of surgical instruments can be achieved through the guidance of infrared light navigation. The operating room currently routinely uses O-ARM combined navigation technology to complete various minimally invasive spine surgeries. In spine surgery, navigation technology was mainly used for the implantation of complex pedicle screws in the early days, including the correction of spine deformities and upper cervical internal fixation. Now, it is not only used for the implantation of pedicle screws, but also can realize the navigation of the entire surgical process, including the design of skin incisions, exposure of the surgical area, resection of lesions, and local repair and reconstruction. Navigation technology has become a very important method and means in spine surgery. The navigation-guided posterior cervical endoscopic technology currently being carried out can achieve full-process navigation guidance from skin positioning to the implantation of surgical channels. In spine surgery applications, navigation technology not only improves the accuracy of surgery, but also avoids radiation damage to clinicians. More importantly, it achieves real-time surgical tracking throughout the entire process, which is more accurate and convenient. Electromagnetic navigation is a navigation technology that has matured in recent years and has its unique advantages. In electromagnetic navigation-assisted percutaneous endoscopic surgery, the instrument puncture and plasty process under electromagnetic navigation can be directly observed.

◎ 分析：

1. "椎弓根螺钉的植入"译作"the implantation of pedicle screws"，国外讲者有时也会讲"the insertion of pedicle screws"；

2. "手术室"此处译作"operating room"，其在英语中有多种表达，包括"operating theater""operating theatre""OR"和"OT"。口译时译员如遇到缩略语，应结合上下文作出判断。

第四节 补充练习

一、中译英

近年来，多现实技术（X-REALITY）也是数字技术中得到迅猛发展和关注的技术。数字虚拟现实（virtual reality，VR）技术已用于日常娱乐中，在多款电子游戏、电影中都有虚拟现实技术的应用。虚拟现实技术实际上是将现实和计算机虚拟的图像、情景交织在一起，从而构成了交互影像。近年来，此类技术在医学中也得到了广泛的关注。多现实技术包含了 VR 技术、增强现实（augmented reality，AR）技术、混合现实（mixed reality，MR）技术。

VR 技术又被称为"虚拟现实技术"，医师戴上特殊的眼镜就会看到我们在现实中见不到的情景和人物，它实际上是计算机模拟出来的场景。VR 技术在医学教育中非常重要。基于上述技术而开发出来的教育系统，有关节镜虚拟教育系统、椎间孔镜教育系统等，都能让医生不需要在大体标本上面进行学习和训练。通过这种虚拟的场景可以进行术前培训和计划。

AR 技术是在虚拟现实的基础上将虚拟和现实结合在一起，又可被称为"增强现实技术"。AR 技术实际上是将虚拟和现实重叠起来，在临床上可以定位病灶，医生可以透过皮肤直接观察到身体内部的骨骼结构和脏器，其中包括投影式、叠加式等多种应用。

MR 技术，即混合现实技术，它是虚拟和现实不断交互、混合的技术。它的虚拟产生于现实，现实又用于虚拟。其在医学中同样具有巨大的应用价值。例如 X 公司开发出的 MR 技术，能够帮助医生通过一种特殊的眼镜看到术前计划，同时也能实现包括病灶的定位、切除，甚至椎弓根螺钉的植入等操作。此项技术目前尚处于研究阶段。由于医师要戴上特殊眼镜，不便于手术操作，目前这类技术已从头戴式发展为屏幕式，甚至未来可以在空气中就可以实现图像的术前、术中，甚至未来手术中的各种各样图像的转化。

◎ **参考译文**：In recent years, multi-reality technology (X-REALITY) is also a technology that has developed rapidly and received attention in digital technology. Digital virtual reality (VR) technology has been used in daily entertainment, and virtual reality technology has been applied in many electronic games and movies. Virtual reality technology actually interweaves real and computer virtual images and scenes to form interactive images. In recent years, this type of technology has also received widespread attention in medicine. Multi-reality technology includes VR technology, augmented reality (AR) technology, and mixed reality (MR) technology.

VR technology is called virtual reality technology. Doctors only need to wear special glasses to see scenes and characters that we cannot see in reality. It is actually a scene simulated by a computer. VR technology is very important in medical education. Education systems developed based on the above technology include arthroscopic virtual education system and foraminal endoscopic education system, which can enable doctors to learn and train without using gross specimens. Preoperative training and planning can be carried out through this virtual scene.

AR technology combines virtuality and reality on the basis of virtual reality, which is called augmented reality technology. AR technology actually overlaps virtuality and reality. It can locate lesions clinically, and doctors can directly observe the bone structure and organs inside the body through the skin. It includes various applications such as projection and superposition.

MR technology, or mixed reality technology, is a technology that continuously interacts and mixes virtual and real. Its virtuality is generated from reality, and reality is used for virtuality. It also has great application value in medicine. For example, the MR technology developed by Company X can help doctors see the preoperative plan through a special pair of glasses, and can also achieve operations including lesion location, resection, and even pedicle screw implantation. This technology is still in the research stage. Since doctors need to wear special glasses, it is not convenient for surgical operations. At present, this type of technology has developed from head-mounted to screen-mounted, and in the future, it can even realize the conversion of various images before, during, and even in future surgeries in the air.

二、英译中

When describing fractures, the acute care surgeon must use precise language and avoid vague terminology. Essential descriptive terminology includes the anatomic location of the injury, fracture pattern, the amount of displacement and whether the fracture is open or closed. Anatomic locations include articular, metaphyseal or diaphyseal injuries. An intra-articular fracture extends into the joint space. Fracture patterns include transverse, spiral, oblique, comminuted and segmental. A transverse fracture is perpendicular to the bone's line of axis. Spiral and oblique are often confused. Both can be the result of a rotational force applied to the bone. A true spiral fracture involves a fracture line that traverses in two directions while an oblique fracture extends in a single plane. A comminuted fracture has multiple fragments and a segmental fracture is a type of comminuted fracture in which there are well-defined fragments. Certain fractures may be complicated by associated bone loss, which often occurs in the setting of an open fracture.

Fracture displacement occurs when one fragment shifts in relation to the other through translation, angulation, shortening or rotation. Typically, descriptions of displacement of hand and wrist fractures include the terms volar and dorsal instead of anterior and posterior and ulnar and radial instead of medial and lateral. The amount of translation should also be reported, as this may be a surrogate for the amount of energy required to create the fracture. Two millimeters or less of translation is considered "minimally displaced". When describing angulation, the direction of which the apex of the angle is pointing should be stated, that is, medial angulation or volar angulation, as well as the degree of angulation, which can be measured using a goniometer (a protractor-like device). Shortening or rotation of the bone should be noticed on clinical examination and likewise reported.

Initial management for a fracture is realignment and splinting. Realignment and splinting improve pain control, arterial flow, venous drainage and decreases soft tissue tension caused by displaced fractures. Furthermore, realignment and splinting can decrease the potential volume around the fracture diminishing the amount of bleeding. Displaced fractures may also result in nerve impingement that can be relieved with realignment. A dislocated joint should be urgently reduced to prevent further damage to the ligaments, tendons, neurovascular structures and the inner chondral surfaces. Splints are non-circumferential and are molded or otherwise secured around a limb to accommodate swelling. Casts are circumferential, made from plaster or synthetic material. Focal pressure over a bony prominence can cause skin and soft tissue pressure necrosis, hence the need for careful application and extra padding over threatened skin.

Traction improves alignment, reduces fracture motion and can be used as a temporary measure until definitive fixation. An example of this would be the multiple-injured patient with a severe head injury with elevated intracranial pressures and a femur fracture. Length and alignment of the femur fracture can be maintained in traction until the brain injury improves enough for the patient to tolerate non-cranial invasive procedures. Both skeletal and cutaneous traction may be used in a safe manner, however skeletal traction is typically preferred over cutaneous, especially for prolonged delays.

Multiply injured patients with fractures are co-managed by acute care surgeons and orthopedic surgeons. In most centers, orthopedic surgeons definitively manage fractures, but preliminary management, including washouts, splinting, reductions, and external fixations, may be performed by selected acute care surgeons. The acute care surgeon should have a working knowledge of orthopedic terminology to communicate with colleagues effectively. They should have an understanding of the composition of bone, periosteum, and cartilage, and their reaction when there is an injury. Fractures are usually fixed urgently, but some multiply injured patients are better served with a damage control strategy. Extremity compartment syndrome should be suspected in all critically injured patients with or without fractures and a low threshold for compartment pressure measurements or empiric fasciotomy maintained. Acute care surgeons performing rib fracture fixation and other chest wall injury reconstructions should follow the principles of open fracture reduction and stabilization.

◎ **参考译文**：描述骨折时，急诊外科医生必须使用精确的语言，避免使用模糊的术语。基本描述术语包括损伤的解剖位置、骨折类型、位移量以及骨折是开放性还是闭合性。解剖位置包括关节、干骺端或骨干损伤。关节内骨折延伸到关节间隙。骨折类型包括横向、螺旋、斜向、粉碎性和节段性。横向骨折垂直于骨轴线。螺旋和斜向经常被混淆。两者都可能是施加在骨上的旋转力的结果。真正的螺旋形骨折涉及沿两个方向横穿的骨折线，而斜向骨折则在一个平面上延伸。粉碎性骨折有多个碎片，而节段性骨折是一种有明确碎片的粉碎性骨折。某些骨折可能因相关的骨质流失而变得复杂，这通常发生在开放性骨折的情况下。

骨折移位是指一个骨折块通过平移、成角、缩短或旋转相对于另一个骨折块发生移位。通常，在描述手部和腕部骨折移位时，会使用掌侧和背侧而不是前侧和后侧，以及尺侧和桡侧而不是内侧和外侧。还应报告平移量，因为这可能代表造成骨折所需的能量。两毫米或更少的平移被认为是"最小位移"。描述成角时，应说明角度顶点指向的方向，即内侧成角或掌侧成角，以及成角的程度，可使用测角仪（一种类似量角器的装置）测量。临床检查时应注意骨骼的缩短或旋转，并同样进行报告。

骨折的初步治疗是复位和夹板固定。复位和夹板固定可改善疼痛控制、动脉血流、静脉引流并降低由移位骨折引起的软组织张力。此外，复位和夹板固定可减少骨折周围的潜在体积，从而减少出血量。移位骨折也可能导致神经受压，可通过复位缓解。应紧急复位脱臼关节，以防止进一步损伤韧带、肌腱、神经血管结构和内软骨表面。夹板不是环形的，而是模制或以其他方式固定在肢体周围以适应肿胀。石膏是环形的，由石膏或合成材料制成。骨突处的局部压力会导致皮肤和软组织压力性坏死，因此需要小心使用并在受威胁的皮肤上加垫。

牵引可改善对齐，减少骨折移动，并可用作最终固定前的临时措施。例如，多重受伤的患者头部严重受伤，颅内压升高，股骨骨折。牵引可保持股骨骨折的长度和对齐，直到脑损伤得到改善，患者能够耐受非颅内侵入性手术。骨骼牵引和皮肤牵引均可安全使用，但骨骼牵引通常优于皮肤牵引，尤其是在长时间延迟的情况下。

伴有骨折的多重损伤患者由急诊外科医生和骨科医生共同管理。在大多数中心，骨科医生负责骨折的最终治疗，但初步治疗，包括冲洗、夹板固定、复位和外固定，可能由选定的急诊外科医生进行。急诊外科医生应具备骨科术语的应用知识，以便与同事进行有效沟通。他们应该了解骨骼、骨膜和软骨的组成，以及它们在受伤时的反应。骨折通常需要紧急固定，但一些多重损伤患者最好采用损伤控制策略。所有严重受伤的患者，无论有无骨折，都应怀疑有肢体筋膜室综合征，并保持较低的筋膜室压力测量阈值或经验性筋膜切开术。进行肋骨骨折固定和其他胸壁损伤重建的急诊外科医生应遵循开放性骨折复位和固定的原则。

参 考 书 目

[1] 鲍刚. 口译理论概述[M]. 北京：中国对外翻译出版有限公司，2011.
[2] 梅德明. 高级口译教程[M]. 上海：上海外语教育出版社，2006.
[3] 齐涛云. 商务英语翻译教程（口译）（第三版）[M]. 北京：中国水利水电出版社，2022.
[4] [瑞士]让·艾赫贝尔. 口译须知[M]. 孙慧双，译. 北京：外语教学与研究出版社，1982.
[5] 冯庆华，梅德明. 英语口译教程[M]. 北京：高等教育出版社，2008.
[6] 王逢鑫. 高级汉英口译教程[M]. 北京：外文出版社，2004.